EVIDENCE-BASED EYE CARE

Edited by

Peter J. Kertes, MD, CM, FRCS (C)

The University of Toronto
Sunnybrook Health Sciences Center
Toronto, Ontario, Canada

T. Mark Johnson, MD, FRCS (C)

The National Retina Institute
Chevy Chase, Maryland, USA

 Lippincott Williams & Wilkins
a Wolters Kluwer business
Philadelphia · Baltimore · New York · London
Buenos Aires · Hong Kong · Sydney · Tokyo

Acquisitions Editor: Jonathan Pine
Managing Editor: Jean McGough
Associate Director of Marketing: Adam Glazer
Project Manager: Bridgett Dougherty
Manufacturing Manager: Kathleen Brown
Design Coordinator: Risa Clow
Production Services: Laserwords Private Limited, Chennai, India
Printer: Gopsons Papers Limited

530 Walnut Street
Philadelphia, PA 19106 USA
LWW.com

Library of Congress Cataloging-in-Publication Data
Evidence-based eye care / edited by Peter J. Kertes and T. Mark Johnson.
 p. ; cm.
 Includes bibliographical references and index.
 ISBN-13: 978-0-7817-6964-8
 ISBN-10: 0-7817-6964-7
 1. Eye—Diseases—Treatment. 2. Evidence-based medicine.
3. Ophthalmology. I. Kertes, Peter J. II. Johnson, T. Mark
(Thomas Mark), 1969- .
 [DNLM: 1. Eye Diseases. 2. Evidence-Based Medicine. 3. Eye
Diseases—therapy. 4. Randomized Controlled Trials. WW 140
E93 2007]
 RE48.E95 2007
 617.7—dc22
                                    2006022739

Care has been taken to confirm the accuracy of the information presented and to describe generally accepted practices. However, the authors, editors, and publisher are not responsible for errors or omissions or for any consequences from application of the information in this book and make no warranty, expressed or implied, with respect to the currency, completeness, or accuracy of the contents of the publication. Application of this information in a particular situation remains the professional responsibility of the practitioner.

The authors, editors, and publisher have exerted every effort to ensure that drug selection and dosage set forth in this text are in accordance with current recommendations and practice at the time of publication. However, in view of ongoing research, changes in government regulations, and the constant flow of information relating to drug therapy and drug reactions, the reader is urged to check the package insert for each drug for any change in indications and dosage and for added warnings and precautions. This is particularly important when the recommended agent is a new or infrequently employed drug.

Some drugs and medical devices presented in this publication have Food and Drug Administration (FDA) clearance for limited use in restricted research settings. It is the responsibility of the health care provider to ascertain the FDA status of each drug or device planned for use in their clinical practice.

To purchase additional copies of this book, call our customer service department at (800) 638-3030 or fax orders to (301) 223-2320. International customers should call (301) 223-2300.

Visit Lippincott Williams & Wilkins on the Internet: at LWW.com. Lippincott Williams & Wilkins customer service representatives are available from 8:30 am to 6 pm, EST.

10 9 8 7 6 5 4 3 2 1

This book is dedicated to the loving memory of Hilda Kertes (1922–2005). Her smiling eyes and limitless love will stay with me always.

CONTRIBUTORS

Sophie J. Bakri, MD
Assistant Professor
Department of Ophthalmology
Vitreoretinal Diseases and Surgery
Mayo Clinic College of Medicine
Rochester, Minnesota

Anna Ells, MD, FRCS (C)
Associate Professor
Department of Surgery
Division of Ophthalmology
University of Calgary
Ophthalmologist
Vision Services Eye Clinic
Alberta Children's Hospital
Calgary, Alberta

Dean Eliott, MD
Professor
Director of Clinical Affairs
Doheny Retina Institute
University of Southern California
Keck School of Medicine
Los Angeles, California

Ayad A. Farjo, MD
Assistant Clinical Professor
Department of Ophthalmology
and Visual Sciences
University of Wisconsin
Hospitals and Clinics
Madison, Wisconsin;
Opthalmologist
Brighton Vision Center Institution
Brighton, Michigan

Qais A. Farjo, MD
Director of Corneal and Refractive Surgery
Vision Associates
Toledo, Ohio

Amani A. Fawzi, MD
Assistant Professor
Department of Ophthalmology
Doheny Retina Institute
Doheny Eye Institute
Keck School of Medicine
University of Southern California
Los Angeles, California

Sharon Fekrat, MD, FACS
Associate Professor
Department of Ophthalmology
Duke University Eye Center
Duke University Medical Center
Durham, North Carolina;
Vitreoretinal Surgeon
Department of Ophthalmology
Duke University Medical Center
Durham, North Carolina

Seenu M. Hariprasad, MD
Assistant Professor and Director
of Clinical Research
Department of Ophthalmology
and Visual Science
University of Chicago
Chicago, Illinois

Hussein Hollands, MD, MS (Epid)
Resident
Department of Ophthalmology
Queen's University
Hotel Dieu Hospital
Kingston, Ontario

Jonathan M. Holmes, BM, BCh
Professor and Chair
Department of Ophthalmology
Mayo Clinic College of Medicine
Rochester, Minnesota

Peter K. Kaiser, MD
Director
Digital OCT Reading Center
Cole Eye Institute
Cleveland, Ohio

Raymond T. Kraker, MSPH
Assistant Director
Pediatric Eye Disease Investigator Group
Coordinating Center
Jaeb Center For Health Research
Tampa, Florida

Louise A. Mawn, MD
Assistant Professor
Department of Ophthalmology and Neurological
Surgery
Vanderbilt University Medical Center
Nashville, Tennessee

William F. Mieler, MD
Professor and Chairman
Department of Ophthalmology
University of Chicago
Chicago, Illinois

Louis E. Probst, MD
Medical Director
TLC Laser Eye Centers
Chicago Illinios
Greenville, South Carolina

Paul E. Rafuse, PhD, MD, FRCS (C)
Assistant Professor
Department of Ophthalmology
and Visual Sciences
Halifax, Nova Scotia;
Active Staff
Department of Ophthalmology
Capital District Health Authority
Halifax, Nova Scotia

Michael X. Repka, MD
Professor
Department of Ophthalmology and Pediatrics
Johns Hopkins University
Baltimore, Maryland

Michael A. Samuel, MD
Attending Physician
Retina Service
Wills Eye Hospital
Philadelphia, Pennsylvania

Sanjay Sharma, MD, MS (Epid), FRCS (C), MBA
Associate Professor
Department of Ophthalmology
Assistant Professor
Department of Epidemiology
Queen's University
Kingston, Ontario;
Director, Cost Effective Ocular
Health Policy Unit
Department of Ophthalmology
Hotel Dieu Hospital
Kingston, Ontario

Ernest Rand Simpson, MD, FRCS (C)
Associate Professor
Department of Ophthalmology
University of Toronto
One King's College Circle;
Director, Ocular Oncology
Department of Surgical Oncology
Princess Margaret Hospital
University Health Network
Toronto, Ontario

Jay M. Stewart, MD
Assistant Professor
Department of Clinical Ophthalmology
University of California
San Francisco, California

Jonathan D. Trobe, MD
Professor
Departments of Ophthalmology and Neurology
University of Michigan
Kellogg Eye Center
Ann Arbor, Michigan

Henry Tseng, MD, PhD
Fellow
Department of Ophthalmology
Duke University Eye Center;
Clinical Associate
Department of Ophthalmology
Duke University Health System
Durham, North Carolina

FOREWORD

The practice of medicine has changed in the last several decades with the emerging concepts of "evidence-based medicine." This book, Evidence-based Eye Care edited by Drs. Peter Kertes and T. Mark Johnson, provides a unique and comprehensive evaluation of the major clinical studies conducted in the various disciplines within the field of ophthalmology in the past several decades. It is rare to find a single source that contains the clinical research, particularly the controlled clinical trials pertaining to the anterior segment, glaucoma, pediatric, neuro-ophthalmic, and retinal vascular diseases. In particular, the 3 leading causes of blindness in the developed countries, age-related macular degeneration, diabetic retinopathy, and glaucoma are extensively covered.

With the increase in the scrutiny of our federal government dollars spent on health care, the importance of evidence-based medicine is clearly elevated. What is the definition of evidence-based medicine? Evidence based medicine draws not only from randomized controlled clinical trials, but also involves evidence we can best use for the disease or clinical predicament. Clinical trials, especially well designed, double-masked controlled, however, remain the "gold-standard" that is most likely to inform us whether a treatment has more favorable than adverse effects. However, not every disease lends itself well to the assessment by controlled clinical trials. Some questions about therapy may not require randomized trials. If there are no randomized trials, we must then go beyond and review other types of evidence for the clinical decision making. This may include basic science studies or cohort or case–control studies. It is possible that the only evidence may be cases series. The first chapter in the book nicely describes the different methodology used in clinical research. All residents and practicing physicians should be familiar with this information and read every article, whether it is in the medical journal or in the media, with these guiding principles of clinical research.

Evidence-based medicine however, is not a "cookbook" type of medicine. It requires the clinician to make clinical decisions based on external clinical evidence that can inform and guide, but never replace individual clinical expertise. The external clinical evidence, as well as the patient's clinical state and, of course, the patient's preferences all need to be integrated into this complex web of clinical decision making. This book serves the important role of providing guidance to the practicing clinician and is recommended for all ophthalmologists, either in training or practicing in the community. Congratulations to the authors and the editors for a gem!

Emily Y. Chew, MD
Deputy Director of Division of Epidemiology
and Clinical Research,
Clinical Trials Branch

Since the beginning of clinical medicine, physicians have been charged with the task of providing their patients with the best diagnostic and therapeutic skills available. The goal has always been to optimize the outcome and minimize the risk. The practice of medicine was initially, and remains to a much lesser extent even today, based heavily upon the wisdom and experience of certain experts. Over time, physicians and their patients have demanded increasing validation of diagnostic and therapeutic interventions.

Over the past quarter century, evidence-based medicine has come to the forefront of clinical medicine. The underlying principle of evidence-based medicine is the application of the best basic science and clinical research available to a specific patient complaint. The randomized controlled trial (RCT) has become the most revered component of evidence-based medicine. It represents the ideal model for hypothesis testing in clinical medicine. The RCT has been an important part of ophthalmology since the Diabetic Retinopathy Study validated the role of pan-retinal laser photocoagulation for high-risk proliferative diabetic retinopathy. The RCT continues to play a vital role in all subspecialties in ophthalmology.

Clinical trials in ophthalmology face unique challenges. RCTs have limitations. RCTs are generally able to answer a single research question. The costs and time involved in answering that single question can be significant. It is not always ethical or practical to do an RCT. For example, to be sufficiently powered, RCTs typically require large sample sizes. Ophthalmology is a specialty of relatively rare diseases. Other than glaucoma, cataract, myopia, diabetic retinopathy, and macular degeneration, most ophthalmic conditions are relatively rare from a population point of view. Thus, conducting RCTs on many ophthalmic conditions can be difficult from a recruitment perspective. In addition, RCTs, by their very nature, risk being a little behind the times. From the time a question is formulated, and a study funded, carried out, and analyzed, often some new questions have been asked and new or modified

therapies introduced. Therefore, in ophthalmology we must frequently look to sources other than the clinical trials to case–control studies, small controlled trials and case series for evidence upon which to base our treatment decisions.

The goal of this text is therefore twofold. Firstly, we aim to summarize the major clinical trials in ophthalmology, those RCTs that form the foundation of how we practice ophthalmology. The authors were charged with the task of summarizing the trials in a manner that would allow easy understanding and ready application to clinical practice. The summaries include the specific populations under investigation so that clinicians know to which patients to best apply the findings. The interventions and their results also are summarized and clearly laid out. Finally the limitations of the studies are reviewed. While a clinical trial answers one question, inevitably, there are many questions about a given condition or therapy that remain. The second goal is to highlight the questions that remain after the clinical trial and to provide the reader with a sense of where the field of ophthalmology is headed and the body of evidence that exists to support heading off in another direction.

The text is multi-authored. Each author has an academic and clinical interest in his or her particular subspecialty. All the authors are practicing clinicians and have written the chapters from the perspective of how the results of these clinical trials are applied within the context of patient care. An attempt has been made to provide some uniformity to the chapters, but each has its own unique style.

The genesis of this book lies in the discussions of a junior resident (TMJ) and a senior resident (PJK) on the underlying principles of patient care in ophthalmology. The editors sincerely hope that this book will provide clinicians, residents, and students with a foundation in the therapeutic principles of ophthalmic care and serve as a basis for going beyond our current clinical trials in the future.

Peter J. Kertes, MD, CM, FRCS (C)
T. Mark Johnson, MD, FRCS (C)

ACKNOWLEDGMENTS

Dr. Johnson thanks his mother for teaching him to write, his father for inspiring an interest in science, Lenorah for being a loyal little sister and tolerant first patient, and Joanne for providing endless love and support. He also thanks the contributing authors for their enthusiasm and effort in producing this text. In addition he thanks Dr. Kertes for the coffee and the fundamental ophthalmology training provided in the café of the Ottawa Civic Hospital.

Dr. Kertes thanks his wife and daughters for their love and support; the many medical students, residents, and fellows that he has had the privilege of working with who keep asking the important questions that make the practice of ophthalmology stimulating and gratifying; and the investigators—the contributing authors chief among them—and the brave patients who have tested the bounds of scientific exploration and allowed ophthalmology to progress to its present and future heights.

CONTENTS

XIII

SECTION I

CLINICAL EPIDEMIOLOGY AND HEALTH ECONOMICS

CHAPTER 1

Clinical Epidemiology

Hussein Hollands, MD, MS (Epid) and Sanjay Sharma, MD, MS (Epid), FRCS (C), MBA

Introduction

It is now commonplace for physicians and patients to expect that clinical decisions made by physicians—especially when related to therapy or prevention of disease—are based on sound scientific evidence. New treatments, whether aimed at reducing symptoms, curing disease, or reducing the risk of disease or disease symptoms, must be proved with results from a randomized controlled trial (RCT) to be considered for government approval. In addition, patients are becoming more likely to demand scientific reasoning in the form of valid clinical studies before undertaking therapy.

Clinical epidemiology can be thought of as the science of making predictions regarding individual patients using a sound scientific method.[1] To accurately assess the evidence available for a particular therapy or preventative measure, it is necessary to understand the fundamentals of clinical study design. Depending on the strengths and inherent biases of different study designs, epidemiological evidence varies greatly in value when applied to clinical decision making. Evidence is classified from Class I through V, from the strongest to the weakest, respectively.[1,2] Table 1.1 summarizes the various classes of evidence as described previously.[2]

In this chapter, we will present a review of the common study designs focusing specifically on the important issues in critical appraisal, interpretation of clinical research, and application to patient care.

TABLE 1.1 □ **Summary of Hierarchical Levels of Evidence for Interventional and Observational Studies**[2]

Level of Evidence	Study Design
Level V	Interventional case report
Level IV	Intervention in a series of patients with no comparison group
Level III	Nonrandomized controlled trial (strong level III evidence is a prospective cohort study, moderate level III evidence is a retrospective cohort study or case–control study, and weak level III evidence is a cross-sectional study)
Level II	Randomized controlled trial with high type I error, or low power (high type II error), or both
Level I	Randomized controlled trial with low type I error and high power, or meta-analysis

For each study design, basic statistical tests will be described.

Observational Study Designs

Results from observational study designs are often frowned upon as evidence to support decision making in medicine, but in many situations experimental evidence is not available and an observational study provides important information to support clinical decisions. For instance, observational studies are usually the only possible study design to investigate environmental or dietary risk factors for disease. They are also useful after a treatment becomes commonplace in medicine and it becomes unethical to randomize a patient to not receive that standard treatment. Finally, although clinical trials are ideal, they are expensive and time-consuming and are simply not performed in large numbers. In a typical year, 87% of clinical articles published in the *Archives of Ophthalmology*, *Ophthalmology*, *British Journal of Ophthalmology*, and *Canadian Journal of Ophthalmology* are observational study designs.[3]

Consequently, clinical decisions in ophthalmology are being made using evidence from both clinical trials and observational studies.

Case Reports and Case Series

A case report outlines an interesting or new treatment approach and follows up a patient outcome into the future, whereas a case series simply lists a series of patients treated similarly and followed up during treatment in time. Neither of these study designs employs control groups and is thereby considered the weakest form of clinical evidence (Class V and IV, respectively). In general, clinical decisions should not be made using data only from case reports or case series but these study designs do play an important role in evidence-based medicine by enabling the medical community to stay current with respect to new treatment options and by fueling ideas for more definitive future studies.

Analytic Cross-sectional Studies

An analytic cross-sectional study is used to investigate a risk factor for disease as opposed to a treatment or intervention. In this design, a cross-section of people is investigated, simultaneously in time, as to their exposure status and their outcome or disease status. In the analysis, the prevalence of a given risk factor or exposure to it is compared between those who happen to have the outcome of interest and those who do not. Prevalence is defined as the fraction of people who have the condition at a certain point of time. It is important to distinguish prevalence from incidence; incidence is the fraction of people who *develop* the condition over a certain period of time.

An example of a recent cross-sectional study investigated whether an association exists between the use of angiotensin converting enzyme inhibitors (ACEI) and the prevalence of age-related macular degeneration (AMD).[4] Researchers reported that among a cross-section of 3,654 Australians, 1.3% of ACEI users had late AMD while 2.0% of people not using ACEI had late AMD ($p > 0.05$). A group of patients were observed at one point in time and each patient was defined on the basis of his or her exposure status (i.e., current use of ACEI) and on the basis of their outcome status (i.e., photographic evidence of AMD). Results of a cross-sectional study are generally given as the prevalence rate ratio (PRR), calculated as follows:

$$PRR = \text{Prevalence rate (among the exposed)} / \text{Prevalence rate (among the unexposed)}$$

In the example of AMD among ACEI users, the PRR can be calculated as follows:

$$PRR = \text{Prevalence of AMD (among ACEI users)} / \text{Prevalence of AMD (among ACEI nonusers)} = (73/3,654)/(47/3,654) = 1.53$$

Compared with more intensive observational study designs, a cross-sectional design has the advantage of being less time-intensive and cheaper. In addition, it is usually relatively easy to obtain a representative population using this study design. There are, however, some drawbacks to cross-sectional studies.[5] First, cross-sectional studies are designed to look at one point in time and cannot determine the temporal sequence (or cause and effect) between risk factor and disease. Second, since the outcome measure of a cross-sectional study is prevalence, there is a potential for incidence–prevalence bias whereby transitory or fatal disease may be preferentially missed. Third, associations made using current exposure status may not be indicative of past exposure status and therefore may not fit with the established pathophysiology of the disease. Consequently, cross-sectional studies are considered weak Class III evidence for clinical decision making and should only be employed to study preliminary hypotheses.[2]

Case–Control Studies

Unlike in cross-sectional studies, case–control studies employ a true control group and can thereby make valid comparisons between groups of patients. In a case–control design, two sample patient populations are identified: Those with the disease outcome in question (the cases) and those without the outcome (the controls). The study then looks backward in time to measure the frequency of past exposure.

Although case–control studies are considered retrospective, patients are theoretically followed forward from the time of exposure in the past to the time of known disease outcome in the present.[5] In the analysis, cases are compared to controls with respect to the frequency of the exposure of interest to determine if a cause and effect relationship occurs between exposure and outcome.

An example of a recently published case–control study looked for an association between the use of cholesterol-lowering agents and AMD among a group of 15,792 people enrolled in the Atherosclerosis Risk in Communities study between 1987 and 1989.[6] Cases were initially identified as those people found to have AMD after applying a standard definition to their fundus photographs. Controls were participants with no evidence of AMD on fundus photographs. Researchers then established previous exposure to cholesterol-lowering agents through a questionnaire. Exposed patients were those who had used cholesterol-lowering agents during the study period while unexposed patients had never used such agents. Of the 871 AMD cases, 11% made use of cholesterol-lowering medications, as compared with 12.3% of the 11,717 controls (unadjusted odds ratio (OR), 0.89; 95% confidence interval (CI), 0.71–1.11).

In a case–control study, selecting appropriate controls is perhaps the most difficult, yet important, methodological consideration since the control group defines what is normal and provides a basis for comparison. A control group ideally should be picked from a population that is similar to the group of cases in all ways except that they do not have the disease in question. Another methodological consideration in case–control studies is the accurate determination of exposure status. Objective exposures should be used whenever possible to minimize the chance of recall bias* and interviewers should be blinded to minimize the chance of observer bias.[†]

Since case–control studies are not randomized, there is potential for confounding variables to affect the results of the study. Confounding variables go with the risk factor being investigated and are significantly associated with the disease in question. Therefore, it may look as though the exposure in question causes the disease, when, in fact, the exposure is simply associated with a confounding factor, which causes the disease. The most common example of a confounder in most clinical studies is age. In the example above, age is associated with AMD, and older people are also more likely to be on cholesterol-lowering agents. When designing the study and interpreting the results one must take care to tease out whether cholesterol-lowering agents are

---

*Recall bias can occur because cases preferentially remember past exposures better than controls.
[†]Observer bias can occur if observers in the study consciously or unconsciously record observations differently depending on the outcome status of the participant.

TABLE 1.2 ☐ Standard 2 × 2 Contingency Table

	Cases	Controls
Exposure (+)	a	b
No exposure	c	d

temporally associated with AMD after accounting for the effect of age.

Case–control studies are usually reported as a 2 × 2 contingency table (Table 1.2) and an OR (defined in Equation 1.1). Table 1.3 shows the contingency table for the case–control study of cholesterol-lowering agent use and risk of developing AMD. The OR calculation for this example is shown in Equation 1.2.

(Equation 1.1:)
$$OR = (a/c)/(b/d) = ad/bc$$
(Equation 1.2:)
$$OR = (96/775)/(1441/10276) = 0.89$$

The interpretation of the unadjusted OR in the example described is as follows: The odds of having a history of using cholesterol-lowering agents among patients with AMD were 0.89 times greater than those among patients without AMD. The OR is a measure of the strength of association between two variables; an OR of 1.0 or close to 1.0 indicates no or little relationship between the variables being studied, whereas a large OR, or an OR close to zero indicates a strong association between the variables.

In addition to the strength of association, one must consider the precision of the reported results.

TABLE 1.3 ☐ Case–Control Study of Lipid-Lowering Agents and Risk of AMD

	AMD Cases	Control Group
History of lipid-lowering agent use	96	1,441
No history of lipid-lowering agent use	775	10,276
Total	871	11,717

Precision describes how confident we are that the reported strength of association is due to a true effect as opposed to chance.[5] Statistical tests are used for this purpose and reported as either a p value or a 95% CI. The appropriate statistical test to use in a case–control study is the chi-squared test.

Confounding variables can be controlled for in a case–control study during the design phase by matching cases and controls on the basis of known prognostic (or confounding) factors. Stratification is a process of separating a sample into two or more subgroups on the basis of the specified level of a third variable (i.e., the potentially confounding variable) and can be used during the analysis phase of a study to assess the role of confounding. If stratified data are presented in a report, a Mentel Haenszel OR, which is a combined measure of the stratum-specific ORs, should be reported. Most introductory epidemiology textbooks will provide additional information on this test. An alternative way of accounting for potentially confounding variables is to use a multivariate regression analysis. In a case–control study where the outcome of interest is dichotomous, a multivariate logistic regression analysis should be used. In this case, an adjusted OR with 95% CIs should be reported. In the case–control study described in the preceding text, potentially confounding factors including age, gender, and ethnicity were controlled for in a second analysis and the study revealed a statistically significant association between AMD and the use of cholesterol-lowering agents after accounting for these variables (adjusted OR, 0.79; 95% CI, 0.63–0.99).

Case–control studies are most helpful in assessing cause and effect relationships. Logistically, these studies tend to be relatively inexpensive and quick to perform. They are especially well suited for studying rare diseases where incidence rates are low because cases can be selected at the outset. Furthermore, multiple potential risk factors may be studied simultaneously among the same group of cases and controls.

Case–control studies have a number of important weaknesses. First, true incidence rates in exposed and unexposed participants cannot generally be determined.[5] Second, case–control studies are not useful in studying rare exposures. Third, information on past exposures or potential confounders may be unknown, incomplete, or available information may be different among cases and controls. Finally, it may be difficult to obtain a comparable group of control subjects.

Given these inherent weaknesses, well-designed case–control studies are considered moderate level III evidence.[2] However, they can be very useful in clinical decision making regarding cause and effect when used with caution. The case–control study design is appropriate for hypothesis testing, leading to future definitive research and making inferences about risk factors for rare diseases when controlled clinical trials are unethical or impractical.

Cohort Studies

A cohort is a group of people with a common exposure who are followed up to look for an outcome of interest. In a cohort study, groups of people are identified at the start of the study and are classified as to their exposure status. The exposure of interest could be an environmental factor, dietary factor, pharmaceutical treatment, or any intervention.

After the exposure status of each person in the study has been established, two cohorts are naturally formed: A cohort of exposed persons and a cohort of unexposed persons. The two cohorts are then followed up in time to assess the outcome. The outcome measure in a cohort study is the rate or incidence of disease, or the fraction of the cohort that develops disease over a certain period of time. This design differs from a cross-sectional study where the exposure and disease are identified simultaneously and from a case–control study where the outcome is identified first and the presence of past exposure status is compared between the groups.

Cohort studies may be either prospective cohort studies (PCS) or retrospective cohort studies (RCS). In a PCS, exposure status is obtained at the beginning of the study and the cohort is observed forward in time for outcomes of interest to occur. At the beginning of the study, participants must be free from the disease outcome and be at risk for developing the outcome sometime in the future. An RCS is similar to a PCS except for the fact that in the exposed cohort the exposure occurred in the past and participants are then traced from the past to the present for disease development. Constructing an RCS requires historical records of exposure status from the past and appropriate follow-up to obtain outcome status through medical records or disease registries.

In a PCS, the control group is usually the portion of the cohort that is not exposed; this represents an internal comparison. If an internal comparison

group is not possible (for example, among a group of people exposed to an infectious pathogen), then an external comparison group can be used. In an RCS, the comparison group is usually external because a group of exposed persons from the past is followed up to act as the basis for the study. When an external comparison group is used in any study, it is essential that this unexposed group be similar to the exposed group in all ways except for the exposure of interest.[5]

An example of a recently published PCS investigated the association between C-reactive protein (CRP) levels (exposure) and the development of AMD (outcome).[7] A cohort of 261 patients who had some signs of nonexudative AMD was identified. Inflammatory biomarkers were then collected on each patient and the cohort was grouped into quartiles on the basis of the CRP level. Patients within the highest quartile of CRP level were defined as exposed, whereas those within the lowest quartile of CRP level were defined as unexposed. The outcome was the incidence of progression of AMD, confirmed on the basis of standardized fundus photographs followed up over a period of 4.6 years.

When critiquing a cohort study, as with any nonrandomized study design, the potential for bias and confounding should be sought out. Bias is minimized by using objective exposure and outcome measures, blinding to exposure and/or outcome status during data collection, and using uniform methods to collect information. Confounding factors must be clearly identified in the study design phase, and data for these factors must be obtained either prospectively or through available records. Confounding variables should then be controlled for either during the design phase of the study or through stratification in the analysis phase with multivariate regression analysis.

The results of a cohort study are reported using a relative risk ratio (RRR), which is simply the rate of disease outcome among the exposed group divided by the rate of disease outcome among the unexposed group. The precision of the RRR is calculated using a chi-squared test and reported as either a p value or 95% CI. In the PCS example described above, CRP was associated with progression of AMD. A multivariate adjusted relative risk of 2.10 (95% CI, 1.06–4.18; p value = 0.046) was found after controlling for body mass index, smoking status, and other confounding cardiovascular risk factors.

A properly conducted PCS or RCS can determine the temporal sequence between cause and effect. The cohort study design is particularly useful for studying rare exposures or clinical interventions in a nonrandomized fashion. Indeed, multiple outcomes may be assessed. Cohort studies also allow for the calculation of a disease incidence rate without underestimating transitory or fatal disease processes. A true relative risk of disease between the unexposed and exposed groups can be calculated.

The disadvantages of cohort studies are as follows.[5] First, PCSs generally require large sample sizes and a long follow-up period, and can therefore have significant rates of follow-up loss and expense. Second, in a PCS there is the possibility of exposure misclassification because of changes in exposure status or in disease detection techniques during the follow-up period. In an RCS, inadequate information regarding exposure status throughout the course of the follow-up can be a problem.

Overall, although prospective and retrospective cohort designs have similar theoretical disadvantages, a PCS is considered much stronger evidence. This is because a PCS can be designed to avoid potential biases and to collect all necessary information, whereas an RCS relies on previously collected data. Cohort studies are considered moderate to strong observational level III evidence.[2] In particular, they are helpful in supporting clinical decision making in situations such as identifying rare risk factors for disease or studying the effect of a treatment or intervention where randomization cannot ethically or practically be employed.

Randomized Controlled Trials

Experimental Design

An (RCT) is similar to a PCS in that a group of people are assembled and followed up in time to look for an outcome event of interest. However, a clinical trial is superior in that it is experimental. Rather than merely observing exposure and outcome, clinical trials manipulate an exposure of interest in two randomly assigned groups of patients. The experimental arm receives a treatment hypothesized to lead to better outcomes than standard therapy. The control arm receives only standard therapy. Direct comparison with the control arm ensures that any observed treatment effect in the experimental arm cannot be explained by a placebo effect or regression toward the mean.

A clinical trial may be a preventive trial (e.g., using vitamin supplementation to prevent wet AMD), an interventional trial (e.g., trial of a lipid-lowering agent to prevent heart disease), or a therapeutic trial (e.g., treatment of neovascular AMD with pegaptanib sodium injection [Macugen]). However, randomization is the crucial element in any RCT that distinguishes experimental evidence from observational evidence. Each patient enrolled in the trial has an equal chance of being placed in the experimental or control arm. In other words, the process of randomization makes certain that all variables (other than the experimental manipulation or treatment) are distributed randomly between the two groups to effectively eliminate selection bias.

The major drawback in an observational study design is the risk of confounding—the chance that study groups will differ with respect to known or unknown prognostic variables and that the treatment effect is actually due to a systematic difference between the study groups as opposed to a true treatment effect. Since an RCT is an experiment such systematic errors are avoided. Theoretically, any treatment difference between arms should be due to chance alone or the treatment effect being studied. As a result, RCTs provide the best evidence available from the primary medical literature for guiding clinical decisions and are considered level I or II evidence, depending on study methodology and sample size.[2]

Although an RCT is considered the best available study design it can still have large methodological flaws, an inadequate sample size, or a nonrepresentative sample population. Therefore, evaluating experimental evidence from RCTs requires a step-wise approach: Appraisal of study validity, interpretation of results, and application of results to individual patient care. To illustrate these steps practically, we will work through a critical appraisal and interpret the results of a recent clinical trial evaluating dietary supplementation of antioxidants and zinc to slow the advancement of AMD.[8]

Appraising the Validity of a Clinical Trial

Validity reflects whether we believe the treatment effect reported by a study to be true or whether we believe the treatment effect to be falsely influenced by systematic errors in study design.[9] The internal validity of any trial should be appraised before the results are interpreted or applied to patient care.

Sample

The first important aspect to address is the sample of patients being studied. A population of interest should be targeted by outlining clear inclusion and exclusion criteria. Pharmaceutical RCTs are usually designed with very rigorous inclusion and exclusion criteria to ensure that the sample of people participating in the study are compliant and therefore the most likely to benefit from treatment. Indeed, many pharmaceutical trials employ an initial open label phase whereby patients who are noncompliant with medications can be identified and dropped from further study. Both inclusion and exclusion criteria as well as the method of sampling play into how well the targeted population is represented in an RCT and help us to assess the generalizability of the study. We will discuss the idea of generalizability in greater detail in the sections to follow.

A sample size calculation ensures that an appropriate number of subjects are recruited to answer the specified study question. The sample size should be calculated *a priori*. Obtaining adequate power in a study depends on the following: (a) Alpha or Type I error (concluding that a treatment is effective when it is not), (b) beta or Type II error (concluding a truly effective treatment to be not effective), (c) treatment effect that is considered clinically significant, and (d) the nature of the data in the study.

Type I error is customarily set at 0.05 and Type II error is set at 0.20 (representing 80% power). A clinically relevant treatment effect should be determined such that the study is designed to detect a statistically significant result if the reported treatment effect is equal to or greater than the predetermined effect. It would require a very small sample size to detect a dramatic treatment effect (for example, surgery for senile cataracts) but this is rare in clinical trials today. Most new RCTs are designed to detect relatively small treatment effects and therefore require large sample size. Equivalency trials, which attempt to show that two treatments are equally effective within a certain range of error, tend to require large sample sizes. This is because, to show equivalency, a higher methodological rigor must be met.

Sample size also depends on the nature of the data in the study. If the outcome measure is a continuous variable such as intraocular pressure, then the sample size will depend on the variation in intraocular pressure among patients in the study. If the natural variation is large, then a large sample size will be required, whereas if the variation is small then a smaller sample size will be adequate. If the outcome measure is an event such as the progression of the disease, then the sample size required will depend on the number of events rather than the number of patients entered. Consequently, studying a rare event outcome in an RCT will require a much larger sample size than studying a common event.[10]

A study with too few patients recruited runs the risk of not having the power to detect a treatment effect, even if a treatment effect truly exists. For example, the results of a study may show a 50% risk reduction that is not statistically significant because of an inadequate sample size. This is a problem because this 50% risk reduction may be a clinically important treatment effect that is reported as an insignificant result simply because too few people were studied. The same study with a larger sample size and equivalent treatment effect would potentially show a significant result. In addition to not answering the question intended, the results of low-powered studies are often misinterpreted as "the treatment was found to be ineffective," when the correct interpretation is that "no significant association was found."

In conclusion, an RCT should report an *a priori* sample size calculation and the assumptions used in that calculation. When interpreting the results of a trial, if the treatment effect was clinically but not statistically significant, then an error was made in the assumptions of the sample size calculation and too few people were recruited to adequately power the study.

Randomization

The method of randomization should be reported. Before randomization, patients may be stratified according to one or more prognostic variables identified during the design phase of the study. Stratification of patients in a randomized trial produces a truly *equal* distribution (as opposed to a random distribution) of these variables between the treatment arms, and is especially useful when the sample size is small and there are known variables that are highly prognostic.

Intervention

The methodology of the treatment being examined in an RCT should be described to a reproducible extent. An ideal treatment is one that can be realistically and straightforwardly implemented into clinical practice if benefit is demonstrated.[10] Often large pharmacological RCTs use complex drug protocols with intensive patient monitoring to ensure that patients are receiving optimal therapy. This is appropriate in an *efficacy* trial when the treatment is being tested under tightly regulated situations. However, the clinical *effectiveness* is the effect of the treatment in the real-world setting. Results of an effectiveness trial are more useful for making clinical decisions, particularly when treatment protocols become complex.

Control Group and Blinding

The therapy administered to the control group should coincide with the current standard of care. If there are no standard treatments being offered for a particular condition, then a placebo is employed. The Hawthorne effect states that patients who are observed or treated intensely do clinically better than patients who are not. Also, patients given a placebo therapy with conviction do better than patients given no treatment.[10] Therefore, aspects of the experimental and control treatments, other than the obvious biologic differences, should be minimized as much as possible.

Blinding attempts to retain a similar prognosis between the two treatment arms after the treatment protocol begins.[9] Trials may be single-, double-, or triple-blinded depending on the nature of the treatment and the flexibility of the study design. In single-blinded trials, only the patients are kept unaware of their treatment arm. Double-blinded trials blind the patients as well as the treating physician or observer to eliminate the opportunity for observer bias. Triple-blinded trials also mask statisticians during the analysis phase.

Although blinding is difficult, and sometimes impossible, in many cases, in sound methodological studies every reasonable attempt is made to minimize bias. For example, in a recent trial demonstrating that pegaptanib sodium injection (Macugen) is effective in treating neovascular AMD[11] a subconjunctival anesthetic was used in both control and experimental groups to blind the patient to the treatment arm. Also, a second nontreating ophthalmologist performed all postinjection assessments.

Differences between Treatment Arms

Generally, randomization in a clinical trial results in two treatment arms that are similar in every way except for the treatment or intervention being studied. The success of randomization is confirmed by comparing basic demographic variables and known prognostic variables between treatment arms. These variables should be reported in the published study. Any differences that do exist are explainable either by a systematic error in randomization or bad luck. If known prognostic variables are different between the treatment arms, statistical adjustments can be made but such manipulation should raise serious concerns as to the validity of the randomization process.

As the clinical trial progresses, all patients should receive equivalent follow-up and be treated identically except for the therapeutic intervention under study. Cointervention can occur when a clinician not involved in the RCT prescribes an intervention known to affect the outcome or when the trial physician prescribes additional therapy for the condition in question because of a changing medical picture. Potential cointerventions should be predicted before the study starts and a rule should be established as to how to deal with various situations.

For example, in the recent trial studying Macugen for the treatment of wet AMD, photodynamic therapy could be administered to patients freely at the treating physician's discretion. As long as the treating ophthalmologist is blinded to the patient's treatment arm, this is an appropriate means of dealing with this issue. If patients in the treatment arm receive more effective cointerventions more frequently than patients in the control arm, the study results will have questionable validity despite adjustments made during data analysis. In the Macugen trial[11] there was no significant difference in the administration of photodynamic therapy (PDT)—a cointervention known to be effective in treating wet AMD—between treatment arms and, in fact, patients in the control arm received more PDT than patients in the Macugen arm.

Follow-up

A published RCT should display a flow-chart outlining the number of patients recruited, included and excluded, randomized, treated, and lost to follow-up. Researchers must make a reasonable effort to track down people who are lost to follow-up irrespective of the treatment arm. Although there is no set level of acceptable loss to follow-up, any loss can introduce bias if there is a reason as to why one arm is affected preferentially.

In many trials, noncompliance can be a problem and many patients may be randomized to one treatment but end up essentially receiving intervention from the other study arm. In these cases patients should be analyzed in the groups to which they were originally randomized, the so-called intention-to-treat method. This allows the RCT to answer the question of primary interest to clinicians: *What treatment option is best at the time the decision must be made?* If an intention-to-treat method is not employed, then the validity of the trial must be questioned since the randomization process becomes compromised and there is room for systematic differences between treatment groups.[10]

Throughout the patient follow-up period, adverse events and side effect data must be collected and periodically reported. These data are an important component in the overall interpretation of the study results.

Interpretation of Results

Size of Treatment Effect

In most trials, the primary outcome is a dichotomous event (e.g., a 15-letter loss in visual acuity or mortality). The incidence rate of the primary outcome is measured in both treatment arms for the duration of the follow-up period. The size of the treatment effect is generally reported as an RRR defined as the incidence rate of the outcome in the treatment group divided by the incidence rate of the outcome in the control group. If the treatment arm is effective in preventing disease, then the RRR will be less than 1.0; a smaller RRR corresponds to a larger treatment effect. If confounding variables are controlled for in the analysis phase, then a multiple logistic regression analysis should be employed and an adjusted OR should be reported.

In many clinical trials the primary outcome is the time until an event, or survival. Survival is a more powerful outcome as it incorporates the time elapsed until outcome ascertainment as opposed to simply whether or not the disease outcome occurred. RCTs will often report survival analyses such as Kaplan Meier curves, log-rank statistics, or Cox Proportional Hazards models. Although statistically they are more powerful, survival analyses may not be as intuitive to the clinician. Even if a variable is time dependent in nature, an RCT should report the raw data needed for a reader to calculate more intuitive basic statistics such as the incidence rates and RRR.

Precision of Treatment Effect

Along with a measurement of the size of the treatment effect statistical tests are used to measure the precision as either a *p* value or 95% CI. A *p* value represents the probability that an observed treatment effect is due to sampling error and by convention a *p* value of less than 5% is considered statistically significant. A 95% CI indicates the level of certainty that the true treatment effect lies within a range of treatment effects. As such, if the 95% CI of an RRR includes 1.0 then we cannot confidently exclude the possibility that no treatment effect exists and we cannot consider the treatment effect statistically significant.

Clinical Significance

In addition to the statistical significance of a treatment effect, it is important to look at the *clinical* significance of that effect. The *clinical* significance of a result refers to the level of effectiveness of a treatment at which a clinician feels adoption of the treatment would be justified in clinical practice. For instance, an ophthalmologist may feel that to justify the risk of adverse events for a particular treatment it should confer an RRR of 0.5 or less for a loss of 15 or more letters of distance visual acuity. However, a larger sample size (and thereby more outcome events) leads to more confidence in the results and hence more precision. Practically, this means a smaller *p* value or a narrower 95% CI. In fact, any treatment effect, in theory, can be found to be "statistically significant" through an RCT if enough people are studied. Therefore, when interpreting a result, the clinician should decide on an RRR that is practically significant for the clinical application of the study. Then, if the results show a statistically significant treatment effect equal to or greater than the practically significant cutoff point, the clinical intervention can be considered for use. As discussed in the section on sample size calculations, if a given treatment effect is practically but not statistically significant, then the study is inadequately powered and no useful conclusion can be made.

Absolute Risk Reduction and Number Needed to Treat

The absolute risk reduction (ARR) is the rate of outcome in the control group minus the rate of outcome in the treatment group and can be a useful and intuitive statistic since it accounts for the absolute incidence of disease. For example, a treatment that reduces disease incidence from 20% to 10% over 5 years has the same treatment effect (RRR = 2) as a treatment that reduces disease incidence from 4% to 2% over 5 years. However, more patients will benefit from the first treatment (ARR = 10% vs. 2%).

The ARR can also be mathematically described in an intuitive statistic called the *number needed to treat* (NNT). The NNT is simply the inverse of ARR and is the number of patients that need to be treated with the intervention to prevent one outcome event. Again, this measure can be useful when deciding whether or not to implement the use of a particular therapy among the patients in clinical practice. The RRR, ARR, and NNT are useful statistics but they need not be reported formally. However, raw data should be available such that they can be calculated by hand.

Generalizability to Patient Care

There are two main factors to be considered when deciding if study results are generalizable to the individual patient. First, most RCTs outline detailed inclusion and exclusion criteria that reflect a very specific target population. In real life, physicians are often faced with the decision of whether to apply evidence from these studies to their own patients who may not precisely match the study criteria. A practical way to determine if the results of a particular clinical trial are applicable to the patient is to ask if the patient is different from the study population in any way that would logically affect the treatment result. Second, large RCTs are designed to provide optimal study conditions to maximize any treatment effect that does exist because it is easier to prove efficacy than it is to prove effectiveness. High compliance rates and intensive follow-up may make a large difference to study results, yet may be impractical in regular clinical practice. The physician must evaluate how realistic the treatment—as administered in the RCT—will be for a given patient.

Outcome Measures

Primary and secondary outcome measures should be clearly defined *a priori* and be clinically meaningful. This includes clearly defining a time frame for the primary analysis. If outcome measures are not defined *a priori*, the possibility of data dredging cannot be excluded. If enough analyses are conducted (i.e., over different time frames and using different outcome

measures), then there is a high likelihood of finding a statistically significant clinical outcome through chance alone. In general, multiple comparisons should be avoided, or if they are unavoidable the *p* value considered to be statistically significant in the study should be adjusted downward, using appropriate statistical methodology.

Surrogate measures of disease are less powerful evidence of clinical effectiveness. For example, in a study investigating an antihypertensive agent for the treatment of heart disease, all-cause mortality or cardiac-specific mortality is a much more meaningful outcome measure than blood pressure reduction (a surrogate marker). An analogous situation in ophthalmology is the use of intraocular pressure as a surrogate marker in glaucoma trials. We do know that decreasing the intraocular pressure in patients with glaucoma will result in better visual outcomes. However, using a primary outcome of visual acuity loss or visual field loss is a much more powerful measure in a glaucoma trial than using intraocular pressure measurements.

Value of Intervention

Finally, the clinician must consider whether the treatment benefits are worth the potential costs of treatment. The RCT provides substantial information on the hard medical outcomes of treatment but little information on the true economic and biopsychosocial cost of treatment. The RCT will provide information about the frequency of treatment side effects and the rate of more serious adverse events. However, when initiating treatment there are other costs to the patient that could negatively affect quality-of-life, including the monetary cost of treatment, the label of disease, and the hassle of taking medication or undergoing a procedure. Clearly, the decision as to whether to recommend treatment will depend highly on the individual circumstances of each patient encounter.

Example-Critical Appraisal

In 2001, the age-related eye disease study (AREDS) Research Group demonstrated that supplementation with antioxidants plus zinc was effective in reducing the risk of progression of neovascular AMD.[8] The following text go through a brief appraisal outlining the key points in appraising the validity of an RCT and interpreting the results appropriately.

CRITICAL APPRAISAL OF THE VALIDITY OF THE AGE-RELATED EYE DISEASE STUDY

Sample of Patients

Patients with evidence of dry AMD were recruited from the offices of 11 retinal surgeons over a six-year period. Broad inclusion criteria were used and patients were categorized according to the severity of dry AMD (categories 1−4). Exclusion criteria were minimal. Patients had to be between 55 and 80 years of age and have at least one eye with the best-corrected visual acuity of 20/32 or better. Consequently, the study sample was broad and generalizable to a typical ophthalmic practice. A sample size calculation was reported to ensure adequate power to detect a 25%−50% treatment effect in progression to advanced AMD. This calculation appropriately accounted for some patients discontinuing treatment medication and some patients in the placebo arms beginning to take new supplementation.[8]

Intervention and Randomization

Four treatment arms were used: Antioxidants (vitamins C and E), zinc, both antioxidants and zinc, and placebo. Patients within the less severe AMD category at baseline were randomized with a 50% probability of placebo or antioxidants. Those patients with more severe AMD at baseline (categories 2−4) had a 25% percent probability to be in the four treatment arms. Randomization and masking were described completely and stratified by study center and AMD severity. Eligible patients were given a 1-month trial with placebo to demonstrate compliance with the treatment regimen before beginning the trial.

Control Group and Blinding

An internal placebo control group was used in this study (placebo controlled). Patients were blinded to the treatment arm through the use of identical medication containers, similar pill appearance, and similar-tasting supplements. This technique also ensured that physicians and other observers were blinded. It did not explicitly state whether the statistician was blinded.

Differences between Treatment Arms

Randomization seemed to be successful as the two treatment arms were similar with respect to baseline variables. Specifically, they were similar with respect to variables that could have potentially influenced study outcome (confounding variables) such as age, gender, and dietary intake and supplementation. Cointervention was an important methodological issue in this trial. Patients who were taking supplements before the study (57%) had to agree to supplement their diet with the multivitamin Centrum only. Ninety-five percent of this group continued to take Centrum. Although not encouraged, 13% of people who had not taken supplements before the study began also started to take Centrum during the study. Supplementation other than with the study treatments was recorded in detail; no significant difference in additional supplementation was noticed among the treatment arms. The original randomization assignments were kept for analyses (i.e., an intention-to-treat analysis was employed).

Follow-up

There were identical follow-up procedures between both groups as the trial progressed. A full ophthalmic exam was done at baseline and every 6 months during the trial. Fundus photographs were taken initially and then annually beginning 2 years after randomization and were centrally graded. Visual acuity was measured using standard Early Treatment Diabetic Retinopathy Study (ETDRS) protocol. Adverse events were assessed through serum level measurements, medical histories, and mortality rates and monitored by a data and safety monitoring committee on an annual basis. Follow-up was clearly described and only 2.4% of study participants were lost to follow-up.

INTERPRETATION OF AGE-RELATED EYE DISEASE STUDY RESULTS

Outcome Measures

The primary outcomes were (a) chance of progression to or treatment for advanced AMD and (b) at least moderate visual acuity loss from baseline (≥ 15 letters). These primary outcomes included a primary time frame (5 years) and are described clearly and were clinically relevant (i.e., not surrogate markers). The statisticians considered the issue of multiple comparisons (because of repeated measure analyses and in-term analyses) during the study design phase and calculated that results should only be considered statistically significant at a level of $p = 0.01$. This p value should be considered equivalent to $p = 0.05$ if multiple comparisons had not been made.

Statistical Analysis

Comparisons were made using an intention-to-treat analysis. The primary analysis was done using repeated-measures logistic regression to account for the fact that the outcome of progression of AMD could come and go in time. This statistical analysis was clearly described and associations were reported as adjusted odd ratios. The results section of the report contained enough primary information to allow the reader to calculate simple RRRs, ARRs, and NNT.

Treatment Effect

Less than 0.5% of patients in AMD Category I (essentially free from AMD abnormalities) developed advanced AMD during the study and were therefore excluded from the analysis. The primary outcome showed a significant odds reduction for the development of advanced AMD with antioxidants plus zinc (adjusted OR of 0.72; 99% CI, 0.52–0.98) over placebo among patients in AMD Categories II–IV. When patients with more severe AMD at baseline (AMD categories III and IV) were analyzed the odds reduction increased (adjusted OR of 0.66; 99% CI, 0.47–0.91).

Although not calculated in the report, the paper presented enough primary data for the reader to calculate RRRs, ARRs, and an NNT for patients who had more advanced AMD at baseline (AMD categories III and IV). Although not as statistically comprehensive as the repeated-measures

logistic regression, these statistics are very useful for grasping the practical effectiveness of this treatment. These simple statistics are calculated as follows:

> Risk of AMD advancement in placebo group at 5 years = 0.278
>
> Risk of AMD advancement in the antioxidants/zinc group at 5 years = 0.202
>
> Relative risk ratio = 0.202/0.278 = 0.726
>
> Relative risk reduction = 100% × (0.278 − 0.202)/0.278 = 27%
>
> Absolute risk reduction = 0.278 − 0.202 = 0.076 = 7.6%
>
> NNT = 1/0.076 = 13 people

Practical Significance

Assessing the practical significance of a treatment effect will depend on many factors specific to the practicing ophthalmologist. Certainly, in many circumstances a relative risk reduction of 27% (see preceding text) for developing advanced AMD would be considered a practically significant clinical effect. However, this risk reduction is over a 5-year period and is only applicable to patients at the highest risk of developing advanced AMD. In addition, although there is a substantial relative risk reduction over 5 years, the ARR attributable to the treatment is only 7.6%. The practical or clinical significance of this treatment should be assessed on a patient-to-patient basis.

Generalizability

This study included a large sample with fairly broad criteria for inclusion and as such the results should be fairly generalizable to a typical ophthalmic practice. One weakness with respect to generalizability was that the study participants were assessed for their ability to comply with the study protocol before randomization. Therefore, the study was more of an efficacy trial as opposed to an effectiveness trial. An ophthalmologist in clinical practice could not be as sure that his or her patients would comply as well with vitamin supplementation when compared to the patients accrued for this trial. A second weakness for generalizability was that the main results of the study were among a subset of patients at higher risk for development of advanced

AMD. Therefore, when applying these results to patient care, an ophthalmologist must assess the risk of advancement when determining if a patient should begin supplementation.

Cost of Intervention

The efficacy of supplementation has been clearly shown through this RCT. However, when beginning a patient on high dose antioxidant supplementation to prevent progression of AMD the costs of intervention must also be considered. In addition to the monetary expense of long-term supplementation, taking four large pills per day may lead to non-compliance and therefore loss of treatment effect among some patients in the real-world setting.

Overall Assessment

This RCT employed very sound methodology and provided clear results to a common clinical problem. Methodological strengths of the study included a large and broad sample size allowing easy generalization to ophthalmic practice. Cointervention with supplementation had the potential to cause problems in this study but the authors did a good job to account for this problem through a well-thought-out study design. The authors showed a modest treatment effect for preventing advancement of AMD (adjusted OR = 0.72) among patients at higher risk for disease advancement. Thirteen patients among those at higher risk would have to be treated over 5 years to prevent one case of advancement of AMD. One weakness of the study—from the standpoint of its applicability to being applied in a general ophthalmic practice—was that it was more of an efficacy trial than an effectiveness trial. Specifically, compliance may be more of an issue in the real-world setting. As with any study, these results should be applied on an individual basis to an ophthalmologist's individual patient population.

References

1. Sackett DL, Haynes RB, Tugwell P. *Clinical epidemiology a basic science for clinical medicine.* Toronto: Little, Brown and Company; 1988.
2. Sharma S. Levels of evidence and interventional ophthalmology. *Can J Ophthalmol.* 1997;32: 359–362.
3. Albiani D, Sharma S. Canadian Ophthalmological Society Conference. *Poster presentation.* Toronto;June 2001.
4. Wu KH, Wang JJ, Rochtchina E, et al. Angiotensin-converting enzyme inhibitors (ACEIs) and age related maculopathy: Cross-sectional findings from the Blue Mountains Eye Study. *Acta Ophthalmol Scand.* 2004;82:298–303.
5. Oleckno WA. *Essential epidemiology principles and applications.* Prospect Heights. IL: Waveland Press; 2002.
6. McGwin G, Xie A, Owsley C Jr. The use of cholesterol-lowering medications and age-related macular degeneration. *Ophthalmology.* 2005;112(3):488–494.
7. Seddon JM, George S, Rosner B, et al. Progression of age-related macular degeneration: Prospective assessment of C-reactive protein, interleukin 6, and other cardiovascular biomarkers. *Arch Ophthalmol.* 2005;123(6):774–782.
8. AREDS Report No. 8. A randomized, placebo-controlled, clinical trial of high-dose supplementation with vitamins C and E, Beta Carotene, and Zinc for age-related macular degeneration and vision loss. *Arch Ophthalmol.* 2001;119:1417–1436.
9. Guyatt GH, Sackett DL, Cook DJ. Users' guides to the medical literature. II. How to use an article about therapy or prevention. A. Are the results of the study valid? *JAMA.* 1993;270(21):2596–2601.
10. Fletcher RW, Fletcher SW. *Clinical epidemiology the essentials.* 4th ed. New York: Lippincott Williams & Wilkins; 2005.
11. Gradoudas ES, Adamis AP, Cunningham ET Jr, et al. Pegaptanib for neovascular age-related macular degeneration. *N Engl J Med.* 2004;351(27):2805–2816.

CHAPTER 2

Health Economics

Hussein Hollands, MD, MS (Epid) and Sanjay Sharma, MD, MS (Epid), FRCS (C), MBA

Introduction

Economic evaluation in medicine has the potential to greatly influence policy decisions both in the public and private sectors of society, thereby impacting many facets of health care. Recently, both government agencies and academic researchers have realized the need for collaboration between policy makers and academics. Specifically, policy makers and governing bodies are becoming increasingly interested in basing their policy decisions on rigorous scientific evidence, while academics are trying to make their research more relevant to the people who will eventually be applying it.

An economic evaluation of a health care program is meant to aid in a decision regarding whether, from a particular perspective, a program should be undertaken, when compared to another available use of resources. A basic assumption is that the cost-effective analysis (CEA) is being performed to optimize the total health of a target population with access to a finite amount of resources. Consequently, this technique is not appropriate for individual physicians making decisions about their patients since it is a physician's duty to maximize the health of his or her individual patients.[1] However, an economic evaluation and analysis in health care, if performed using rigorous scientific methods, is arguably one of the most relevant research studies available to a policy maker as an aid to decision making. There have been a number of good books on CEA in health care;[2-4] it is the purpose of this chapter to give only an overview of the important aspects of an economic evaluation.

When referring to a health care program we refer to any intervention that will cost money and is being considered for implementation for the purpose of improving health. This definition is purposefully broad and could include, for example, a public health safety program, a governmental health policy, or a decision by a third-party insurer or government agency to fund a certain drug or medical treatment. Before a particular health program is taken up for an economic evaluation, it should have been previously proved both safe and efficacious, usually through a well-designed randomized controlled trial (RCT).[2]

A full economic evaluation has two key elements that distinguish it from a partial evaluation.[2] First, it measures the cost-effectiveness of a health care program against another option—preferably against the next best available alternative or another option that could potentially be implemented. Second, it evaluates both the health outcomes of the program (effectiveness) and the cost simultaneously.

A CEA, as first described by Weinstein, forces decision makers to be explicit with respect to the benefits and values that underlie a resource allocation decision.[3] It is important that a CEA is broad and comprehensive, and oriented toward outcomes. The ratio of incremental cost per unit of health outcome gained through a health program is referred to as the cost-effectiveness ratio and can be used to compare the cost-effectiveness of different health programs. League tables are lists of cost-effectiveness ratios whereby the cost-effectiveness of different health programs or interventions can be compared.

Full evaluations can be classified into four subgroups: Cost-effectiveness analyses, cost-minimization analyses, cost–benefit analyses, and cost–utility analyses. A full economic evaluation will compare both the effectiveness and cost of two or more health care programs. In each subgroup the cost of the program is measured but it is the measurement of effectiveness that distinguishes the different types of analyses. We will briefly examine each of the subtypes of CEAs.

Cost-effective Analysis

A CEA is the most general, full, economic evaluation and can be distinguished from the other subgroups because the effectiveness of the health program being evaluated is measured in natural units of effect. The most common unit of effect is length of life, such that an analysis would compare the cost per life year saved between two potential health programs. In medicine, many clinical trials measure survival as the primary outcome, and are therefore well suited to be used in a CEA. However, life years saved may not be the most appropriate outcome measure if the program is designed to improve quality of life (QOL), such as is the case in ophthalmology. It is possible to base a CEA on a natural outcome measure that is assumed to be associated with better health. For instance, the cost per vision-year saved could be calculated in a CEA. Irrespective of the natural outcome unit chosen for the analysis, the purpose of a CEA is to compare the cost per natural health outcome between the health programs under consideration.

Cost-Minimization Analysis

In a cost-minimization analysis (CMA), one assumes that the effectiveness of the health programs under consideration is equivalent. In a CMA, the cost of two or more health programs is compared and the program with the lower cost is considered the "preferred" option from the health policy maker's perspective. For example, consider a situation in which an equivalence trial had shown that there was no statistically significant difference between two drugs for the treatment of glaucoma. An equivalence trial is a type of (RCT) specifically designed to test the hypothesis that a treatment option is as good as another alternative that has previously been proved to be efficacious. Here, the treatment option with the lower cost would be preferred.

Cost–Benefit Analysis

In the real world there are many situations where a number of important health outcomes such as length of life, QOL, and potential complications or consequences with treatment must be considered simultaneously to fully assess the effectiveness of a program. In addition, it may be necessary to directly compare programs that provide drastically different health benefits. Cost–benefit analysis (CBA) and cost–utility analysis (CUA) have been designed to account for different health outcomes and may be important in evaluating the true cost-effectiveness of a program and to allow for the comparison of programs or treatment interventions designed to effect health in different ways.

A CBA is also a special form of CEA, except that in this case the effectiveness of a program is measured monetarily. Costs can clearly be measured monetarily, but to measure the effectiveness in this way it is necessary to convert health outcomes into dollars. Consequently, a monetary value must be placed on all health outcomes pertinent to the analysis including length of life, QOL, and other health consequences. If the outcome of interest is simply years of life, then annual earnings per life year saved can be defined as a monetary measure of effectiveness. However, when other factors such as QOL and potential complications must be considered, effectiveness is generally measured using a willingness-to-pay method. In this technique, a separate study would be conducted and subjects would be asked how much money they would be willing to pay to completely avoid a certain negative health outcome. A CBA should report results in the form of a net benefit in dollars, or the difference between the monetary values of the health benefits derived minus the cost of the health program.[4]

The major advantage with using a CBA is that health programs with widely varying health outcomes can be compared to each other. In addition, by definition a CBA compares the net benefit versus the net cost of a health program so that one can determine whether the benefits outweigh the costs of initiating the program. However, assigning a price of a health outcome is a very difficult and controversial task that may only be possible in a limited number of situations. The main disadvantage with this method is that people from different sociodemographic backgrounds may be willing to pay vastly different dollar amounts for the same health outcome. In addition, whether a person lives in a country with a universal health care system or whether the person has full health insurance will dramatically affect a person's willingness to pay. These differences can drastically bias a study toward or against a certain demography of the population. Also, these differences make it very difficult to compare CBAs with each other.

Cost–Utility Analysis

A CUA is another type of CEA that allows different health outcomes of a program to be combined into one overall measure of effectiveness, thereby allowing for health programs designed to achieve different health outcomes to be compared. In addition, the difficult task of assigning monetary values to health outcomes is avoided. The effectiveness measure for a CUA is usually a quality adjusted life year (QALY) where years of life are adjusted using utilities as a weighting factor. Measuring a health outcome in terms of QALYs allows for incorporation of both morbidity and mortality into one measure. Therefore, a CUA can investigate the cost per quality of life (QOL) adjusted year gained from the implementation of a particular health program compared to an alternative.

A utility is a measure of the strength of preference for a particular health outcome and has a theoretical foundation in economics and decision theory. Essentially, a utility is a measure of the value that a person places on a certain outcome or health state. Using utilities, the QOL associated with a particular health state that may have many important aspects can be measured using one method, and can be reported with one value. Common methods of utility valuation are the time trade-off (TTO) technique, standard reference gamble (SRG), and rating scale. We will examine the details of utility theory later in the chapter.

Important Aspects of an Economic Evaluation

Cost-effectiveness Ratio

A true CEA must measure both the cost and effectiveness of a health program against the next best alternative. As mentioned above, the cost-effectiveness of a health program will usually be expressed in terms of an incremental cost-effectiveness ratio (ICER). Ideally, this will be defined as the difference in cost between the health program under question and the next best alternative (the numerator, or cost) divided by the difference in effectiveness between the health program under question and the next best alternative (the denominator, or effectiveness). It is important to differentiate between a marginal ICER and an average ICER. In the former, the cost and effectiveness both represent differences in costs and effectiveness between the treatment in question and the next best alternative, whereas in the latter the

costs and effectiveness are measured independently of any alternative strategy.[1] Through the use of an ICER, it is possible to discern the true opportunity cost of a program, or the health outcomes that could be achieved by implementing the program of interest as opposed to the next best available option. By examining health policy in this way, it is possible to compare the cost-effectiveness of various health interventions in a consistent manner.

Perspective

The first fundamental question that must be answered in an economic evaluation is the perspective that the decision maker is taking when conducting the analysis. For instance, the decision of whether photodynamic therapy for patients with age-related macular degeneration is cost-effective could be drastically different depending on whether the decision is being made from the perspective of a for-profit third-party insurer or society at large. The insurer's viewpoint may simply take into account the incremental cost of treatment and a health outcome in terms of vision-years saved or QALYs gained. However, society's viewpoint may have to consider the cost of blindness that could include the utilization of many social and disability services provided by a government. The conclusion of a CEA could easily be different depending on the perspective taken. Unless a CEA is inherently being undertaken from a specific viewpoint (e.g., from the perspective of a third-party insurer or hospital) it has been recommended that the most general societal perspective be used.[4] However, if the evaluation is undertaken from a societal viewpoint, it may be relatively easy and informative to provide other viewpoints in a CEA.

Designing the Study

In designing a CEA, a clear problem that can be realistically answered through the analysis must be identified. The objective, method, and target population of the program alternatives must also be clear. A description of the effectiveness of the health intervention should be included as it is not logical to investigate the cost-effectiveness of something that has not been proved to be effective. To visualize health outcomes being modeled in the analysis, it may be useful to draw a flow diagram using a hypothetical cohort of people who begin the program, and follow that cohort through every possible event outcome. Consultation with medical and economic experts is usually required.

Measuring Effectiveness

Survival is a basic and very useful outcome measure in a CEA and can be the sole outcome or it can be incorporated with other data. If survival does not fully explain the health outcome that is conferred by a program, then another method to measure effectiveness must be used. It is often easy and useful to base a CEA on an intermediate outcome measure that is assumed to be associated with better health. For instance, the cost per vision-year saved could be calculated for an ophthalmic intervention. If an intermediate health outcome is being used, a strong link with QOL or survival must be established.

Real-world situations commonly arise where a number of important health outcomes such as survival, QOL, and potential complications or consequences of treatment must be considered simultaneously to fully determine the effectiveness of a program. It is also desirable to be able to compare programs that provide drastically different health benefits. When the effectiveness of a health outcome is measured in dollars, the economic evaluation is known as a CBA. The most critical aspect in a CBA is valuing health using money; often the value of a health outcome, health state, or health scenario is measured by the willingness to pay or by annual earnings on the basis of expected length of life. As mentioned earlier in the chapter, there are many inherent biases involved in doing this.

The most comprehensive measure of health outcome combines both length and QOL into a QALY. A QALY can be conceptualized further by examining Figure 2.1, where the y-axis represents health-related quality of life (HRQL), the x-axis represents duration of life, and the curve represents various health states that a hypothetical person could potentially go through within a certain period. The area under the curve represents the QALYs associated with that particular set of health states over the specified time frame.

Measuring Health-Related Quality of Life

It has been generally accepted that QOL should be measured with a broad-based definition of health, accounting for physical/mobility function, emotional/psychological function, sensory function, cognitive function, pain, dexterity, and self-care.[5] However, there remain many alternatives in measuring HRQL. HRQL measurement tools can be classified as generic, which attempt to measure overall HRQL, or specific, which focus on certain aspects of health such as disease, population, or function.[6]

Specific HRQL instruments such as the 51-item National Eye Institute Visual Function Questionnaire[7] and the Visual Function 14 (VF-14)[8] in ophthalmology give more information about certain aspects of health (i.e., visual function) and are considered more responsive to changing health states. Generic HRQL instruments use one measure to encompass all aspects of HRQL and are comparable across different health conditions. One example of a generic HRQL instrument is a health status profile. Health status profiles are single instruments that can detect differential effects on various aspects of health status. Examples of health status profiles include the Medical Outcomes Short Form-36 (SF-36)[9] and the Sickness Impact Profile.[10]

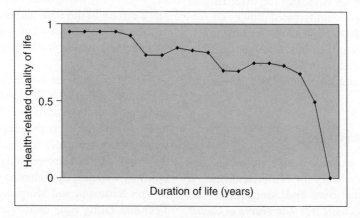

FIGURE 2.1 ■ Graphic depiction of a quality-of-life adjusted year. The area under the curve represents QALYs associated with this particular set of health states.

HRQL measurement tools can also be classified as preference based or nonpreference based. Health status profiles are nonpreference based and do not account for a patient's judgment on how disease affects them. In contrast, preference-based methods allow for a person's values toward the consequences of various health outcomes to be determined according to what is personally important. The measure of HRQL using patient preferences is called a *utility* and is considered the most appropriate HRQL weighting factor for use in a CEA.[4]

Sources for Utility Valuation

Utilities can be obtained from people who have the disease state in question (such as current patients or former patients) or from those who do not (including the general public, patients with other disease, or health care professionals). It has been shown empirically that people in the health state in question respond with higher utilities than people not in the health state and are making hypothetical utility assessments.[11] Additionally, these differing responses can dramatically affect the outcome of commonly accepted decision analyses.[12] The main argument for using current patients to derive utilities is that they have first-hand knowledge of the disease. However, using current patients can limit the number of disease states investigated simultaneously and can bias the results against the ill, disabled, or elderly.[4] In addition, using community-derived utility values allows for more consistent comparisons across studies performed in different fields.

The final decision as to whose utilities to use in a CEA will eventually depend on the specific situation, the availability of data, and the preference of the investigators. Community-based utilities are recommended as the default and should be used unless there are specific reasons to choose another sample. Using utilities derived from health professionals is not recommended and should only be used as a last resort.[4]

Techniques for Eliciting Utilities

Utilities were first introduced and applied in economics and game theory by Von Neumann, a Hungarian mathematician, and Morgenstern, an economist, in their classic text *The Theory of Games and Economic Behavior*.[13] They described a method of decision making under conditions of *uncertainty*

that enables a reasonable decision maker to make the best decision in accordance with his or her fundamental preferences. From a health care perspective, the first fundamental axiom states that a person can quantify a probability (p) of indifference between the following two outcomes: (a) A sure outcome of the health state which is to be evaluated; and (b) a gamble with probability p of the best possible outcome (perfect health), and $(1 - p)$ for the worst possible outcome (death). This probability (p) is defined as the SRG utility for a particular outcome. The SRG is said to measure utilities under *risky*, or *uncertain*, conditions because an individual is forced to quantify a probability, but is not assured of any particular outcome (i.e., the individual is playing a game of chance).

Popular riskless utility instruments (measured under conditions of *certainty*) include the TTO and a rating scale. The TTO method was initially developed by Torrence et al. [14] and requires a patient to hypothetically trade off years of remaining life in exchange for perfect health to quantify the QOL of the particular disease state. Two pieces of information are needed to quantify the utility of an individual in a particular disease state: (a) An expected life span (x) available for trading; and (b) the number of years (y) that an individual is willing to trade off out of the x available years, in return for restoring perfect health. TTO utility is calculated as [(number of years expected to live (x) − number of years willing to trade (y))/ number of years expected to live (x)]. For example, if a patient expects to live for 12 years and is willing to trade off 4 years for perfect health, then the utility of the current health state is [(12 − 4)/ 12] = 0.67. The rating scale requires a participant to rate a certain health state (either a hypothetical state or the state that they are currently in) between two set extremes, usually death (utility = 0) and perfect health (utility = 1).

Different utility elicitation techniques are known to produce different utility values[5,15,16] and consequently the decision about what utility instrument to use in an analysis is important. TTO and rating scale utilities are easier to understand and obtain than SRG utilities. However, only the SRG method of utility elicitation is equivalent to the axiom put forth by Von Neumann and Morgenstern and, therefore, TTO and rating scale utilities are approximations. Regardless of the method used, in a given situation, utilities should be valid, reliable, and responsive to changing health states. In 1996, the Panel on Cost-Effectiveness in Health and Medicine was unable to come to a conclusion on the best utility assessment technique.[17] The decision of which utility assessment tool is appropriate will therefore differ, depending on the population of participants, the nature of the study, the preferences of the researchers, and the nature of the current QOL literature in the particular field of interest.

Outcome Probabilities

Ideally, a full prospective study that measures the health outcome of interest and relevant costs associated with the program in a randomized fashion would be employed. In this way, the study would be designed to answer the study question and the results would be easily transferable to a cost-effective model. In the absence of a randomized prospective CEA, level I evidence in the form of a well-designed RCT or meta-analysis should be used to estimate outcome probabilities (or treatment effect) and adverse reactions in a CEA. If a suitable RCT is not available, outcome probabilities may be based on observational studies such as prospective cohort designs. However, this introduces the potential for bias and is less than ideal. In many situations, a trade-off between the level of evidence (or internal validity) and generalizability to the situation and population of interest will exist and will need to be considered. Again, it is important to emphasize that before studying the cost-effectiveness of a health intervention, the intervention must have been shown to be clinically effective.

Estimating Costs

To assess the true opportunity cost of an intervention, cost should be valued as the difference in resource use between an intervention and an alternative intervention. Consequently, costs should refer to the incremental resources consumed or saved rather than the total resources used.[18] Although it is difficult to measure true opportunity costs, costs in a competitive economy are thought to reflect the opportunity cost of resources. Costs should be measured in dollars during a specific year, and a broad long-term societal outlook should be taken when relevant costs are being identified. When measuring costs in an economic evaluation, four main classifications have been identified as important:[4] (a) Health care resources, (b) nonhealth care resources, (c) informal caregiver's time, and (d) patient time.

It is useful to classify costs as direct costs or productivity costs (also known as indirect costs). Direct costs are defined as the value of all goods, services, and other resources that are consumed in the provision of an intervention or in dealing with the side effects or other current and future consequences linked to it.[4] Direct health care costs can include costs of tests, pharmaceuticals, and other medical treatments relating to the procedure, as well as any potential costs in the future that result from the health program or intervention. Direct nonhealth care costs can include such items as the cost of child care needed to complete an intervention or transportation. Changes in the use of informal caregiver's time should also be considered a direct cost, and can be measured using average wages in the community. Finally, direct costs due to patients' time associated with the intervention should be considered a cost, and can also be measured using average wages from the community.

When determining which health care costs to include in a cost analysis, any health care costs in the future that are associated with the disease should be considered. However, health care costs unrelated to the intervention should not necessarily be included. Productivity costs are associated with the loss (or gain) in productivity because of a health program or intervention and by convention are not counted in a CEA because they are inherently incorporated into the effectiveness component of the CEA.

Modeling the Problem

Unless a fully prospective economic evaluation is being performed, relevant cost and effectiveness data must be combined through analytic modeling to determine an ICER. Clearly an economic evaluation can be very complex and incorporate a large number of variables; consequently, the purpose of modeling the problem is to simplify reality to a level where it is of practical use. The first task in modeling a problem is to decide on a time horizon. It is usually advisable to perform a short-term analysis where data are available, and a longer-term analysis where data are modeled into the future. All health outcomes and costs will be discounted to their net present value, therefore health outcomes and costs that are incurred in the distant future will have a smaller effect on the outcome than those incurred at the beginning of the analysis.

The most common method for modeling is to employ expected value decision analysis to the problem. There is a large body of literature on medical decision analysis, and the reader is recommended to read Sox[19] for a detailed description of modeling methods and points of consideration. Decision analysis has its roots in economics and game theory, and is useful in aiding decision making when the consequences of actions are uncertain. In essence, decision tree models are a sequence of chance events and decisions over time where every chance event is assigned a probability.[20] Each path through the tree consists of a combination of chance and decision nodes and is associated with a final outcome, or utility. Each decision alternative is evaluated with an expected utility value, and the preferred decision choice is defined as the alternative with the largest expected utility. If a problem is simple and does not have to be modeled into the future, then a simple decision tree will often be adequate.

Modeling becomes more difficult when recurrent events over time are considered in the analysis. In this case a transition-state model is required, and is commonly performed using a Markov-cycle decision tree. In a Markov model a hypothetical participant will have the option of changing health states at the end of each time period, or cycle, according to predefined transition probabilities. The hypothetical patient is then given appropriate credit in the form of a utility for each cycle they spend in a given Markov state. An expected utility for each decision alternative can then be calculated mathematically.

A CEA should employ the simplest modeling technique possible that incorporates all relevant data and can adequately represent the problem.[4] There are a number of decision analysis software programs available that can be useful in formulating the decision tree and performing the CEA.

Discounting

The rationale for discounting costs in an economic analysis is derived from the idea that a dollar today is worth more than a dollar tomorrow. This time preference of money is due to a number of factors including inflation, rate of return on investment, and degree of risk associated with the investment being considered. Discounting is a simple calculation and can be described easily through an example. If $1,000 dollars is spent n years from now, and we assume a fixed rate of interest of 10%, then that $1,000 is worth $1,000/(1.10)^n$ today. This follows from the idea that this value ($1,000/(1.10)^n$), invested at a 10% annual return for n years, will yield $1,000 at the end of the n years. Therefore, if something of value is gained in the future it is worth less than if it was obtained today.

It is widely understood that costs should be discounted to reflect the time value of money; however, it is the discount rate that is controversial. Many discount rates have been proposed, but the Panel for Cost-Effectiveness in Health and Medicine recommended 3% as a riskless real discount rate to be used in economic evaluations. In sensitivity analyses, this rate should be varied between 0% and 7%.

In an economic evaluation, QALYs should be discounted at the same rate as costs. The reason for discounting future life years is not that years of life lived in the future are less valuable than years of life lived earlier, or that a year of life in the present can be invested today (analogously to a dollar) to produce an increase in life at a later date. The reason is that QALYs are being valued relative to the dollar and since the dollar is being discounted so must the QALY. Weinstein[3] walks readers through a simple scenario demonstrating the fundamental break in logic that will occur if years of life are not discounted at the same rate as cost in an economic evaluation.

Sensitivity Analysis

When modeling a health intervention versus an alternative, there are many potential uncertainties that must be considered. The most important uncertainties are associated with point estimates used in the model. These can include health outcomes (such as length of life, QOL, or other intermediate health outcomes), costs, probabilities, or discount rates. To access the robustness of a model, one-, two-, three-, or n-way sensitivity analyses can be performed by varying one or more parameters in the model simultaneously. If the model is large and complex there will be many sensitivity analyses possible. Sensitivity analyses should be reported on variables that will have a large impact on the study outcome when varied.

Another method for assessing the robustness of a cost-effectiveness model is to perform a Monte Carlo simulation. Most decision analysis software programs have a Monte Carlo simulation procedure whereby a hypothetical trial of the model is performed. In a primary Monte Carlo simulation, the model is performed using the reference-case point estimates, and a hypothetical cohort is put through the model using random number generators at each chance node. The outcome is an "observed" ICER that will be similar to the expected value ICER. The average "observed" ICER will be very close to the expected ICER if the simulation is performed a large number of times. Through the use of this method, a measure of uncertainty in the model can be determined, and statistical tests can be employed. A primary Monte Carlo simulation does not, however, consider the inherent variability of the point estimates (such as outcome probabilities, costs, or survival) in the model. In a secondary Monte Carlo simulation, during each simulation, some of the variables will be sampled from their respective distributions and then random number generators will be used to determine an expected ICER. In a complicated analysis with good effectiveness and outcome data, it is possible for a large number of variables to be defined statistically as distributions and sampled in this manner. Secondary Monte Carlo simulation generates a more accurate estimate of the inherent variability in the model.

Roles and Limitations

Limitations

There are a number of limitations with current economic evaluations that account for why CEA is not more readily applied in the field of health policy. An economic evaluation is not an exact science, and the methods used are not always systematic among analysts. An economic evaluation is by definition a multidisciplinary study design requiring input from the fields of economics, epidemiology, public policy, and mathematics. Methodological controversies such as the decision perspective, the method for measuring QOL, or the rate used to account for the time preference of money have led to inconsistent study designs being employed.

Varying methodologies in evaluating cost-effectiveness in health care have made it necessary to define guidelines. The broadest sets of guidelines were developed by the Panel for Cost-Effectiveness in Health and Medicine in 1996, and discuss a reference case, which is a standard set of methodological practices. However, economic evaluations are performed for a number of reasons, and consequently, different procedural guidelines have been defined for these different purposes. The multidisciplinary nature of an economic evaluation along with potentially differing methodological guidelines depending on the perspective of the study and the intended audience provides another challenge for researchers in the field.

Another limitation of CEA is the varying quality of resources available. Most economic evaluations rely heavily on previously published data because performing a fully prospective evaluation with sufficient power to detect a meaningful effect would be prohibitively expensive. Consequently, it may be difficult to follow commonly used guidelines when there is a limited amount of previously published research available on a subject.

In addition to methodological limitations, there are distributional consequences inherent in allocation decisions that are based on CEA. A basic assumption of CEA in health care is that the decision maker has the sole objective of maximizing the net health benefit of a target population with limited resources, and that all persons in the target population are valued equally by the decision maker. When decisions are based on this method, then although the net health benefit of the population will be maximized, some groups of individuals will benefit and some will lose. For example, if a Health Maintenance Organization (HMO) uses CEA results to relinquish funding of photodynamic therapy for patients with macular degeneration in favor of funding a novel treatment for diabetic retinopathy on the basis of a more favorable ICER, then those beneficiaries with diabetic retinopathy will gain at the expense of those with macular degeneration.

A CEA, by definition, values incremental QALYs equally for all persons. However, a particular decision maker may value QALYs gained by a particular group of people over QALYs gained by another group. For instance, QALYs gained by unidentified people who benefit from a prevention program or those with mental illness may be valued less than QALYs gained by a group of people suffering from a widely publicized disease such as cancer, AIDS, or heart disease. In addition, QALYs gained by children are considered more valuable by decision makers and the public than QALYs gained by adults.[1] In these situations, the net health of the population may not be maximized as determined by the CEA.

Uses

CEA has been used increasingly to evaluate health interventions over the past decade. This increase can be attributed to a number of sources including interest from pharmaceutical companies in demonstrating the value of their products and the advancement of the scientific methods used in evaluating cost-effectiveness.

Most formulary committees for hospitals, HMOs, and Medicaid programs in the United States require data on the cost-effectiveness of a pharmaceutical company before funding it through their insurance plan. In the province of Ontario, Canada, the Ministry of Health and Long-term Care requires any pharmaceutical company submitting a request to have their drug funded through the provincial formulary (which covers drug costs for seniors and those on social assistance) to submit a cost-effectiveness analysis that meets a certain set of criteria. However, formulary committees generally use these submissions subjectively in making final decisions. In addition, other funding agencies such as the federal and state or provincial government, nonprofit research organizations, universities, and insurers are increasingly interested in the cost-effectiveness of current medical treatments and are subsequently funding this research more heavily.

In recent years, the scientific interest in CEA has also increased, thereby allowing more scientifically rigorous studies to be performed and published. The financial support of agencies with an inherent interest in the potential results of economic evaluations—including insurers, pharmaceuticals, and government—has facilitated this academic interest. In addition, the relative abundance of effectiveness trials being published has allowed for full economic evaluations to be performed more easily. The increase in computing power in recent years has also played an important role by allowing more sophisticated computer programs to be designed and more iterations and complex analyses to be performed more quickly.

Although there has been an increasing interest in the economic evaluation of health interventions, the actual applications of scientifically rigorous studies have not been well documented. The most common application of rigorous full economic evaluations is likely to be in the decision by a formulary committee on whether to fund a new drug or medical treatment. Even in this case, the CEA is used subjectively in the decision making process. CEA can also be used by private or government insurers but it is difficult to know how often this is being done or how important the CEA is in the decisions being made; it is presently not good public relations to announce that

a medically effective treatment is not being funded because it is not cost-effective.

As the scientific methods of CEA develop and become more systematic, and the public begins to understand the importance of basing funding decisions on the *value* of a medical treatment, there will be many more potential applications of CEA in health policy. For instance, the cost-effectiveness of a treatment or medical practice is not currently considered when agencies determine best practice guidelines for medical or public health. In future, these guidelines could consider not only the effectiveness of medical treatments but also their value when compared to comparable alternatives. In addition, as cost-effective literature becomes more systematic and easily comparable, it will be possible to create valid league tables, or lists of health interventions along with their respective ICER. If the cost-effectiveness of the various programs in a league table has been measured rigorously using similar methods, then the cost-effectiveness of a wide variety of health interventions could potentially be compared, and difficult resource allocation decisions could be aided.

In conclusion, as the costs and complexities of health care in North America continue to rise faster than available budgets, assessing the value of health care interventions will become increasingly important. At present, CEA in health care offers a method that combines available data in a logical way, and forces decision makers to consider both the costs and benefits of different resource allocation alternatives. Resource allocation decisions in the real world will never be based solely on CEA but as the methodologies used in economic evaluations improve, they will begin to play a more important role as an aid in making difficult funding decisions in health care.

References

1. Detsky AS, Naglie IG. A clinician's guide to cost-effectiveness analysis. *Ann Intern Med.* 1990; 113:147–154.
2. Drummond MF, O'Brien B, Stoddart GL, et al. *Methods for the economic evaluation of health care programmes.* 2nd ed. Toronto: Oxford University Press; 1997:305.
3. Weinstein MC, Stason WB. Foundations of cost-effectiveness analysis for health and medical practices. *N Engl J Med.* 1977;296:716–721.

4. Gold MR, Siegel JE, Russell LB, et al., eds. *Cost-effectiveness in health and medicine.* New York: Oxford University Press; 1996:425.
5. Torrance GW, Feeny D. Utilities and quality-adjusted life years. *Int J Technol Assess Health Care.* 1989;5:559–575.
6. Guyatt GH. A taxonomy of health status instruments. *J Rheumatol.*1995;22:1188–1190.
7. Mangione CM, Berry S, Spritzer K, et al. Identifying the content area for the 51-item National Eye Institute Visual Function Questionnaire: Results from focus groups with visually impaired persons. *Arch Ophthalmol.* 1998;116:227–233.
8. Steinberg EP, Tielsch JM, Schein OD, et al. The VF-14. An index of functional impairment in patients with cataract. *Arch Ophthalmol.* 1994; 112:630–638.
9. Ware JE, Sherbourne CD Jr. The MOS 36-item short-form health survey (SF-36). I. Conceptual framework and item selection. *Med Care.* 1992;30:473–483.
10. Bergner M, Bobbitt RA, Carter WB, et al. The sickness impact profile: Development and final revision of a health status measure. *Med Care.* 1981;19:787–805.
11. Clarke AE, Goldstein MK, Michelson D. et al. The effect of assessment method and respondent population on utilities elicited for Gaucher disease. *Qual Life Res.* 1997;6:169–184.
12. Boyd NF, Sutherland HJ, Heasman KZ, et al. Whose utilities for decision analysis? *Med Decis Making.* 1990;10:58–67.
13. Neumann JV, Morgenstern O. *Theory of games and economic behaviour.* 2nd ed. London: Princeton University Press; 1947:641.
14. Torrance GW, Thomas WH, Sackett DL. A utility maximization model for evaluation of health care programs. *Health Serv Res.* 1972;7: 118–133.
15. Read JL, Quinn RJ Berwick DM, et al. Preferences for health outcomes. Comparison of assessment methods. *Med Decis Making.* 1984;4: 315–329.
16. Bakker C, van der Linden S. Health related utility measurement: An introduction. *J Rheumatol.* 1995;22:1197–1199.
17. Weinstein MC, Siegel JE, Gold MR, et al. Recommendations of the panel on cost-effectiveness in health and medicine [see comments]. *JAMA.* 1996;276:1253–1258.
18. Weinstein MC, Siegel JE, Gold MR, et al. Recommendations of the panel on cost-effectiveness in health and medicine. *JAMA.* 1996;276:1253–1258.
19. Sox HC, Blatt MA, HM C, et al. *Medical decision making.* Toronto: Butterworths; 1988:406.
20. Pauker SG, Kassirer JP. Decision analysis. *N Engl J Med.* 1987;316:250–258.

CHAPTER 3

Anterior Segment: Cornea and External Diseases

Ayad A. Farjo, MD and Qais A. Farjo, MD

Herpes Simplex Virus Eye Disease of the Anterior Segment

Introduction and Epidemiology

Herpes simplex virus type 1 (HSV-1) constitutes the vast majority of herpetic ocular infections of the anterior segment. Diagnosis is typically made clinically, although serologic and molecular testing is available.[1,2] Humans are the only natural reservoir, and an estimated 50% to 80% of the adult population has antibodies to HSV-1.[3] After primary infection by HSV, which typically manifests with nonspecific upper respiratory symptoms, the virus may achieve latency in the trigeminal ganglion. Any structure in the anterior segment can be involved and the infection presents, sometimes simultaneously, in several major forms: Blepharoconjunctivitis, infectious epithelial keratitis, neurotrophic keratopathy, stromal keratitis, endotheliitis, iridocyclitis, and trabeculitis.

There is considerable variation in the literature regarding incidence, presentation, and recurrences of herpetic keratitis, which may be the result of differing study populations, disease definitions, length of follow-up and/or other factors. In the United States, estimates from a relatively homogenous white population in the upper Midwest indicated the prevalence to be 149 per 100,000 population with an incidence of 8.4 per 100,000 person-years.[4] Bilateral involvement is less common, usually associated with atopy or other systemic immunosuppression and, depending on the definition used, can range from 3% to 12%.[3,5] In one study, primary ocular HSV presented as infectious epithelial keratitis in 15% of patients and stromal keratitis in only 2% of patients.[6] Another study found that initial episodes involved the eyelids or conjunctiva in 54% of cases, the superficial cornea in 63%, the deep cornea in 6%, and the uvea in 4%.[4] In susceptible individuals, recurrence of the virus can lead to blinding keratitis or uveitis. In patients who suffered from primary ocular HSV followed up from 2 to 15 years, 32% had recurrences, with 51% of those patients having multiple recurrences,[7] but most of the recurrences did not involve the cornea. Recurrence

rates for any form of ocular HSV have been estimated at 9.6% at 1 year, 22.9% to 33% at 2 years, 36% to 40% at 5 years, and 63.2% at 20 years.[4,8−10]

Herpetic Eye Disease Studies (HEDS) I and II were a set of six trials, supported primarily by the National Eye Institute of the United States National Institutes of Health (NEI/NIH), whose goals were to answer clinical questions about the treatment and recurrence of HSV keratitis and uveitis (see Tables 3.1–3.6). The studies were well-designed and monitored, with intervention by the Data and Safety Monitoring Committee in three of the trials. One systematic review (see Table 3.7) details available therapeutic interventions for infectious epithelial keratitis.[11] Taken together, the HEDS and systematic

---

TABLE 3.1 ◻ The Herpetic Eye Disease Studies (HEDS) I – The Herpetic Eye Disease Studies-Stromal Keratitis, not on Steroid Trial (HEDS-SKN)

Study question	Efficacy of topical corticosteroids in treating herpes simplex stromal keratitis in conjunction with topical trifluridine
Study design	Prospective, multicenter, randomized, double-masked, placebo-controlled trial. Nine clinical centers and a data coordinating center
Inclusion/exclusion criteria	1. Active HSV stromal keratitis, diagnosed clinically, with no topical steroids in the preceding 10 d 2. Age over 12 y 3. No active HSV epithelial keratitis 4. No prior keratoplasty of the involved eye 5. Not pregnant
Interventions	1. All patients received topical trifluridine as prophylaxis 2. Randomized to treatment with topical prednisolone phosphate 1% drops or topical placebo drops. Schedule started with eight drops/d for 1 wk and tapered over 10 wk so that patients received one drop/d of 0.125% prednisolone for last 3 wk. Placebo drops were given using the same schedule.
Primary outcome measure	Time to the development of treatment failure in corticosteroid and placebo groups during the 26-wk period of examination
Major findings	1. Faster resolution of stromal keratitis and fewer treatment failures with prednisolone phosphate therapy 2. Delay in initiation of corticosteroids did not affect eventual visual outcome at 26 wk. 3. The trial was terminated before the completion of the planned enrollment due to a statistically significant difference in the primary outcome between treatment groups, no convincing evidence of increased recurrence in either group, and little chance that additional data would alter the study conclusions.
Unanswered questions	It is unclear whether a longer treatment schedule, in conjunction with oral antiviral coverage, would have shown a benefit over placebo

HSV, herpes simplex virus.

TABLE 3.2 ◻ The Herpetic Eye Disease Studies (HEDS) I — The Herpetic Eye Disease Studies-Stromal Keratitis, on Steroid Treatment (HEDS-SKS)

Study question	Evaluation of the efficacy of oral acyclovir in treating herpes simplex stromal keratitis in patients receiving concomitant topical corticosteroids and trifluridine
Study design	Prospective, multicenter, randomized, double-masked, placebo-controlled trial. Eight clinical centers and a data coordinating center
Inclusion/exclusion criteria	1. Active HSV stromal keratitis, diagnosed clinically, already being treated with topical steroids 2. Age over 12 y 3. No active HSV epithelial keratitis 4. No prior keratoplasty of the involved eye 5. Not pregnant
Intervention	1. All patients received topical trifluridine as prophylaxis 2. Randomized to either 400 mg 5 times/d ACV (200 mg capsules) for 10 wk or identical frequency of placebo capsules 3. Prednisolone phosphate 1% drops or topical placebo drops. Schedule started with eight drops/d for 1 wk and tapered over 10 wk so that patients received one drop/d of 0.125% prednisolone for the last 3 wk
Primary outcome measure	Time to the development of treatment failure in acyclovir and placebo groups during the 26-wk period of examination
Secondary outcome measures	1. Proportion of patients who were treatment failures at 16 wk 2. Proportion of patients whose stromal keratitis had resolved at 16 wk 3. Best-corrected visual acuity at 26 wk and change from randomization
Major findings	Over 16 wk, no difference between treatment groups suggesting no apparent benefit to adding oral ACV to corticosteroid + trifluridine
Unanswered questions	In the absence of topical antiviral therapy, one would expect oral ACV to have benefit

ACV, acyclovir; HSV, herpes simplex virus.

review provide valuable insight into the clinical management of HSV keratitis (see Table 3.8).

Infectious Epithelial Keratitis

The initial phase of HSV-1 epithelial disease presents as minute corneal vesicles that stain negatively with fluorescein dye.[1] This may progress to a dendritic keratitis (see Fig. 3.1), a geographic keratitis (see Fig. 3.2), or a marginal keratitis with limbitis (see Fig. 3.3). Although these conditions may resolve spontaneously without therapy, antiviral therapy is generally indicated to accelerate resolution. Rates of healing appear equivalent between acyclovir (ACV), trifluridine, and vidarabine.[11] Debridement alone does not appear effective, but in conjunction with antiviral therapy may speed epithelial healing rates.[11] The addition of a 3-week course of oral ACV to trifluridine was found by the HEDS epithelial keratitis trial (EKT) (Table 3.4) to provide no additional benefit in epithelial healing rates or prevention of stromal keratitis or iridocyclitis.[12] In spite of the injury invoked by episodes of disease activity, most patients affected will have a final visual outcome that remains acceptable.[4]

Stromal Keratitis and Endotheliitis

Manifestations of HSV-1 stromal disease include immune stromal keratitis (see Fig. 3.4) and necrotizing keratitis. While the latter is potentially devastating in the acute period, immune stromal keratitis leads to corneal blindness through a chronic relapsing and remitting course (see Fig. 3.5). Endotheliitis can accompany stromal keratitis and manifests with

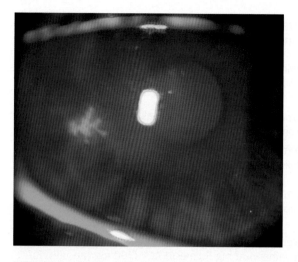

FIGURE 3.1 ◻ Dendritic herpes simplex virus keratitis.

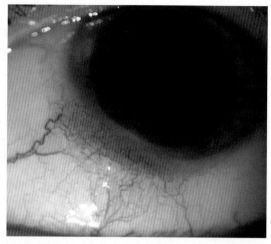

FIGURE 3.3 ◻ Herpes simplex virus limbitis and marginal keratitis.

microcystic corneal edema and keratic precipitates (Fig. 3.4). The value of corticosteroid treatment of stromal keratitis was assessed in the HEDS stromal keratitis, not on the steroid (SKN) trial (Table 3.1).[13] The main conclusion was that a 10-week course of topical corticosteroid treatment contributes to a faster visual recovery, although a delay in therapy does not affect final visual outcome at six months.

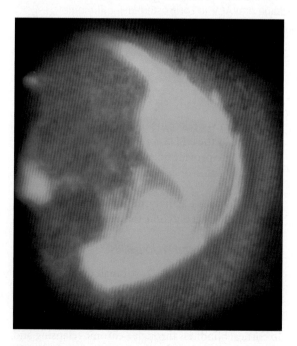

FIGURE 3.2 ◻ Geographic herpes simplex virus keratitis.

The major question that remains unanswered by this study was whether a 10-week course was sufficient. Half of the patients in the corticosteroid group of the study who "failed treatment" did so in the 6 weeks after discontinuation of the topical steroid. Currently, in clinical practice, topical steroids may be continued for many months, and perhaps indefinitely at low dosages and frequencies, often in conjunction with chronic oral ACV therapy. Although the final visual outcome was not affected by delay in treatment, it should be noted that 76% of the placebo group failed treatment, and 72% of the placebo group that showed visual improvement was eventually treated with topical corticosteroids. In fact, by 16 weeks after randomization, the total duration of topical corticosteroid usage was similar in both the placebo and corticosteroid groups. It is important to note, however, that 22% of patients had resolution of stromal keratitis with only topical antiviral treatment.

Iridocyclitis and Trabeculitis

HSV iridocyclitis and trabeculitis are uncommon conditions. The HEDS iridocyclitis, receiving topical steroid (IRT) trial (Table 3.3) was stopped because of low recruitment, with only 50 of the planned 104 patients recruited over 4 years.[14] These conditions can occur concomitantly with other forms of HSV infections, as noted in the HEDS-SKN trial in which 34% and 16% of the eyes with stromal keratitis had concomitant iridocyclitis and trabeculitis, respectively. The iridocyclitis can be either granulomatous

TABLE 3.3 ▣ **The Herpetic Eye Disease Studies (HEDS) I—The Herpetic Eye Disease Studies-Iridocyclitis, Receiving Topical Steroids (HEDS-IRT)**

Study question	Evaluate the efficacy of oral acyclovir in treating herpes simplex iridocyclitis in conjunction with topical corticosteroids and trifluridine.
Study design	Prospective, multicenter, randomized, double-masked, placebo-controlled trial. Eight clinical centers and a data coordinating center
Inclusion/exclusion criteria	1. Active iridocyclitis, with HSV diagnosed clinically or with the presence of serum antibodies 2. Age over 12 y 3. No active HSV epithelial keratitis 4. No prior keratoplasty of the involved eye 5. Not pregnant
Intervention	1. All patients received topical trifluridine as prophylaxis 2. Randomized to either ACV 400 mg five times/d (200 mg capsules) for 10 wk or an identical frequency of placebo 3. Prednisolone phosphate 1% drops or topical placebo drops. Schedule started with eight drops/d for 1 wk and tapered over 10 wk so that patients received one drop/d of 0.125% prednisolone for the last 3 wk.
Primary outcome measure	Time to the development of treatment failure in acyclovir and placebo groups during the 26-wk period of examination
Major findings	1. Treatment failures occurred at a higher rate in the placebo group compared to the ACV group, but trial too small to be statistically significant 2. Trial stopped due to slow recruitment (only 50 of planned 104 patients enrolled over 4 y)
Unanswered questions	Unclear benefit of adding ACV to corticosteroid + trifluridine

ACV, acyclovir; HSV, herpes simplex virus.

or nongranulomatous. Intraocular pressure (IOP) increase from trabeculitis, when stromal keratitis or iridocyclitis is present, may easily be misinterpreted as being a steroid-induced glaucoma. In fact, HSV should be included in the differential diagnosis of any iridocyclitis associated with increase in IOP. Owing to its small sample size, the HEDS iridocyclitis, receiving topical steroid (IRT) trial (Table 3.3.) suffered from low recruitment, between the ACV and placebo groups in the rates of treatment failure in patients treated with corticosteroids and trifluridine. There was a trend, however, toward a reduction of treatment failures in patients treated with oral ACV.

Prevention of Recurrence

It had been previously demonstrated in a small, prospective randomized series that oral ACV reduced recurrences of HSV keratitis and improved graft survival after penetrating keratoplasty (PKP).[15] The reduction in recurrence rate was confirmed by the HEDS acyclovir prevention trial (APT) (Table 3.5) and yielded, perhaps, the most important results from the HEDS. It demonstrated that not only was oral ACV 400 mg, taken twice daily, able to reduce the recurrence rate of any form of ocular HSV compared to placebo, it also reduced nonocular recurrences.[16] Given that recurrent stromal keratitis leads to progressive corneal scarring and potential corneal blindness, it was clinically significant that oral ACV reduced stromal recurrence by 50% among patients who had stromal keratitis in the previous year.

However, lingering questions remain, such as whether a lower dosage would have been equally efficacious or whether a higher dosage would be more successful in preventing recurrences.[17] Likewise the end point for treatment with oral ACV remains unclear, as recrudescence occurs upon discontinuation of the medication.[18] As the HEDS-EKT demonstrated a low risk of developing stromal keratitis or iridocyclitis after a primary episode of

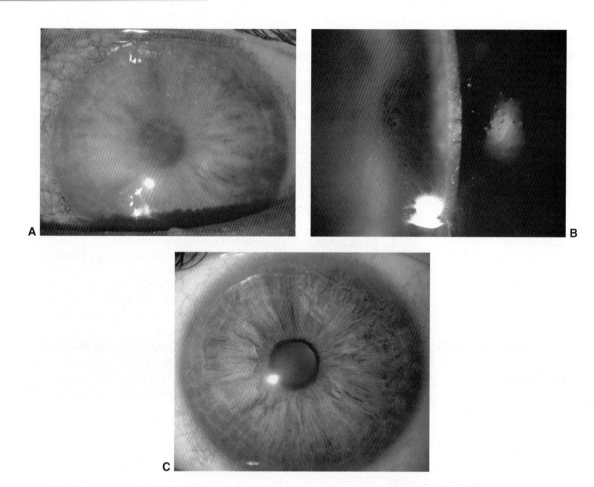

FIGURE 3.4 ▢ Pretreatment stromal keratitis and endotheliitis **(A)** with microcystic corneal edema **(B)**. Posttreatment with topical steroids and oral acyclovir **(C)**.

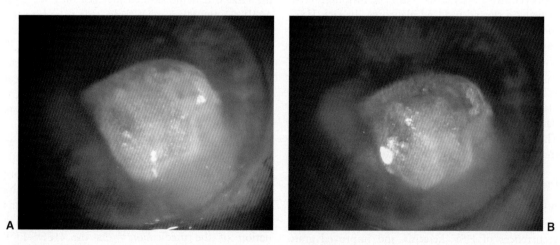

FIGURE 3.5 ▢ Chronic stromal keratitis leading to lipid keratopathy **(A)**. The lipid will be slowly reabsorbed with prolonged disease inactivity **(B)**.

TABLE 3.4 ◻ The Herpetic Eye Disease Studies (HEDS) II – The Herpetic Eye Disease Studies-Epithelial Keratitis Trial (HEDS-EKT)

Study question	Determine whether early treatment of HSV epithelial keratitis ulceration with oral ACV prevents blinding complications of stromal keratitis and iridocyclitis.
Study design	Prospective, multicenter, randomized, double-masked, placebo-controlled trial. One national coordinating center, eight regional coordinating centers, 60 clinical sites (university and community based practices)
Inclusion/exclusion criteria	1. Dendritic or geographic epithelial ulceration clinically consistent with HSV with less than 1 wk onset 2. Age over 12 y 3. No active HSV stromal keratitis or iritis 4. No prior keratoplasty or refractive surgery of the involved eye 5. Not pregnant or nursing 6. No history of immune dysfunction or immunosuppression
Intervention	1. Patients received topical trifluridine 1% drops eight times/d until epithelial ulcerations resolved, then decreased to four times/d for 3 d and stopped (Three patients were treated with vidarabine 3% ointment due to trifluridine allergy). 2. Randomized to either ACV 400 mg 5 times /d (200 mg capsules) for 3 wk or identical frequency of placebo
Primary outcome measure	Time to the development of first occurrence of HSV stromal keratitis or iridocyclitis in the study eye
Major findings	1. Recruitment stopped at 287 of planned 502 patients because of lack of any suggestion of efficacy of treatment protocol. 2. No benefit from the addition of oral ACV to treatment with trifluridine in preventing stromal keratitis or iritis 3. Risk of stromal keratitis or iridocyclitis was low in the year following an episode of epithelial keratitis treated with trifluridine alone (7% if first episode, 26% if multiple episodes) 4. At 3 wk of treatment, 99% of epithelial keratitis had resolved.
Unanswered questions	Can oral ACV be used instead of trifluridine? Would a longer duration of therapy with ACV have shown a benefit? Should these patients receive long term oral ACV?

HSV, herpes simplex virus; ACV, acyclovir.

epithelial keratitis, it does not seem necessary to begin therapy, perhaps lifelong, with oral ACV in these patients. Unfortunately, ACV prophylaxis is relatively cost-ineffective and a theoretic model for treatment, targeting patients with stromal keratitis, found no increase in cost-effectiveness compared with targeting any patient with a history of HSV ocular disease.[19] Long-term treatment may therefore be best reserved for patients with recurrent disease or cases in which visual acuity is already threatened or compromised.

Although long-term oral ACV therapy was found helpful in the HEDS-APT, other HEDS trials could not definitely elicit a benefit of high-dose short-term therapy with oral ACV in patients already taking trifluridine 1% drops concomitantly. In the HEDS stromal keratitis, on steroid treatment (SKS) trial (Table 3.2), no apparent benefit of a 10-week course of oral ACV (400 mg 5 times daily) was found over placebo.[20] Likewise, the HEDS-IRT and HEDS-EKT (Tables 3.3 and 3.4) trials did not find significant advantages in using short-term courses of oral ACV in conjunction with trifluridine. It should also be noted that in the HEDS, some patients had recurrences in spite of treatment with oral ACV and/or topical trifluridine.

TABLE 3.5 ☐ **The Herpetic Eye Disease Studies (HEDS) II – The Herpetic Eye Disease Studies-Acyclovir Prevention Trial (HEDS-APT)**

Study question	Determine efficacy of oral ACV in preventing recurrent HSV eye infection in patients with previous episodes of herpetic eye disease.
Study design	Prospective, multicenter, randomized, double-masked, placebo-controlled trial. One national coordinating center, eight regional coordinating centers, 60 clinical sites (university and community based practices)
Inclusion/exclusion criteria	1. Any kind of ocular HSV infection (blepharitis, conjunctivitis, keratitis, or iridocyclitis) in preceding year. Inactive infection and untreated for at least 30 d. 2. Age over 12 y 3. No prior keratoplasty of the involved eye 4. Not pregnant
Intervention	1. Randomized to either ACV 400 mg two times/d (200 mg capsules) for 1 y or identical frequency of placebo
Primary outcome measure	Time to first recurrence of any type of HSV eye disease in either eye
Major findings	1. Oral ACV reduced by 41% the probability that any form of herpes of the eye would return in patients who had the infection in the previous year. 2. Oral ACV reduced stromal recurrence by 50% among patients who had stromal keratitis in the past year. 3. Oral ACV reduced the incidence of epithelial keratitis from 11% to 9% and the incidence of stromal keratitis from 13% to 8%. 4. Four percent of patients in the ACV group and 9% in placebo group had more than one recurrence.
Unanswered questions	When does one discontinue ACV?

ACV, acyclovir; HSV, herpes simplex virus.

Risk Factors

On the basis of the study of 260 patients enrolled in the HEDS-SKN, HEDS-SKS, and HEDS-IRT, it was suggested that during treatment for stromal keratouveitis there was a greater risk of recurrent epithelial keratitis in nonwhite patients and patients with a previous history of HSV epithelial keratitis.[21] Identifying potential triggering factors for HSV ocular disease was attempted by the HEDS recurrence factor study (RFS). The goal was to ascertain whether any specific external or behavioral factors such as psychological stress, exposure to sunlight, menstrual cycle, contact lens wear or eye injury could be determined as definitive risk factors. From self-reported questionnaires, high-stress did not appear to be associated with recurrence.[22] Likewise, none of the other factors studied were noted to be associated with recurrence; however, this trial had limited power to detect true differences between these factors. In addition, measures such as "sunlight exposure"

proved difficult to quantitate. Interestingly, a recall-bias was observed in patients who had onset of symptoms, but did not complete their exposure log in a timely manner, with over-reporting of high stress and systematic infection.

Alternative Therapies and Future Directions

Development of better diagnostic and therapeutic options for HSV, and other *herpesviruses*, is essential, given the morbidity of these viruses and the chronic nature of these infections. It is unknown as to how many cases of ocular HSV are undiagnosed or misdiagnosed. Likewise, although oral ACV is assumed to be an effective treatment for most patients, ACV-resistant HSV strains have been found in 7% of immunocompromised individuals.[23] As such, various medical and alternative therapies are under investigation. There is mixed evidence on the usage of oral or topical forms of lysine in the management

TABLE 3.6 ☐ Herpetic Eye Disease Studies (HEDS) II—HEDS-RFS (recurrence factor study)

Study question	Determine the role of external factors (UV light or trauma) and behavioral factors (e.g., stress) on ocular recurrences of HSV eye infections and disease.
Study design	Prospective, multicenter trial. Fifty-eight clinical centers and a data coordinating center
Inclusion/exclusion criteria	1. History of HSV ocular infection within the preceding year 2. Age over 18 y and immunocompetent
Intervention	Questionnaire completed every Sunday for 52 wk to track acute and chronic stressors
Primary outcome measure	Development of recurrent HSV ocular disease
Major findings	1. Higher levels of psychological stress were not associated with an increased risk of recurrence. 2. No association was found between any of the other exposure variables and recurrence. 3. When an analysis was performed including only the recurrences for which the exposure week log was completed late and after symptom onset, there was a clear indication of retrospective over-reporting of high stress and systemic infection.
Unanswered questions	What are the risk factors for HSV recurrence?

HSV, herpes simplex virus.

of herpes labialis.[24,25] A proposed mechanism of action is that high intracellular concentrations of lysine competitively inhibit arginine, which is necessary for HSV reproduction.[26] Currently, there are no available topical ophthalmic preparations of lysine. If there is a beneficial effect from oral lysine supplementation, it will likely need to be administered as a chronic treatment at high dosages (1000–3000 mg/day) to help prevent recurrences. Newer drugs, such as CTC-96, that inhibit the ability of HSV to enter noninfected cells may offer hope for prevention of disease acquisition.[27]

It has become apparent that virus-specific Th1 cytokines and active innate immunity can prevent HSV recurrence.[28] This knowledge has been incorporated into new vaccine strategies and a recent vaccine reduced the clinical symptoms of primary HSV-2 infection by over 70%, but only in women who were both HSV-1 and HSV-2 seronegative.[28–30] Although there are still no clinical vaccines available for HSV and significant challenges remain, these results suggest the eventual development of more effective options. Through a better understanding of the biology of HSV, either new medications or vaccines should be able to interfere with the acquisition of the primary infection, recurrence of the infection, or possibly eradicate the virus altogether.

Corneal Transplantation

Indications and Epidemiology of Penetrating Keratoplasty

The rates of PKP in the United States have slowly declined since 1995, with increasing numbers of tissue being exported internationally.[31] Studies on the indications for PKP vary depending on the time frame assessed, classifications used, region of origin, and specific practice-style sampled.[32] For example, in the United States, pseudophakic bullous keratopathy (PBK) is the leading indication for PKP[31] but regional and practice variations place either repeat grafts or Fuchs corneal endothelial dystrophy as the next most common indication and keratoconus (KC) as either the second or the third most common indication.[32–34] Worldwide, the leading indications for PKP are PBK in Canada and France,[35–37] KC in Israel, Saudi Arabia, Australia, and New Zealand,[38–41] corneal scarring in India, Nepal, and Taiwan[42–44] and regrafting at one center in the United Kingdom.[45] Changes in indication over time were noted in many series.[32,34,38,39,46] The significance of HSV as an indication for PKP appears to be decreasing.[38,47]

KC continues to be an important indication for corneal transplantation worldwide (see Fig. 3.6). The

TABLE 3.7 ▢ Herpes Simplex Virus (HSV)

Therapeutics

Topical antivirals
1. Increase healing rates of epithelial keratitis
2. No significant differences between vidarabine, trifluridine, or ACV

Topical interferons
1. Increase healing rates of epithelial keratitis

Topical corticosteroids
1. Reduce stromal inflammation and lessen the duration of stromal keratitis
2. May induce epithelial keratitis if not given concomitantly with an antiviral

Oral ACV
1. Effective in treating epithelial and stromal keratitis
2. Long-term oral ACV (400 mg twice daily) is effective in preventing recurrence of HSV keratitis
3. May offer additional benefit to patients with HSV iridocyclitis
4. Does not offer any additional ocular benefit to immunocompetent patients already on trifluridine for the treatment of epithelial or stromal keratitis

Treatment recommendations for disease subsets

Dendritic or geographic epithelial keratitis
1. Treatment with a topical or an oral antiviral is sufficient
2. For initial episodes, long-term ACV usage is unnecessary for most patients.
3. For patients with a history of multiple recurrences, long-term oral ACV prophylaxis may be more valuable.

Stromal keratitis
1. Resolution of symptoms is more rapid with corticosteroids
2. Recurrence is reduced with long-term oral ACV prophylaxis
3. If topical steroids are used, many patients require greater than 10 wk of therapy

Iridocyclitis
1. It is unclear whether short-term high-dose oral ACV is beneficial, but there are few negative side effects and there is a suggestion of benefit to this regimen.

Corneal Transplantation
1. Oral ACV prophylaxis appears to reduce HSV recurrence and improve graft survival.

ACV, acyclovir; HSV, herpes simplex virus.

prevalence and incidence, as well as disease severity, appear to vary with ethnicity. In the United Kingdom, patients aged 10 to 44 with an Asian origin had a prevalence of 229 per 100,000 as compared with 57 per 100,000 in white patients.[48] In the same age-group, Asians had an annual incidence of 19.6 per 100,000 versus 4.5 per 100,000 in white patients. Age at diagnosis and age at corneal transplantation were also lower in Asians. In the United States, the prevalence of KC in a mainly white population was 54.5 per 100,000 with an annual incidence of 2.0 per 100,000.[49] The disease process tends to be bilateral and asymmetric, with roughly 50% of clinically normal fellow eyes progressing to KC over a 16-year time span.[50] Occasionally, breaks occur

in the Descemet's membrane, leading to corneal hydrops (see Fig. 3.7), which then resolve with associated corneal scarring. Although mechanical factors may play a role in its development, KC is felt to have a genetic origin based in part on studies examining the videokeratography of family members with KC.[51–54]

The Collaborative Longitudinal Evaluation of Keratoconus (CLEK) study (see Table 3.9) is an ongoing prospective observational study intended to describe the clinical course of KC and identify predisposing or protective factors influencing the severity and progression of the disease. It is primarily funded by the NEI/NIH and conducted mainly through academic optometric sites. In early results, KC has been found to be bilateral and asymmetric with a

TABLE 3.8 ▢ Interventions for Herpes Simplex Virus Epithelial Keratitis

Study question	Compare the effects of various treatments for dendritic or geographic herpes simplex virus epithelial keratitis.
Study design	Systematic review
Inclusion/exclusion criteria	1. Comparative clinical trials that assessed 1-wk and/or 2-wk healing rates of topical ophthalmic or oral antiviral agents and/or physical or chemical debridement in people with active epithelial keratitis 2. Age over 18 y and immunocompetent
Intervention	Sources searched for relevant studies were the Cochrane Central Register of Controlled Trials — CENTRAL, MEDLINE (1966 to August 2002), EMBASE (1980 to August 2002), LILACS (up to 2002), Index Medicus (1960 to 1965), Excerpta Medica Ophthalmology (1960 to 1973)>, reference lists of primary reports and review articles, and conference proceedings pertaining to ocular virology.
Primary outcome measure	Interventions were compared by the proportions of participants healed at seven days and at 14 d after trial enrollment.
Major findings	1. Compared to idoxuridine, the topical application of vidarabine, trifluridine, or acyclovir generally resulted in a significantly greater proportion of participants healing within one week of treatment. 2. Insufficient placebo-controlled studies were available to assess debridement and other physical or physicochemical methods of treatment. 3. Interferon was very useful combined with debridement or with another antiviral agent such as trifluridine.
Unanswered questions	Is debridement useful in treating HSV epithelial keratitis?

greater asymmetry and corneal steepening in patients with a history of eye rubbing or ocular trauma.[55] Not unexpectedly, this trial has found that corneal scarring in KC is also significantly associated with decreased high- and low-contrast visual acuity.[56] Perceived visual function in the CLEK study, as measured by the NEI Visual Function Questionnaire (VFQ), has been found to be disproportionately lower than measured visual acuity.[57] This is similar to a previous article suggesting that the best predictors of patient satisfaction after PKP were subjective outcomes rather than objective measures such as visual acuity.[58] While the CLEK study will contribute to the understanding of KC, it is unclear whether it is possible to generalize the patient population being studied to ophthalmology practices or different ethnic populations.

Graft Survival After Penetrating Keratoplasty

Graft failures after PKP may be due to immunologic rejection, recurrence of the original disease process (see Fig. 3.8), nonimmunologic late endothelial failure, surface problems, infection, glaucoma, or other factors. Primary graft failure, defined as a diffusely edematous corneal graft that fails to clear in the early postoperative period, is uncommon, and as many as 33% of cases may be due to HSV.[59] The leading cause of graft failure within the first 1 to 3 years after transplantation is immunologic rejection,[60] whereas late failures are more attributable to nonimmunologic endothelial failure.[61,62] The risk factors for graft failure can be primarily divided into host factors, including ancillary intraoperative procedures, and donor factors. Postoperative immunosuppression and surgical complications are also important factors in maintaining a clear corneal graft.

With current eye banking standards, the greatest predictive role in determining graft survival are host factors, with presenting diagnosis, in particular, as the most significant factor. PKP for KC has the best graft survival results with >90% survival from 5 to 12 years after transplantation.[42,60,62−68] Five-year or longer graft survival for an initial diagnosis of Fuchs corneal endothelial dystrophy (see Fig. 3.9) ranges from 81% to 98%,[60,62,67−69] interstitial keratitis ranges from 95% to 100%,[67,68] herpes simplex

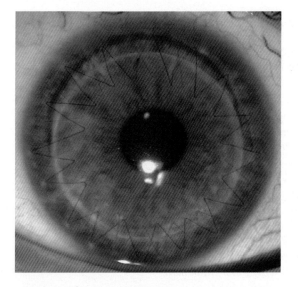

FIGURE 3.6 ◻ Penetrating keratoplasty for keratoconus with a double-running suture technique. Larger donor grafts are commonly used and arcus senilis, as in this photograph, may be evident.

keratitis ranges from 65.3% to 89.5%,[60,63,68,70] and PBK ranges from 50% to 76%.[60,63,68,71] As recurrence of corneal stromal dystrophies is known to occur after PKP,[72] phototherapeutic keratectomy is emerging as an alternative treatment option given its efficacy and shorter recovery period, although recurrences occur after that procedure as well.

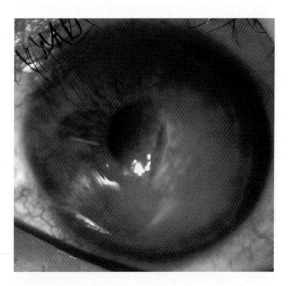

FIGURE 3.7 ◻ Keratoconus with hydrops.

The recipient age may also play an important role. Young children have lower graft survival rates, roughly 66% to 80% at one year,[73,74] varying again with the indication for transplantation.[75–78] In younger patients a more vigorous healing or immune response, in addition to greater difficulty with compliance to the prescribed postoperative regimen, may contribute to worse outcome. Even with a clear transplant, visual outcome may be limited by amblyopia in young children.[73] Outside of the pediatric population, there is no apparent relationship between graft clarity and recipient age.[79]

Graft survival rates of PKP also vary depending on whether the graft is combined with secondary procedures. Exchange of an anterior chamber intraocular lens (IOL) during PKP for PBK has been reported to increase graft survival (see Fig. 3.10), as well as the placement of an IOL in cases of aphakic bullous keratopathy.[62] Studies of implantation of secondary anterior chamber IOLs during PKP have reported survivals of 87% to 95% at 2 to 3 years[80,81] and 65% at 8 years.[80] Grafts with secondary scleral-sutured IOLs have an 87% survival at three years[82] and iris-sutured IOLs have survival rates of 89% to 91.2% at 2 years and 81% at 5 years.[83,84] There does not appear to be a clear superiority of one lens type over another during PKP.[85,86]

Although graft survival decreases when PKP is combined with glaucoma surgery, the combined procedures may offer better long-term graft survival and IOP control than staged procedures.[87,88] Corneal transplants with glaucoma drainage devices have reported survivals of 50% at 3 years with adequate IOP control in 86%,[89] as compared to trabeculectomy with mitomycin-C with 60% graft survival at 2 years and adequate IOP control in 50% of the cases.[90] Placement of the drainage device into the vitreous cavity, rather than the anterior chamber, may improve graft survival[91] but may also be associated with greater posterior segment complications.[92]

When PKP is combined with a temporary keratoprosthesis and vitreoretinal surgery, graft survival is relatively poor[93,94] but may be more successful if the etiology is ocular trauma (see Fig. 3.11) and surgical intervention is performed relatively proximal to the injury.[95,96] Labeling of these cases as "successes" is more difficult as it requires a clear graft, control of IOP, and a good anatomic retinal result. Even in successful cases, visual acuity may be severely limited and most articles gauge the

TABLE 3.9 ▫ Collaborative Longitudinal Evaluation of Keratoconus (CLEK)

Study question	1. Describe the clinical course of KC. 2. Describe relationships among its visual and physiological manifestations, including high- and low-contrast visual acuity, corneal curvature, slit lamp findings, cornea scarring, and quality of life. 3. Identify risk factors and protective factors that influence the severity and progression of KC.
Study design	Prospective, multicenter (15 clinical optometry centers), observational study of 1,209 KC patients
Inclusion/exclusion criteria	1. 12 y or older 2. Irregular cornea as determined by keratometry, retinoscopy, or direct ophthalmoscopy in at least one eye 3. Vogt's striae,Fleischer's ring, or corneal scarring characteristic of KC in at least one eye 4. Available for 3 y of follow-up 5. Ineligible if they had bilateral corneal transplants or bilateral nonkeratoconic eye disease (cataract, IOLs, macular disease, or optic nerve disease other than glaucoma)
Intervention	Annual examinations for 3 y
Outcome measures	Visual acuity, patient-reported quality of life, manifest refraction, keratometry, photodocumentation of central corneal scarring, photodocumentation of the flattest contact lens that just clears the cornea, slit lamp biomicroscopy, corneal topography, photodocumentation of Rigid Gas-Permeable lens fluorescein staining pattern if patient is wearing them
Major findings	1. Ongoing study 2. KC patients with more severe disease are also more asymmetric in disease status. 3. Corneal scarring in KC is significantly associated with decrease in high- and low-contrast visual acuity. 4. Corneal scarring is associated with corneal staining, contact lens wear, Fleischer's ring, a steeper cornea, and increasing age. 5. KC is not associated with increased risk of connective tissue disease.
Unanswered questions	1. These patients were recruited from optometric centers and may not be applicable to patients seen in ophthalmology practices (most patients in the study had mild to moderate KC). 2. KC in the United States may not have a similar course as elsewhere in the world.

KC, keratoconus; HSV, herpes simplex virus.

percentage of eyes with improvement in vision rather than the final visual result. If patients are adequately prepared for the postoperative regimen and limited outcomes, these complex procedures can be worthwhile undertakings as the results exceed the natural history of the untreated conditions.

Multiple factors have been suggested to be "high risk" for graft failure after PKP. From published studies, the most important of these factors is an earlier corneal transplant failure (see Fig. 3.12). Repeat transplantation has a reported 2-year survival of 76%,[97] a reported 5-year survival of 21.2% to 45.6%,[42,98] and, in other series, a reported 10-year survival of 41% to 46%.[60,62] Deep stromal vascularization of greater than one quadrant is also highly associated with graft failure.[42,62,63]

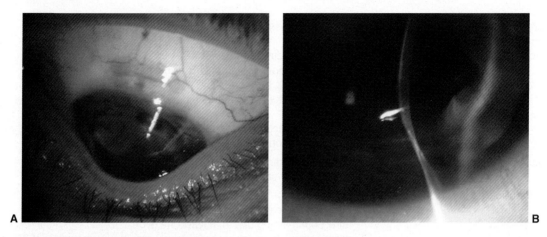

A   B

FIGURE 3.8 □ Recurrence of keratoconus after penetrating keratoplasty, performed 30 years earlier. A Munson's sign is present **(A)** with thinning and ectasia of the donor, graft-host junction and host cornea **(B)**.

Collaborative Corneal Transplantation Studies

Collaborative Corneal Transplantation Studies (CCTS) (see Tables 3.10 and 3.11) were designed to assess whether histocompatibility (HLA) matching improved corneal graft survival in high-risk patients. *High-risk patients* were defined as patients who had two or more quadrants of neovascularization and/or a history of allograft rejection. Specifically excluded

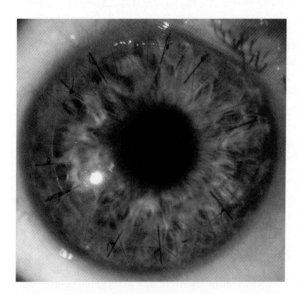

FIGURE 3.9 □ Penetrating keratoplasty for Fuchs corneal endothelial dystrophy with a combination of interrupted and running sutures. At 1 year, with selective suture removal uncorrected visual acuity measured 20/20 in this eye.

were the patients with conditions that may be predisposed to higher levels of nonimmunologic graft failure (e.g., patients with severe ocular surface disorders). Patients in the CCTS were recruited into either the Antigen Matching Study (AMS) or the Crossmatch Study (CS) based on the absence or presence of preexistent lymphocytotoxic antibodies to a standardized panel. Patients in the CS were further segregated into "positive" or "negative" groups, indicating whether preformed antibodies against the specific donor tissue to be transplanted were present. The strongest risk factors for immunologic graft failure at three years postoperatively in these high-risk patients included a younger recipient age (<40 years old), the number of previous failed transplants, and previous anterior segment surgery.[99] Race did not appear to be a risk factor for graft failure in these patients, in agreement with a previous study.[100] The AMS found that in these patients donor-recipient tissue typing HLA-A, -B, and -DR had no significant long-term effect on the success of the transplant,[101] but ABO blood type incompatibility appeared to incur a greater risk of graft failure. The CS did not find a higher rate of corneal graft failure in patients with a positive donor–recipient crossmatch, although lymphocytotoxic antibodies were associated with immune graft rejection.[102] Interestingly, the 65% graft survival rate at 3 years was much higher than expected and was felt to be due to intensive topical steroids, good patient compliance, and close patient follow-up.

The CCTS raised important questions regarding the etiology of immunologic graft failures after

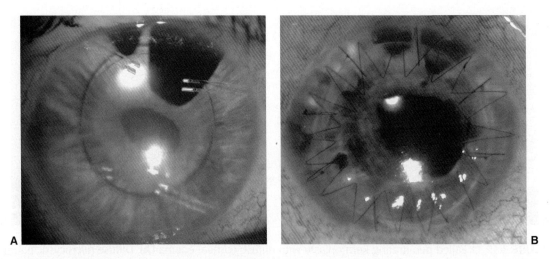

FIGURE 3.10 ☐ Pseudophakic bullous keratopathy with a closed loop anterior chamber IOL **(A)**. One week postoperative appearance after penetrating keratoplasty, IOL exchange with an iris-sutured posterior chamber lens implant, anterior vitrectomy, and pupilloplasty **(B)**.

corneal transplantation. If neither HLA-A, -B, and -DR antigens, nor preexistent lymphocytotoxic antibodies explain the immunologic failures then other factors must exist. Although it has been suggested that the multicenter and multisurgeon protocol in the CCTS may have led to differing surgical and clinical management, graft failure rates were not substantially different among the centers. The CCTS also did not assess whether these factors improved graft survival in non-high-risk patients. A more recent study of non-high-risk corneal transplantation performed at a single institution found a 92% graft survival at 4 years with 0 to 2 mismatches versus a 66% graft survival in patients with 3 to 6 mismatches in the A/B/DR loci, respectively.[103] Given that PKPs in non-high-risk patients have generally high success rates, it remains questionable whether the time and expense of HLA matching appears to be of benefit to these patients.

Cornea Donor Study

The issue of ABO incompatibility as a risk factor of graft failure was raised by the CCTS but is

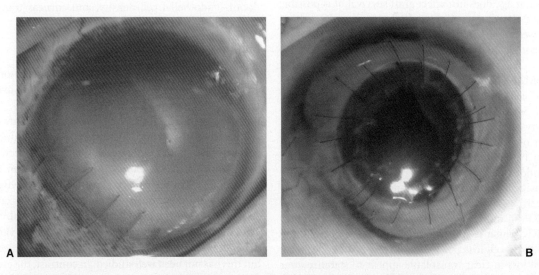

FIGURE 3.11 ☐ Corneal blood staining from trauma **(A)**. Three-month postoperative appearance after penetrating keratoplasty combined with a temporary keratoprosthesis and vitreoretinal surgery **(B)**.

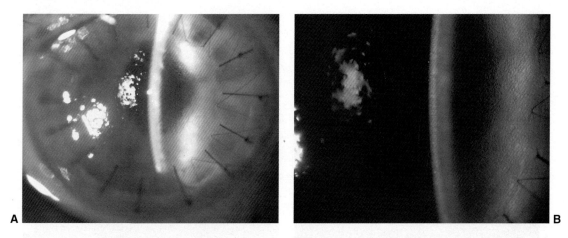

FIGURE 3.12 ☐ Failed penetrating keratoplasty with diffuse corneal edema **(A)**. Diffuse microcystic edema is present **(B)**.

currently not routinely assessed preoperatively in the United States. The Cornea Donor Study (CDS) (see Table 3.12) is an ongoing trial that will readdress this topic as well as determine whether donor age affects graft survival. Donor age has been suggested to be an independent risk factor for graft failure,[60,104–106] while other studies have not indicated significant incurred risk.[107–110] One hypothesis for lower graft survival may be that older donors begin with a decreased endothelial cell density relative to younger donors. Alternatively, other tissue factors may be found to play a role and it may be that for older recipients the effects of donor age are negligible. If donor age does not affect graft survival, it is possible that the donor pool could be increased, perhaps offsetting concerns about a loss of donors due to keratorefractive surgical procedures.

The Specular Microscopy Ancillary Study (SMAS), nested within the CDS, will follow endothelial cell counts prospectively. One finding from the CDS-SMAS has been the identification of variation between local eye banks and the central reading center of >10% in 38% of cases,[111] emphasizing a need for better standards and training among eye banks. Endothelial cell loss between 1 and 3 years after PKP has been reported in the range of 8% to 13% per year,[84] 7.8% per year between 3 to 5 years after PKP,[112] and 4.2% per year between 5 to 10 years after PKP, which is still roughly 7 times the normal rate of 0.6% cell loss per year.[60] The rates of endothelial cell loss in clear transplants appear to stabilize after 10 years with similar rates of cell loss relative to normal eyes.[61,113] Increased donor storage time appears

to reduce endothelial cell density and delay corneal reepithelialization.[114]

Loss of endothelial cells appears to follow a biexponential decay function that implicates preoperative endothelial cell density as a factor in late endothelial failure.[115] One study found risk factors for late endothelial failure to be relatively lower endothelial cell counts preoperatively and at two months postoperatively, suggesting the importance of developing better corneal preservation methods and techniques.[116] Another study found factors predictive of greater cell loss at one year to be corneas obtained from older donors, corneas with higher donor–endothelial cell density, and corneas transplanted to older recipients.[104]

Immunosuppression

Topical corticosteroids are the mainstay of postoperative care after corneal transplantation and may need to be continued indefinitely (see Fig. 3.13). As noted in the CCTS, close patient follow-up and intensive topical corticosteroid therapy appeared to reduce corneal graft failure to rates lower than expected by natural history alone. Additionally, topical cyclosporine 2% appears to improve graft survival after pediatric keratoplasty[117] and reduce allograft rejection[118] and possibly improve graft survival.[119] The effectiveness of topical cyclosporine 2% may vary depending on the vehicle in which it is compounded, but this has not been well studied. In contrast, the evidence of benefit of systemic cyclosporine is mixed. In patients with deep stromal vascularization, systemic

TABLE 3.10 ◻ **Collaborative Corneal Transplantation Studies (CCTS) – Antigen Matching Study (AMS)**

Study question	Determine the effectiveness of HLA-A, -B and -DR donor-recipient matching in high-risk patients who had no lymphocytotoxic antibodies.
Study design	Prospective, randomized, double-masked multicenter trial. Six university-based clinical centers
Inclusion/exclusion criteria	1. Age 10 y or older 2. Two to four quadrants of corneal stroma vascularization or a history of allograft rejection in the eye considered for surgery 3. Willing to participate in 3 y of follow-up 4. No condition that would greatly increase the risk of nonrejection graft failure (e.g., xerophthalmia or severe exposure) 5. No patients with systemic disease or with medication usage that might alter their immune response 6. Not pregnant
Intervention	Patients received corneas of negatively crossmatched donors and were grouped into "high" or "low" antigenic matching for HLA-A, HLA-B, and HLA-DR antigens.
Primary outcome measure	Time to irreversible failure of corneal allograft due to any cause
Secondary outcome measures	1. Time to first immunological graft reaction 2. Time to irreversible graft failure due to allograft rejection 3. Visual acuity
Major findings	1. Donor–recipient tissue typing had no significant long-term effect on the success of corneal transplantation. 2. Matching patient and donor blood types (ABO compatibility) might be effective in improving patient outcome. 3. High-dose topical steroids, good patient compliance and close patient follow-up appear to be important factors to successful transplantation in high-risk patients. 4. Lymphocytotoxic antibodies, especially directed against donor class I HLA antigens following corneal transplantation in high-risk patients, are associated with immune graft rejection and can be an indicator of allograft rejection.
Unanswered questions	What is the mechanism of immunologic reactions after penetrating keratoplasty and what are the important factors?

cyclosporine may reduce the rate of immunologic rejection and graft failure;[120] however, other studies suggest no additional benefit relative to topical steroids alone.[121–123] This variability may be due to patient selection and/or increased graft failure from nonimmunologic mechanisms such as surface reepithelialization.[124] Newer agents such as tacrolimus (FK506) appear to be effective in reducing immunologic graft reactions both topically[125] and systemically.[126] Mycophenolate mofetil may reduce allograft rejection episodes[127] and have similar or greater efficacy than oral cyclosporine.[128]

All forms of immunosuppression carry risks and the regimen to be utilized must be individualized for each patient. Topical agents may mask infectious keratitis, and corticosteroids are well known to contribute to increased IOP and cataracts. Topical cyclosporine and tacrolimus ointments have been associated with HSV epithelial keratitis.[129,130] Systemic administration of cyclosporine, tacrolimus, and other agents can be associated with significant complications including hypertension, systemic infection, irreversible renal failure, and lymphoproliferative disorder (see Table 3.13).[126,131]

TABLE 3.11 ▫ **Collaborative Corneal Transplantation Studies (CCTS)—Crossmatch Study (CS)**

Study question	Determine the effectiveness of crossmatching in preventing graft rejection among high-risk patients with lymphocytotoxic antibodies.
Study design	Prospective, randomized, double-masked multicenter trial. Six university-based clinical centers
Inclusion/exclusion criteria	1. Age 10 y or older 2. Two to four quadrants of corneal stroma vascularization or a history of allograft rejection in the eye considered for surgery 3. Willing to participate in 3 y of follow-up 4. No condition that would greatly increase the risk of nonrejection graft failure (e.g., xerophthalmia or severe exposure) 5. No patients with systemic disease or with medication usage that might alter their immune response 6. Not pregnant 7. CCTS Central Laboratory confirmation of lymphocytotoxic antibodies on two separate occasions
Intervention	Patients received a cornea from either a positively or negatively crossmatched donor.
Primary outcome measure	Time to irreversible failure of corneal allograft due to any cause
Secondary outcome measures	1. Time to first immunological graft reaction 2. Time to irreversible graft failure due to allograft rejection 3. Visual acuity
Major findings	A positive donor—recipient crossmatch was not found to increase the risk of corneal graft failure.
Unanswered questions	Low prevalence of detectable lymphocytotoxic antibodies limited recruitment and study only had an 80% power to detect a 50% difference in groups.

Evolving Techniques and Future Directions

Advances in corneal transplantation will hopefully improve patients' functional and visual outcomes while hastening recovery and reducing complications. Currently, rates of endophthalmitis appear to be on the decline.[132] Endothelial replacement techniques, such as Deep Lamellar Endothelial Keratoplasty (see Fig. 3.14) and Descemet's Stripping Endothelial Keratoplasty (see Fig. 3.15), can reduce or eliminate induced surface astigmatic error and improve visual acuity,[133,134] although long-term data are lacking. Other endothelial-sparing anterior lamellar keratoplasty techniques may reduce the risk of donor rejection and improve graft survival.[135] The use of a femtosecond laser to assist in corneal transplantation may further refine these techniques.[136–139] It may be possible to prevent or delay corneal transplantation for KC by collagen-cross—linking therapies.[140] New tissue adhesives may also reduce suture-related complications.[141] Bioengineered corneas may eventually reduce or eliminate the need for donor tissue altogether.[142] A better understanding of corneal genetics and proteonomics may lead to medical therapies and/or corneal gene therapy. Ultimately, in spite of these advances, the assessment of the utility of techniques and interventions will require better measures of outcome.

Bacterial Keratitis

Introduction and Risk Factors

The diagnosis and management of bacterial keratitis can be challenging, and varying opinions exist within the ophthalmic community as to the best approach for these cases.[143] Although the keratitis can be eradicated in many circumstances, visual acuity is frequently diminished as a consequence of the infection.[144] The damage to the visual function is determined by the virulence of the organism, the inoculum, host defenses, adequacy of therapy, and the proximity of the keratitis to the central

TABLE 3.12 ▫ Cornea Donor Study (CDS)

Study question	1. Determine whether the graft-failure rate over a 5-y follow-up period following corneal transplantation is the same when using corneal tissue from donors older than 65 y compared with tissue from younger donors. 2. Assess the relationship between donor/recipient ABO blood type compatibility and graft failure due to rejection. 3. To assess corneal endothelial cell density as an indicator of the health of the cornea and as a surrogate outcome measure (in the optional Specular Microscopy Ancillary Study)
Study design	Prospective, randomized, double-masked multicenter observational study of 1,101 patients undergoing corneal transplantation
Inclusion/exclusion criteria	1. Patients must be in the age range of 40 to 80 y. 2. Corneal disease associated with endothelial dysfunction, including pseudophakic corneal edema, Fuchs' dystrophy, posterior polymorphous dystrophy, endothelial failure from another cause, interstitial keratitis (nonherpetic), or perforating corneal injury 3. Donor criteria: Age 10 to 75 y, endothelial cell count 2,300 to 3,300, tissue quality very good to excellent, death to preservation time <12 hr if body refrigerated or eyes on ice and <8 hr if not, and death to surgery time <5 d
Intervention	Routine examinations over 5 y
Primary outcome measure	Time to graft failure defined as a persistent cloudy cornea for 3 m or regrafting of the study eye
Major findings	1. Ongoing study 2. Variation in endothelial cell density between local eye banks and reading center of >10% was found in 38% of cases suggests need for better eye bank standards and technician certification.
Unanswered questions	Ongoing study

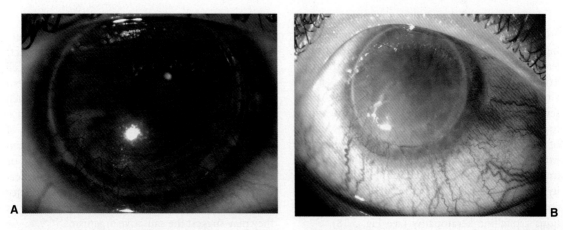

FIGURE 3.13 ▫ Four-month postoperative appearance of an initial penetrating keratoplasty for kerato-conus **(A)**. Florid graft rejection is present at 11 months postoperatively after discontinuation of topical steroids **(B)**.

TABLE 3.13 □ Corneal Transplantation

Epidemiology
1. Rates of PKP are slowly declining in the United States.
2. The leading indications for PKP worldwide are PBK, KC, and corneal scarring.
3. Rates of PKP for HSV appear to be declining.

Keratoconus
1. Prevalence, incidence, and disease severity vary with ethnicity.
2. Mechanical factors, as well as genetic predisposition, play a role in its etiology.
3. Visual function is much lower than measured visual acuity.

Graft Survival after PKP
1. HSV may account for one- third of primary graft failures.
2. Failure within the first couple years is usually immunologic, whereas late failures are generally nonimmunologic in etiology.
3. Graft survival is highest for KC and lowest for repeat PKPs and eyes with deep stromal vascularization.
4. Graft survival is reduced in pediatric populations, and patients requiring concomitant ancillary procedures.
5. Antigen matching and donor-recipient crossmatch do not appear to significant determinants of graft survival in high-risk eyes.
6. ABO incompatibility may be predictive of graft survival.
7. Rates of endothelial cell density loss are greatest within the first few years after PKP and roughly normalize after 10 y.

Immunosuppression
1. Topical corticosteroids are the mainstay of postoperative care.
2. Topical cyclosporine 2% may be an effective adjunct in certain eyes.
3. Oral cyclosporine has questionable effect on graft survival rates.
4. Newer agents such as tacrolimus and mycophenolate mofetil may reduced allograft rejections and improve graft survival.
5. All immunosuppressive agents carry negative, and sometimes severe, side effects.
   Topical and oral tacrolimus may reduce allograft rejection episodes.

HSV, herpes simplex virus; KC, keratoconus; PBK, pseudophakic bullous keratopathy; PKP, penetrating keratoplasty.

visual axis (see Figs. 3.16 and 3.17). For example, highly virulent gram-negative bacterial keratitis may leave little functional impairment if outside the visual axis, whereas a small central corneal scar from a mildly virulent gram-positive organism will have more severe consequences. The ability of the organisms to form biofilms, defined as functional consortiums of microorganisms organized within an extensive extracellular polymer matrix, may inhibit the host immune response as well as limit the bioavailability of antibiotics.[145] This has become more recently recognized in chronic bacterial keratitis, such as infectious crystalline keratopathy (see Fig. 3.18).[145–147]

A variety of inciting or risk factors have been recognized in cases of bacterial keratitis. Surface factors such as contact lens wear, trauma,[148] previous corneal surgery or sutures,[149,150] chronic exposure or irritation, persistent or recurring epithelial defects (see Fig. 3.19), tear deficiency or limbal stem cell deficiency states can predispose to the development of bacterial keratitis. Likewise, systemic factors such as immunosuppression, atopy, diabetes mellitus, or connective tissue diseases increase the risk of infection. Geographic location, medicamentosa, and unusual exposure to animals, contaminated water, or other higher-risk environments (including medical facilities) should always be considered. The presence or absence of these factors is important to elicit as they may suggest the causative organisms.

In North America, as well as in Europe[151] and Asia,[152,153] most cases of microbial keratitis arise from a bacterial etiology. In the western United

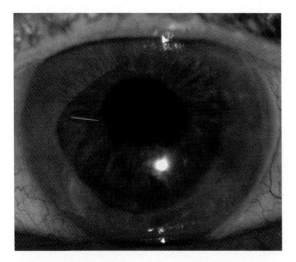

FIGURE 3.14 ◻ Nine-month postoperative appearance after deep lamellar endothelial keratoplasty. Uncorrected visual acuity measures 20/50.

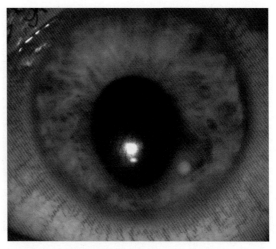

FIGURE 3.16 ◻ Contact lens–associated peripheral bacterial keratitis.

States, gram-positive bacteria, especially the *Staphylococcus* and *Streptococcus* species,[154] were found to be prominent causes. In the southeastern United States although gram-positive bacteria were also prominent, *Pseudomonas* species were more frequently isolated,[155,156] attesting to geographic variability. Other organisms, such as fungi, mycobacteria (see Fig. 3.20), and acanthamoeba (see Fig. 3.21) may

also have geographic variability in frequency.[157] The estimated annual incidence of bacterial keratitis in the United States has been reported to be 5.3 per 100,000 people,[158] with an increasing frequency in the 1980s and associated with contact lens wear in over 50% of cases. More recent studies show a reversal of this trend in the United States.[155] For contact lens wearers in the Netherlands, the estimated annualized incidence of microbial keratitis was 1.1 per 10,000 users of daily-wear rigid gas-permeable lenses (RGP), 3.5 per 10,000 users of daily-wear soft lenses, and 20.0 per 10,000 (10.3 to 35.0) of users of extended-wear soft lenses.[159] This variability in rates of contact

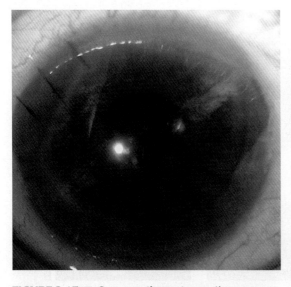

FIGURE 3.15 ◻ One-month postoperative appearance after combined Descemet's stripping endothelial keratoplasty with phacoemulsification and IOL implantation.

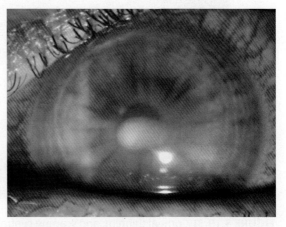

FIGURE 3.17 ◻ Central bacterial keratitis from *propionibacterium acnes*.

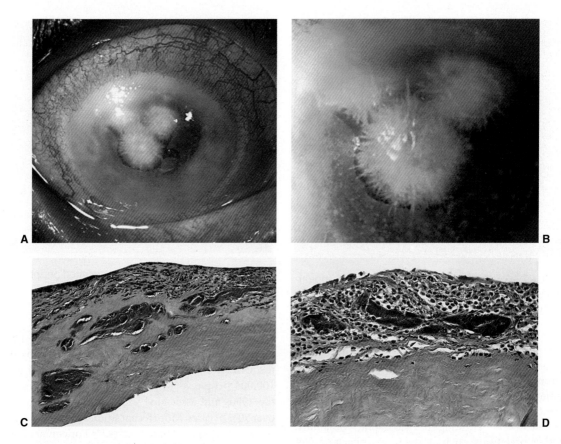

FIGURE 3.18 ▣ Slit lamp biomicroscopic appearance of infectious crystalline keratopathy caused by *streptococcus viridans* **(A and B)**. Histopathologic examination of a lamellar biopsy reveals copious clusters of bacteria with varying levels of inflammatory response **(C and D)**.

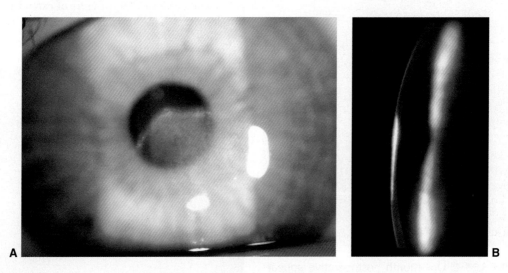

FIGURE 3.19 ▣ Corneal thinning and scarring centrally after bacterial keratitis following a recurrent corneal erosion **(A and B)**.

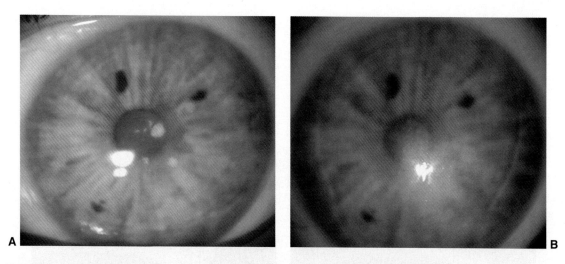

FIGURE 3.20 □ *Mycobacterium chelonae* keratitis presenting one month after laser in situ keratomileusis **(A)**. After flap amputation and three months of topical therapy, residual corneal scarring is evident **(B)**.

lens–related microbial keratitis may be due to contact lens material, design, usage, and/or oxygen transmissibility.[160–164] Contact lenses remain by far the most important risk factor for development of corneal infections.

Diagnosis

Ideally, all corneal ulcers would be cultured and antimicrobial therapy tailored specifically to the organism identified. This does not occur in clinical practice as empiric therapy is typically effective,[165] maintenance of culturing supplies can be costly, and there is a lag in obtaining culture results. A meta-analysis of studies in which culture was performed also found that culture results did not affect 1-week cure rates.[166] However, cultures are valuable in establishing trends in microbial keratitis, especially in regard to resistance to antibiotics. Likewise, when cases demonstrate atypical and/or inadequate response to empiric therapy, as may be seen in a cornea subspecialty practice, cultures should be performed or repeated.[167] It is also important to consider the possibility of a polymicrobial infection in these cases.

Confocal microscopy, although not widely available, may be helpful in diagnosing acanthamoeba and fungal keratitis.[168,169] However, when culture results are negative, deep stromal infiltrates are present, and/or the clinical scenario does not improve in spite of vigorous therapy, a corneal biopsy may be needed to establish a definitive diagnosis. Some surgeons perform an epithelial biopsy alone, but for severe cases a deeper resection not only provides greater tissue for histopathology but also debulks the infectious process, permits greater penetration of antibiotics, and provides more substantive material for culture.

Management

Initial therapy plays an important role in the outcome of bacterial keratitis.[170] For cases of presumed bacterial keratitis, one should combine the knowledge of the most likely causative organism and local antibiotic resistance patterns, with delivery of sufficient antimicrobial(s) to overwhelm bacterial defenses. Aggressive broad-spectrum antibiotic therapy should be promptly initiated with discontinuation of any aggravating or inciting factors such as contact lenses. Although inconvenient for the patient, it is best to begin with a very frequent dosing schedule for loading purposes, such as every 5 to 15 minutes for the first 30 to 60 minutes, then subsequently reduce to a maintenance dosage. If multiple antibiotics are used, it is not necessary to alternate them on different schedules, once a loading dose has been achieved. Patients who cannot comply with the dosing schedule may need hospitalization or home health assistance. Traditional *in vitro* minimum inhibitory concentration (MIC) data do not necessarily apply to topical ophthalmic medications as the generally higher local ocular concentrations can result in clinical response even for organisms deemed "resistant." Newer topical fluoroquinolone antibiotics have contributed to improved success in treatment as they can be used as

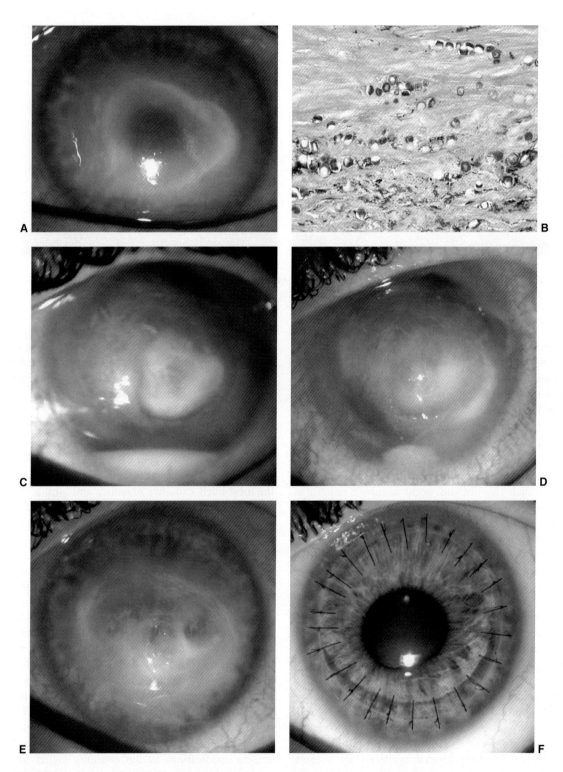

FIGURE 3.21 ◻ Acanthamoeba keratitis. Initial presentation **(A)** with lamellar corneal biopsy revealing numerous cysts **(B)**. Appearance after two months of therapy **(C)**, four months **(D)**, and six months **(E)**. Two months after penetrating keratoplasty, uncorrected visual acuity measures 20/40 **(F)**.

monotherapy and are effective against a broad spectrum of organisms. Unfortunately, resistance to these agents is likely to be inevitable. As such, it is not a good practice to prolong therapy or taper antibiotics after the infection has resolved as this may foster resistant organisms. Likewise, if there is an atypical response, consideration should be given to using fortified antibiotics as guided by cultures and/or the organism(s) most likely to be present.

Topical corticosteroids have an unclear role in the management of bacterial keratitis. The typical objective is to reduce an exaggerated inflammatory response and minimize corneal scarring, while not impairing the healing response. One systematic review (see Table 3.14) found that prior usage of corticosteroids increased the risk of antibiotic treatment failure or other infectious complications.[171] From this review, two recommendations reached "most important" levels. First, topical corticosteroids should be avoided if the causative agent is unknown and, second, topical corticosteroids should be utilized when, after using clinical or laboratory criteria, it is deemed

important to aid reepithelialization or minimize stromal alteration and scarring. In practice, before administering topical corticosteroids, the American Academy of Ophthalmology Preferred Practice Pattern on this subject suggests waiting 2 to 3 days after topical antibiotic therapy has been initiated and in which progress is being made in treating the infection.[172] If topical corticosteroids are initiated, it is important to follow up the patient closely in the initial period to insure against recrudescence of the infectious process.

Concomitant pain management is an important consideration for these patients. One simple measure is the administration of a topical cycloplegic agent in the office. In patients responding to therapy, the pain is typically stabilized or improved by the first day after treatment (although the clinical appearance may appear worsened). Oral narcotics can be used adjunctively, but are frequently unnecessary and can potentially mask clinical worsening or reduce compliance with the treatment regimen. These agents also tend to have an unwanted sedative effect in many

TABLE 3.14 ☐ Corticosteroids for Bacterial Keratitis

Study question	Determine the effects of topical corticosteroids with bacterial keratitis.
Study design	Systematic review
Inclusion/exclusion criteria	1. Bacterial keratitis was defined as a stromal infiltrate with an overlying epithelial defect that warranted intensive antibacterial therapy. 2. All topical corticosteroids studied were considered equivalent.
Intervention	Sources included electronic searching of MEDLINE and EMBASE through 2000; used the text words *keratitis* or *corneal ulcer* combined with *corticosteroid, cortisone, dexamethasone,* or *prednisolone,* without language restrictions. Other sources were identified by manually searching Index Medicus from 1960 through 1965, Excerpta Medica Ophthalmology from 1960 to 1973, and Ophthalmic Literature from 1950 to 1999. Reference lists of primary reports, review articles, and corneal textbooks were searched for additional relevant articles dating from 1950.
Primary outcome measures	Positive and negative effects of corticosteroids used before and during therapy for bacterial keratitis
Major findings	1. Avoid topical corticosteroids if the causative microorganism is unknown. 2. Add a topical corticosteroid if the organism is known and treatment, by clinical, or laboratory criteria, is necessary to aid reepithelialization and/or minimize stromal alteration.
Unanswered questions	If topical corticosteroids have value: 1. Who is a good candidate for therapy? 2. When should topical corticosteroids be initiated? 3. At what frequency and dosage should they be initiated? 4. How long should they be continued?

patients. It may be best to reserve oral narcotics for patients who are expected to have long therapeutic courses. Topical anesthetics are not advisable for these patients, given the potential for abuse and delayed healing. For severe cases of keratitis, as well as those with current or impending perforation, therapeutic PKP may sometimes be a better option than weeks and months of topical therapy (see Fig. 3.22 and Table 3.15).

Future Directions

Multiple advances are anticipated in the management of bacterial keratitis. Of foremost necessity are better preventative measures, particularly in the design, materials, and usage of contact lenses. The introduction of silicone hydrogel lenses appears to be a step in this direction and may reduce the risk of infection for extended-wear contacts.[160] In spite of this, infections associated with silicone hydrogel lenses still occur and can be severe with reported greater adhesion of organisms such as acanthamoeba to this material[173]. Use of extended-wear contacts increases the risk of infection and patient education in this regard remains important. A better understanding of the specific virulence factors of each bacterium, and how these interplay with the host, may lead to medications or devices that reduce the rate of infectious keratitis. From a diagnostic standpoint, the development of rapid, preferably office-based, assays

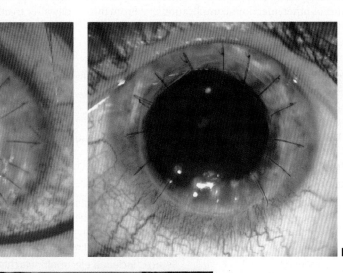

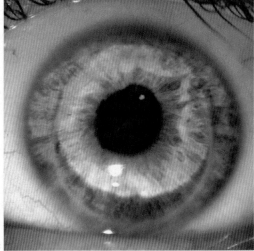

FIGURE 3.22 ❑ Appearance of a therapeutic penetrating keratoplasty performed for a perforated aspergillus corneal ulcer at one day (**A**), six weeks (**B**), and one year (**C**).

TABLE 3.15 ☐ Bacterial Keratitis

Epidemiology
1. Contact lenses are the greatest risk factor for bacterial keratitis
2. Gram-positive bacteria, especially *Staphylococcus,* and *Streptococcus* species, are the most commonly cultured organisms

Diagnosis
1. For primary bacterial keratitis, culture results do not affect 1-wk cure rates
2. Cultures should be performed or repeated when there is an atypical response to therapy
3. Corneal biopsy can establish a definitive diagnosis

Management
1. Aggressive broad-spectrum antibiotic therapy should be initiated promptly
2. Unnecessary prolongation of antibiotic therapy should be avoided as well as tapering of the antibiotics to avoid the possibility of creating resistant organisms
3. Topical corticosteroids have an unclear role in the treatment of bacterial keratitis, but may aid reepithelialization and/or minimization of corneal scarring
4. Severe cases may require therapeutic penetrating keratoplasty

to identify the causative organism and its sensitivities would also be worthwhile. Education regarding the appropriate use of topical antibiotics, especially within the nonophthalmic community, remains an important goal to reduce the spread of resistance. Avoiding long-term treatment at low doses, and avoiding the tapering of antibiotics is important in the prevention of resistance. More research is necessary to understand the appropriate role and timing of corticosteroids in adjunctive therapy. Finally, as microorganisms develop resistance to current antibiotics, a steady supply of alternatives will become necessary.

Acknowledgments

We are grateful and indebted to Patricia Duffel at the University of Iowa Hospitals and Clinics for her assistance with the literature review needed to develop this chapter as well as to Karin R. Sletten, M.D. for her critical review and suggestions.

References

1. Liesegang TJ. Classification of herpes simplex virus keratitis and anterior uveitis. *Cornea.* 1999;18:127–143.
2. Holland EJ, Schwartz GS. Classification of herpes simplex virus keratitis. *Cornea.* 1999;18:144–154.
3. Liesegang TJ. Herpes simplex virus epidemiology and ocular importance. *Cornea.* 2001;20:1–13.
4. Liesegang TJ, Melton LJd, Daly PJ, et al. Epidemiology of ocular herpes simplex. Incidence in Rochester, Minn, 1950 through 1982. *Arch Ophthalmol.* 1989;107:1155–1159.
5. Wilhelmus KR, Coster DJ, Donovan HC, et al. Prognosis indicators of herpetic keratitis. Analysis of a five-year observation period after corneal ulceration. *Arch Ophthalmol.* 1981;99:1578–1582.
6. Darougar S, Wishart MS, Viswalingam ND. Epidemiological and clinical features of primary herpes simplex virus ocular infection. *Br J Ophthalmol.* 1985;69:2–6.
7. Wishart MS, Darougar S, Viswalingam ND. Recurrent herpes simplex virus ocular infection: Epidemiological and clinical features. *Br J Ophthalmol.* 1987;71:669–672.
8. Norn MS. Dendritic (herpetic) keratitis. I. Incidence–seasonal variations–recurrence rate–visual impairment–therapy. *Acta Ophthalmol.* 1970;48:91–107.
9. Ribaric V. The incidence of herpetic keratitis among population. *Ophthalmologica.* 1976;173:19–22.
10. Shuster JJ, Kaufman HE, Nesburn AB. Statistical analysis of the rate of recurrence of herpes virus ocular epithelial disease. *Am J Ophthalmol.* 1981;91:328–331.
11. Wilhelmus KR. Interventions for herpes simplex virus epithelial keratitis. *Cochrane Database Syst Rev.* 2003;2:CD002898. DOI: 10.1002/14651858.CD002898.
12. Herpetic Eye Disease Study Group. A controlled trial of oral acyclovir for the prevention of stromal keratitis or iritis in patients with herpes simplex virus epithelial keratitis. The Epithelial Keratitis Trial. *Arch Ophthalmol.* 1997;115:703–712.
13. Wilhelmus KR, Gee L, Hauck WW, Herpetic Eye Disease Study. A controlled trial of

topical corticosteroids for herpes simplex stromal keratitis. *Ophthalmology*. 1994;101:1883–1896.

14. Herpetic Eye Disease Study Group. A controlled trial of oral acyclovir for iridocyclitis caused by herpes simplex virus. *Arch Ophthalmol*. 1996;114:1065–1072.

15. Barney NP, Foster CS. A prospective randomized trial of oral acyclovir after penetrating keratoplasty for herpes simplex keratitis. *Cornea*. 1994;13:232–236.

16. The Herpetic Eye Disease Study Group. Acyclovir for the prevention of recurrent herpes simplex virus eye disease. *N Engl J Med*. 1998;339:300–306.

17. Hung SO, Patterson A, Rees PJ. Pharmacokinetics of oral acyclovir (Zovirax) in the eye. *Br J Ophthalmol*. 1984;68:192–195.

18. Uchoa UB, Rezende RA, Carrasco MA, et al. Long-term acyclovir use to prevent recurrent ocular herpes simplex virus infection. *Arch Ophthalmol*. 2003;121:1702–1704.

19. Lairson DR, Begley CE, Reynolds TF, et al. Prevention of herpes simplex virus eye disease: A cost-effectiveness analysis. *Arch Ophthalmol*. 2003;121:108–112.

20. Barron BA, Gee L, Hauck WW, Herpetic Eye Disease Study. A controlled trial of oral acyclovir for herpes simplex stromal keratitis. *Ophthalmology*. 1994;101:1871–1882.

21. Wilhelmus KR, Dawson CR, Barron BA, et al. Risk factors for herpes simplex virus epithelial keratitis recurring during treatment of stromal keratitis or iridocyclitis. *Br J Ophthalmol*. 1996;80:969–972.

22. Herpetic Eye Disease Study Group. Psychological stress and other potential triggers for recurrences of herpes simplex virus eye infections. *Arch Ophthalmol*. 2000;118:1617–1625.

23. Stranska R, Schuurman R, Nienhuis E, et al. Survey of acyclovir-resistant herpes simplex virus in the Netherlands: Prevalence and characterization. *J Clin Virol*. 2005;32:7–18.

24. Tomblin FA Jr, Lucas KH. Lysine for management of herpes labialis. *Am J Health Syst Pharm*. 2001;58:298–300, 304.

25. Singh BB, Udani J, Vinjamury SP, et al. Safety and effectiveness of an L-lysine, zinc, and herbal-based product on the treatment of facial and circumoral herpes. *Altern Med Rev*. 2005;10:123–127.

26. Griffith RS, DeLong DC, Nelson JD. Relation of arginine–lysine antagonism to herpes simplex growth in tissue culture. *Chemotherapy*. 1981;27:209–213.

27. Schwartz JA, Lium EK, Silverstein SJ. Herpes simplex virus type 1 entry is inhibited by the cobalt chelate complex CTC-96. *J Virol*. 2001;75:4117–4128.

28. Aurelian L. Herpes simplex virus type 2 vaccines: New ground for optimism? *Clin Diagn Lab Immunol*. 2004;11:437–445.

29. Jones CA, Cunningham AL. Vaccination strategies to prevent genital herpes and neonatal herpes simplex virus (HSV) disease. *Herpes*. 2004;11:12–17.

30. Stanberry LR. Clinical trials of prophylactic and therapeutic herpes simplex virus vaccines. *Herpes*. 2004;11 (Suppl 3):161A–169A.

31. Eye Bank Association of America. *2004 Eye banking statistical report*. Washington DC: Eye Bank Association of America; 2005.

32. Sugar A, Sugar J. Techniques in penetrating keratoplasty: A quarter century of development. *Cornea*. 2000;19:603–610.

33. Cosar CB, Sridhar MS, Cohen EJ, et al. Indications for penetrating keratoplasty and associated procedures, 1996–2000. *Cornea*. 2002;21:148–151.

34. Dobbins KR, Price FW Jr, Whitson WE. Trends in the indications for penetrating keratoplasty in the midwestern United States. *Cornea*. 2000;19:813–816.

35. Maeno A, Naor J, Lee HM, et al. Three decades of corneal transplantation: Indications and patient characteristics. *Cornea*. 2000;19:7–11.

36. Damji KF, Rootman J, White VA, et al. Changing indications for penetrating keratoplasty in Vancouver, 1978-87. *Can J Ophthalmol*. 1990;25:243–248.

37. Poinard C, Tuppin P, Loty B, et al. The French national waiting list for keratoplasty created in 1999: Patient registration, indications, characteristics, and turnover. *J Fr Ophthalmol*. 2003;26:911–919.

38. Yahalom C, Mechoulam H, Solomon A, et al. Forty years of changing indications in penetrating keratoplasty in Israel. *Cornea*. 2005;24:256–258.

39. Al-Towerki AE, Gonnah el-S, Al-Rajhi A, et al. Changing indications for corneal transplantation at the King Khaled Eye Specialist Hospital (1983–2002). *Cornea.* 2004;23:584–588.
40. Williams KA, Muehlberg SM, Lewis RF, et al. How successful is corneal transplantation? A report from the Australian Corneal Graft Register. *Eye.* 1995;9:219–227.
41. Edwards M, Clover GM, Brookes N, et al. Indications for corneal transplantation in New Zealand: 1991-1999. *Cornea.* 2002;21:152–155.
42. Dandona L, Ragu K, Janarthanan M, et al. Indications for penetrating keratoplasty in India. *Indian J Ophthalmol.* 1997;45:163–168.
43. Tabin GC, Gurung R, Paudyal G, et al. Penetrating keratoplasty in Nepal. *Cornea.* 2004;23:589–596.
44. Chen WL, Hu FR, Wang IJ. Changing indications for penetrating keratoplasty in Taiwan from 1987 to 1999. *Cornea.* 2001;20:141–144.
45. Al-Yousuf N, Mavrikakis I, Mavrikakis E, et al. Penetrating keratoplasty: Indications over a 10 year period. *Br J Ophthalmol.* 2004;88:998–1001.
46. Legeis JM, Parc C, d'Hermies F, et al. Nineteen years of penetrating keratoplasty in the Hotel-Dieu hospital in Paris. *Cornea.* 2001;20:603–606.
47. Branco BC, Gaudio PA, Margolis TP. Epidemiology and molecular analysis of herpes simplex keratitis requiring primary penetrating keratoplasty. *Br J Ophthalmol.* 2004;88:1285–1288.
48. Pearson AR, Soneji B, Sarvananthan N, et al. Does ethnic origin influence the incidence or severity of keratoconus? *Eye.* 2000;14:625–628.
49. Kennedy RH, Bourne WM, Dyer JA. A 48-year clinical and epidemiologic study of keratoconus. *Am J Ophthalmol.* 1986;101:267–273.
50. Li X, Rabinowitz YS, Rasheed K, et al. Longitudinal study of the normal eyes in unilateral keratoconus patients. *Ophthalmology.* 2004;111:440–446.
51. Macsai MS, Varley GA, Krachmer JH. Development of keratoconus after contact lens wear. Patient characteristics. *Arch Ophthalmol.* 1990;108:534–538.
52. Jafri B, Lichter H, Stulting RD. Asymmetric keratoconus attributed to eye rubbing. *Cornea.* 2004;23:560–564.
53. Rabinowitz YS, Garbus J, McDonnell PJ. Computer-assisted corneal topography in family members of patients with keratoconus. *Arch Ophthalmol.* 1990;108:365–371.
54. Morrow GL, Stein RM, Racine JS, et al. Computerized videokeratography of keratoconus kindreds. *Can J Ophthalmol.* 1997;32:233–243.
55. Zadnik K, Steger-May K, Fink BA, et al. Collaborative Longitudinal Evaluation of Keratoconus. Between-eye asymmetry in keratoconus. *Cornea.* 2002;21:671–679.
56. Zadnik K, Barr JT, Edrington TB, et al. Corneal scarring and vision in keratoconus: A baseline report from the Collaborative Longitudinal Evaluation of Keratoconus (CLEK) Study. *Cornea.* 2000;19:804–812.
57. Kymes SM, Walline JJ, Zadnik K, et al, Collaborative Longitudinal Evaluation of Keratoconus study group. Quality of life in keratoconus. *Am J Ophthalmol.* 2004;138:527–535.
58. Uiters E, van den Borne B, van der Horst FG, et al. Patient satisfaction after corneal transplantation. *Cornea.* 2001;20:687–694.
59. Cockerham GC, Bijwaard K, Sheng ZM, et al. Primary graft failure: A clinicopathologic and molecular analysis. *Ophthalmology.* 2000;107:2083–2090.
60. Ing JJ, Ing HH, Nelson LR, et al. Ten-year postoperative results of penetrating keratoplasty. *Ophthalmology.* 1998;105:1855–1865.
61. Patel SV, Hodge DO, Bourne WM. Corneal endothelium and postoperative outcomes 15 years after penetrating keratoplasty. *Am J Ophthalmol.* 2005;139:311–319.
62. Thompson RW Jr, Price MO, Bowers PJ, et al. Long-term graft survival after penetrating keratoplasty. *Ophthalmology.* 2003;110:1396–1402.
63. Inoue K, Amano S, Oshika T, et al. Risk factors for corneal graft failure and rejection in penetrating keratoplasty. *Acta Ophthalmol Scand.* 2001;79:251–255.
64. Muraine M, Sanchez C, Watt L, et al. Long-term results of penetrating keratoplasty. A 10-year-plus retrospective study. *Graefes Arch Clin Exp Ophthalmol.* 2003;241:571–576.
65. Paglen PG, Fine M, Abbott RL, et al. The prognosis for keratoplasty in keratoconus. *Ophthalmology.* 1982;89:651–654.

66. Sharif KW, Casey TA. Penetrating kerato-plasty for keratoconus: Complications and long-term success. *Br J Ophthalmol.* 1991;75: 142–146.

67. Price Jr FW, Whitson WE, Collins KS, et al. Five-year corneal graft survival: A large, single-center patient cohort. *Arch Ophthalmol.* 1993;111:799–805.

68. Sit M, Weisbrod DJ, Naor J, et al. Corneal graft outcome study. *Cornea.* 2001;20:129–133.

69. Pineros O, Cohen EJ, Rapuano CJ, et al. Long-term results after penetrating keratoplasty for Fuchs' endothelial dystrophy. *Arch Ophthalmol.* 1996;114:15–18.

70. Epstein RJ, Seedor JA, Dreizen NG, et al. Penetrating keratoplasty for herpes simplex keratitis and keratoconus: Allograft rejection and survival. *Ophthalmology.* 1987;94: 935–942.

71. Sugar A. An analysis of corneal endothelial and graft survival in pseudophakic bullous keratopathy. *Trans Am Ophthalmol Soc.* 1989;87:762–801.

72. Marcon AS, Cohen EJ, Rapuano CJ, et al. Recurrence of corneal stromal dystrophies after penetrating keratoplasty. *Cornea.* 2003;22: 19–21.

73. Dana MR, Moyes AL, Gomes JA, et al. The indications for and outcome in pediatric keratoplasty. A multicenter study. *Ophthalmology.* 1995;102:1129–1138.

74. Aasuri MK, Garg P, Gokhle N, et al. Penetrating keratoplasty in children. *Cornea.* 2000;19:140–144.

75. Schaumberg DA, Moyes AL, Gomes JA, et al. Corneal transplantation in young children with congenital hereditary endothelial dystrophy. Multicenter Pediatric Keratoplasty Study. *Am J Ophthalmol.* 1999;127:373–378.

76. Dana MR, Schaumberg DA, Moyes AL, et al. Corneal transplantation in children with Peters anomaly and mesenchymal dysgenesis. Multicenter Pediatric Keratoplasty Study. *Ophthalmology.* 1997;104:1580–1586.

77. Dana MR, Schaumberg DA, Moyes AL, et al. Outcome of penetrating keratoplasty after ocular trauma in children. *Arch Ophthalmol.* 1995;113:1503–1507.

78. Javadi MA, Baradaran-Rafii AR, Zamani M, et al. Penetrating keratoplasty in young children

with congenital hereditary endothelial dystrophy. *Cornea.* 2003;22:420–423.

79. Chang SD, Pecego JG, Zadnik K, et al. Factors influencing graft clarity. *Cornea.* 1996;15: 577–581.

80. Lois N, Kowal VO, Cohen EJ, et al. Indications for penetrating keratoplasty and associated procedures, 1989–1995. *Cornea.* 1997;16:623–629.

81. Hassan TS, Soong HK, Sugar A, et al. Implantation of Kelman-style, open-loop anterior chamber lenses during keratoplasty for aphakic and pseudophakic bullous keratopathy. A comparison with iris-sutured posterior chamber lenses. *Ophthalmology.* 1991;98:875–880.

82. Djalilian AR, Anderson SO, Fang-Yen M, et al. Long-term results of transsclerally sutured posterior chamber lenses in penetrating keratoplasty. *Cornea.* 1998;17:359–364.

83. Akpek EK, Altan-Yaycioglu R, Karadayi K, et al. Long-term outcomes of combined penetrating keratoplasty with iris-sutured intraocular lens implantation. *Ophthalmology.* 2003;110:1017–1022.

84. Farjo AA, Rhee DJ, Soong HK, et al. Iris-sutured posterior chamber intraocular lens implantation during penetrating keratoplasty. *Cornea.* 2004;23:18–28.

85. Wagoner MD, Cox TA, Ariyasu RG, et al. Intraocular lens implantation in the absence of capsular support: A report by the American Academy of Ophthalmology. *Ophthalmology.* 2003;110:840–859.

86. Schein OD, Kenyon KR, Stenert RF, et al. A randomized trial of intraocular lens fixation techniques with penetrating keratoplasty. *Ophthalmology.* 1993;100:1437–1443.

87. Kirkness CM, Steele AD, Ficker LA, et al. Coexistent corneal disease and glaucoma managed by either drainage surgery and subsequent keratoplasty or combined drainage surgery and penetrating keratoplasty. *Br J Ophthalmol.* 1992;76:146–152.

88. Rapuano CJ, Schmidt CM, Cohen EJ, et al. Results of alloplastic tube shunt procedures before, during, or after penetrating keratoplasty. *Cornea.* 1995;14:26–32.

89. Al-Torbak A. Graft survival and glaucoma outcome after simultaneous penetrating keratoplasty and Ahmed glaucoma valve implant. *Cornea.* 2003;22:194–197.

90. WuDunn D, Alfonso E, Palmberg PF. Combined penetrating keratoplasty and trabeculectomy with mitomycin C. *Ophthalmology*. 1999; 106:396–400.

91. Arroyave CP, Scott IU, Fantes FE, et al. Corneal graft survival and intraocular pressure control after penetrating keratoplasty and glaucoma drainage device implantation. *Ophthalmology*. 2001;108:1978–1985.

92. Sidoti PA, Mosny AY, Ritterband DC, et al. Pars plana tube insertion of glaucoma drainage implants and penetrating keratoplasty in patients with coexisting glaucoma and corneal disease. *Ophthalmology*. 2001;108:1050–1058.

93. Garcia-Valenzuela E, Blair NP, Shapiro MJ, et al. Outcome of vitreoretinal surgery and penetrating keratoplasty using temporary keratoprosthesis. *Retina*. 1999;19:424–429.

94. Gallemore RP, Bokosky JE. Penetrating keratoplasty with vitreoretinal surgery using the Eckardt temporary keratoprosthesis: Modified technique allowing use of larger corneal grafts. *Cornea*. 1995;14:33–38.

95. Roters S, Szurman P, Hermes S, et al. Outcome of combined penetrating keratoplasty with vitreoretinal surgery for management of severe ocular injuries. *Retina*. 2003;23:48–56.

96. Dong X, Wang W, Xie L, et al. Long-term outcome of combined penetrating keratoplasty and vitreoretinal surgery using temporary keratoprosthesis. *Eye*. 2006;20:59–63.

97. Patel NP, Kim T, Rapuano CJ, et al. Indications for and outcomes of repeat penetrating keratoplasty, 1989–1995. *Ophthalmology*. 2000;107:719–724.

98. Weisbrod DJ, Sit M, Naor J, et al. Outcomes of repeat penetrating keratoplasty and risk factors for graft failure. *Cornea*. 2003;22:429–434.

99. Maguire MG, Stark WJ, Gottsch JD, et al. Risk factors for corneal graft failure and rejection in the Collaborative Corneal Transplantation Studies. Collaborative Corneal Transplantation Studies Research Group. *Ophthalmology*. 1994;101:1536–1547.

100. Musch DC, Meyer RF, Sugar A, et al. A study of race matching between donor and recipient in corneal transplantation. *Am J Ophthalmol*. 1988;105:646–650.

101. The Collaborative Corneal Transplantation Studies Research Group. Effectiveness of histocompatibility matching in high-risk corneal transplantation. *Arch Ophthalmol*. 1992;110:1392–1403.

102. Hahn AB, Foulks GN, Enger C, et al. The association of lymphocytotoxic antibodies with corneal allograft rejection in high risk patients. The Collaborative Corneal Transplantation Studies Research Group. *Transplantation*. 1995;59:21–27.

103. Reinhard T, Böhringer D, Enczmann J, et al. Improvement of graft prognosis in penetrating normal-risk keratoplasty by HLA class I and II matching. *Eye*. 2004;18:269–277.

104. Musch DC, Meyer RF, Sugar A. Predictive factors for endothelial cell loss after penetrating keratoplasty. *Arch Ophthalmol*. 1993; 111:80–83.

105. Yamagami S, Suzuki Y, Tsuru T. Risk factors for graft failure in penetrating keratoplasty. *Acta Ophthalmol Scand*. 1996;74:584–588.

106. Böhringer D, Reinhard T, Spelsberg H, et al. Influencing factors on chronic endothelial cell loss characterised in a homogeneous group of patients. *Br J Ophthalmol*. 2002;86:35–38.

107. Jonas JB, Rank RM, Budde WM. Immunologic graft reactions after allogenic penetrating keratoplasty. *Am J Ophthalmol*. 2002;133:437–443.

108. Gain P, Thuret G, Chiquet C, et al. Cornea procurement from very old donors: Post organ culture cornea outcome and recipient graft outcome. *Br J Ophthalmol*. 2002;86:404–411.

109. Williams KA, Muehlberg SM, Lewis RF, et al. Influence of advanced recipient and donor age on the outcome of corneal transplantation. Australian Corneal Graft Registry. *Br J Ophthalmol*. 1997;81:835–839.

110. Palay DA, Kangas TA, Stulting RD, et al. The effects of donor age on the outcome of penetrating keratoplasty in adults. *Ophthalmology*. 1997;104:1576–1579.

111. Cornea Donor Study Group. An evaluation of image quality and accuracy of eye bank measurement of donor cornea endothelial cell density in the Specular Microscopy Ancillary Study. *Ophthalmology*. 2005;112:431–440.

112. Bourne WM, Hodge DO, Nelson LR. Corneal endothelium five years after transplantation. *Am J Ophthalmol*. 1994;118:185−196.

113. Inoue K, Kimura C, Amano S, et al. Corneal endothelial cell changes twenty years after penetrating keratoplasty. *Jpn J Ophthalmol*. 2002;46:189−192.

114. Hu FR, Tsai AC, Wang IJ, et al. Outcomes of penetrating keratoplasty with imported donor corneas. *Cornea*. 1999;18:182−187.

115. Armitage WJ, Dick AD, Bourne WM. Predicting endothelial cell loss and long-term corneal graft survival. *Invest Ophthalmol Vis Sci*. 2003;44:3326−3331.

116. Nishimura JK, Hodge DO, Bourne WM. Initial endothelial cell density and chronic endothelial cell loss rate in corneal transplants with late endothelial failure. *Ophthalmology*. 1999;106:1962−1965.

117. Cosar CB, Laibson PR, Cohen EJ, et al. Topical cyclosporine in pediatric keratoplasty. *Eye Contact Lens*. 2003;29:103−107.

118. Inoue K, Amano S, Kimura C, et al. Long-term effects of topical cyclosporine a treatment after penetrating keratoplasty. *Jpn J Ophthalmol*. 2000;44:302−305.

119. Belin MW, Bouchard CS, Frantz S, et al. Topical cyclosporine in high-risk corneal transplants. *Ophthalmology*. 1989;96:1144−1150.

120. Hill JC. Systemic cyclosporine in high-risk keratoplasty: Long-term results. *Eye*. 1995;9: 422−428.

121. Rumelt S, Bersudsky V, Blum-Hareuveni T, et al. Systemic cyclosporin a in high failure risk, repeated corneal transplantation. *Br J Ophthalmol*. 2002;86:988−992.

122. Poon AC, Forbes JE, Dart JK, et al. Systemic cyclosporin a in high risk penetrating keratoplasties: A case-control study. *Br J Ophthalmol*. 2001;85:1464−1469.

123. Inoue K, Kimura C, Amano S, et al. Long-term outcome of systemic cyclosporine treatment following penetrating keratoplasty. *Jpn J Ophthalmol*. 2001;45:378−382.

124. Reinhard T, Sundmacher R, Heering P. Systemic cyclosporine a in high-risk keratoplasties. *Graefes Arch Clin Exp Ophthalmol*. 1996; 234(Suppl 1):S115−S121.

125. Reinhard T, Mayweg S, Reis A, et al. Topical FK506 as immunoprophylaxis after allogeneic penetrating normal-risk keratoplasty: A randomized clinical pilot study. *Transpl Int*. 2005;18:193−197.

126. Sloper CM, Powell RJ, Dua HS. Tacrolimus (FK506) in the management of high-risk corneal and limbal grafts. *Ophthalmology*. 2001;108:1838−1844.

127. Reinhard T, Mayweg S, Sokolovska Y, et al. Systemic mycophenolate mofetil avoids immune reactions in penetrating high-risk keratoplasty: Preliminary results of an ongoing prospectively randomized multicenter study. *Transpl Int*. 2005;18:703−708.

128. Birnbaum F, Bohringer D, Sokolovska Y, et al. Immunosuppression with cyclosporine a and mycophenolate mofetil after penetrating high-risk keratoplasty: A retrospective study. *Transplantation*. 2005;79:964−968.

129. Field AJ, Gottsch JD. Persisting epithelial herpes simplex keratitis while on cyclosporin-A ointment. *Aust N Z J Ophthalmol*. 1995;23: 333−334.

130. Joseph MA, Kaufman HE, Insler M. Topical tacrolimus ointment for treatment of refractory anterior segment inflammatory disorders. *Cornea*. 2005;24:417−420.

131. Algros MP, Angonin R, Delbosc B, et al. Danger of systemic cyclosporine for corneal graft. *Cornea*. 2002;21:613−614.

132. Taban M, Behrens A, Newcomb RL, et al. Incidence of acute endophthalmitis following penetrating keratoplasty: A systematic review. *Arch Ophthalmol*. 2005;123:605−609.

133. Terry MA, Ousley PJ. Deep lamellar endothelial keratoplasty visual acuity, astigmatism, and endothelial survival in a large prospective series. *Ophthalmology*. 2005;112:1541−1548.

134. Price FW Jr, Price MO. Descemet's stripping with endothelial keratoplasty in 50 eyes: A refractive neutral corneal transplant. *J Refract Surg*. 2005;21:339−345.

135. Anwar M, Teichmann KD. Deep lamellar keratoplasty: Surgical techniques for anterior lamellar keratoplasty with and without baring of Descemet's membrane. *Cornea*. 2002;21:374−383.

136. Seitz B, Brunner H, Viestenz A, et al. Inverse mushroom-shaped nonmechanical penetrating keratoplasty using a femtosecond laser. *Am J Ophthalmol*. 2005;139:941−944.

137. Terry MA, Ousley PJ, Will B. A practical femtosecond laser procedure for DLEK endothelial

transplantation: Cadaver eye histology and topography. *Cornea*. 2005;24:453–459.

138. Sarayba MA, Juhasz T, Chuck RS, et al. Femtosecond laser posterior lamellar keratoplasty: A laboratory model. *Cornea*. 2005;24:328–333.

139. Soong HK, Mian S, Abbasi O, et al. Femtosecond laser-assisted posterior lamellar keratoplasty: Initial studies of surgical technique in eye bank eyes. *Ophthalmology*. 2005;112:44–49.

140. Wollensak G, Spoerl E, Seiler T. Riboflavin/ultraviolet-a-induced collagen crosslinking for the treatment of keratoconus. *Am J Ophthalmol*. 2003;135:620–627.

141. Velazquez AJ, Carnahan MA, Kristinsson J, et al. New dendritic adhesives for sutureless ophthalmic surgical procedures: In vitro studies of corneal laceration repair. *Arch Ophthalmol*. 2004;122:867–870.

142. Carlsson DJ, Li F, Shimmura S, et al. Bioengineered corneas: How close are we? *Curr Opin Ophthalmol*. 2003;14:192–197.

143. McLeod SD, DeBacker CM, Viana MA. Differential care of corneal ulcers in the community based on apparent severity. *Ophthalmology*. 1996;103:479–484.

144. Gudmundsson OG, Ormerod LD, Kenyon KR, et al. Factors influencing predilection and outcome in bacterial keratitis. *Cornea*. 1989;8:115–121.

145. Fulcher TP, Dart JK, McLaughlin-Borlace L, et al. Demonstration of biofilm in infectious crystalline keratopathy using ruthenium red and electron microscopy. *Ophthalmology*. 2001;108:1088–1092.

146. Georgiou T, Qureshi SH, Chakrabarty A, et al. Biofilm formation and coccal organisms in infectious crystalline keratopathy. *Eye*. 2002;16:89–92.

147. Mihara E, Shimizu M, Touge C, et al. Case of a large, movable bacterial concretion with biofilm formation on the ocular surface. *Cornea*. 2004;23:513–515.

148. Upadhyay MP, Karmacharya PC, Koirala S, et al. The Bhaktapur eye study: Ocular trauma and antibiotic prophylaxis for the prevention of corneal ulceration in Nepal. *Br J Ophthalmol*. 2001;85:388–392.

149. Christo CG, van Rooij J, Geerards AJM, et al. Suture-related complications following keratoplasty - A 5-year retrospective study. *Cornea*. 2001;20:816–819.

150. Al-Rajhi AA, Wagoner MD, Badr IA, et al. Bacterial keratitis following phototherapeutic keratectomy. *J Refract Surg*. 1996;12:123–127.

151. Neumaier-Ammerer B, Stolba U, Binder S, et al. Corneal infiltrates and ulcers. A retrospective study of 239 eyes. *Ophthalmologe*. 2004;101:33–38.

152. Kunimoto DY, Sharma S, Garg P, et al. Corneal ulceration in the elderly in Hyderabad, south India. *Br J Ophthalmol*. 2000;84:54–59.

153. Upadhyay MP, Karmacharya PC, Koirala S, et al. Epidemiologic characteristics, predisposing factors, and etiologic diagnosis of corneal ulceration in Nepal. *Am J Ophthalmol*. 1991;111:92–99.

154. Varaprasathan G, Miller K, Lietman T, et al. Trends in the etiology of infectious corneal ulcers at the F. I. Proctor Foundation. *Cornea*. 2004;23:360–364.

155. Alexandrakis G, Alfonso EC, Miller D. Shifting trends in bacterial keratitis in South Florida and emerging resistance to fluoroquinolones. *Ophthalmology*. 2000a;107:1497–1502.

156. Forster RK. Conrad Berens lecture. The management of infectious keratitis as we approach the 21st century. *CLAO J*. 1998;24:175–180.

157. Meier PA, Mathers WD, Sutphin JE, et al. An epidemic of presumed acanthamoeba keratitis that followed regional flooding. Results of a case-control investigation. *Arch Ophthalmol*. 1998;116:1090–1094.

158. Erie JC, Nevitt MP, Hodge DO, et al. Incidence of ulcerative keratitis in a defined population from 1950 through 1988. *Arch Ophthalmol*. 1993;111:1665–1671.

159. Cheng KH, Leung SL, Hoekman HW, et al. Incidence of contact-lens-associated microbial keratitis and its related morbidity. *Lancet*. 1999;354:181–185.

160. Morgan PB, Efron N, Hill EA, et al. Incidence of keratitis of varying severity among contact lens wearers. *Br J Ophthalmol*. 2005;89:430–436.

161. Sankaridurg PR, Sweeney DF, Holden BA, et al. Comparison of adverse events with daily disposable hydrogels and spectacle wear: Results from a 12-month prospective clinical trial. *Ophthalmology*. 2003;110:2327–2334.

162. Grant T, Chong MS, Vajdic C, et al. Contact lens induced peripheral ulcers during

hydrogel contact lens wear. *CLAO J*. 1998a;24: 145–151.

163. Glynn RJ, Schein OD, Seddon JM, et al. The incidence of ulcerative keratitis among aphakic contact lens wearers in New England. *Arch Ophthalmol*. 1991;109:104–107.

164. Schein OD, Poggio EC. Ulcerative keratitis in contact lens wearers. Incidence and risk factors. *Cornea*. 1990;9(Suppl 1):S55–S58; discussion S62-63.

165. McLeod SD, Kolahdouz-Isfahani A, Rostamian K, et al. The role of smears, cultures, and antibiotic sensitivity testing in the management of suspected infectious keratitis. *Ophthalmology*. 1996;103:23–28.

166. Wilhelmus KR, Schlech BA. Clinical and epidemiological advantages of culturing bacterial keratitis. *Cornea*. 2004;23:38–42.

167. Rodman RC, Spisak S, Sugar A, et al. The utility of culturing corneal ulcers in a tertiary referral center versus a general ophthalmology clinic. *Ophthalmology*. 1997;104:1897–1901.

168. Nakano E, Oliveira M, Portellinha W, et al. Confocal microscopy in early diagnosis of Acanthamoeba keratitis. *J Refract Surg*. 2004; 20(5 Suppl):S737–S740.

169. Kaufman SC, Musch DC, Belin MW, et al. Confocal microscopy: A report by the American Academy of Ophthalmology. *Ophthalmology*. 2004;111:396–406. Erratum in: *Ophthalmology*. 2004;111:1306.

170. McLeod SD, LaBree LD, Tayyanipour R, et al. The importance of initial management in the treatment of severe infectious corneal ulcers. *Ophthalmology*. 1995;102:1943–1948.

171. Wilhelmus KR. Indecision about corticosteroids for bacterial keratitis: An evidence-based update. *Ophthalmology*. 2002;109: 835–842.

172. American Academy of Ophthalmology. *Bacterial Keratitis. Preferred practice pattern*. San Francisco: American Academy of Ophthalmology; 2000:10.

173. Beattie TK, Tomlinson A, McFadyen AK, et al. Enhanced attachment of acanthamoeba to extended-wear silicone hydrogel contact lenses: A new risk factor for infection? *Ophthalmology*. 2003;110:765–771.

CHAPTER 4

Refractive Surgery

Louis E. Probst, MD

Refractive surgery has at least two unique characteristics when compared to the other subspecialties of ophthalmology. The preoperative and postoperative refractive evaluations allow calculations of efficacy, predictability, and stability that provide for detailed analysis and comparison. Refractive surgery is a purely elective procedure that the patients continuously evaluate visually for the rest of their lives. This means that the success of refractive surgery is entirely based on the results; patients pleased with the outcomes will refer others while those displeased will not. Understandably, refractive surgeons and the laser providers focus equally on the outcomes to achieve the expectations of the patients.

With the achievement of perfect uncorrected vision, success in refractive surgery has become an obsession for surgeons, equipment manufacturers, and patients. As this chapter demonstrates, there are many studies and comparisons available to evaluate the various refractive procedures, and the results are getting remarkably better particularly in the area of custom wavefront laser in situ keratomileusis (LASIK).

Options for Refractive Surgery

Before discussing the results of the various studies on refractive surgery, it is first necessary to provide a brief outline of each of the procedures available in the armamentarium of the refractive surgeon and the indications for each procedure (see Fig. 4.1). The reader should note that the indications for each refractive procedure are rapidly changing as new technologies become available and replace other procedures.

Conventional *LASIK* and *photorefractive keratectomy (PRK)* remain the mainstay of the armamentarium of refractive surgery. For PRK, the ideal treatment for maximum spherical myopia is −6.0 D (extended range up to −10.0 D). For LASIK, the ideal treatment for maximum myopia treatment is now −10.0 D (extended range −12.0 D). Other factors that influence the amount of correction include corneal thickness, flap thickness, pupil size, and the amount of ocular aberrations. Mitomycin-C is now used intraoperatively with higher myopic PRK to reduce the risk of postoperative haze.[1] The limits of the hyperopic corrections have been reduced because of regression and disturbances in night vision associated with the smaller postoperative hyperopic optical zones noted with corrections over +3.0 D spherical equivalent.

Custom wavefront PRK and LASIK are now being performed for the same refractive range as conventional LASIK . Currently, wavefront treatments are available for up to −11.0 D of myopia and −4.0 D of astigmatism. Custom procedures are rapidly gaining popularity because of their superior results as compared with those of conventional LASIK and PRK.

Laser epithelial keratomileusis (LASEK) has emerged as a hybrid of PRK and LASIK. LASEK utilizes an epithelial flap created by exposing the cornea to ethanol. Proponents of LASEK believe that it reduces the risk of intraoperative flap complications and preserves posterior corneal stroma. Critics are concerned about the slow visual recovery and the risks of corneal haze. Only short-term data on LASEK has been reported at this point.[2]

Epi-LASIK has recently emerged as a variation of LASEK. For epi-LASIK, the epithelial flap is created with a modified microkeratome. Proponents state that the flaps created in this manner heal faster and the results are comparable to LASIK. Others have had less success with this technique, and it is yet to gain widespread acceptance.

Conductive keratoplasty (CK)[3] has been approved by the U.S. Food and Drug Administration (FDA) for the treatment of hyperopia. The thermal corneal

Options for refractive surgery

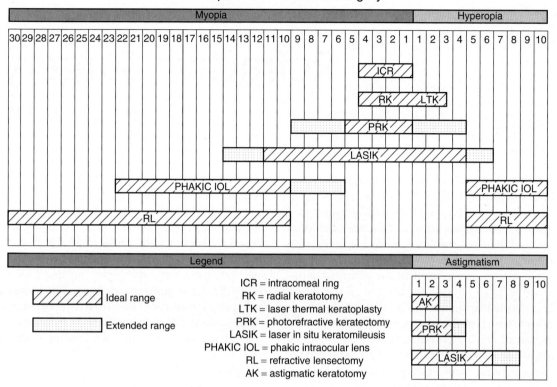

FIGURE 4.1 ◻ The options for refractive surgery demonstrate the ideal and extended ranges for treatment of the various refractive options for myopia, hyperopia, and astigmatism. The indications for each of these procedures is constantly changing as more experience is gained and other options become available.

burns are applied with a radio frequency probe down to about 90% of the corneal depth (500 μm). It is hoped that the deeper corneal penetration will help avoid the problems with regression associated with laser thermal keratoplasty (LTK).[4,5] CK is no longer performed by most refractive surgeons; however, it is occasionally used to create "blended vision" in one eye for the correction of presbyopia.

Intracorneal rings (ICRs) or *Intacs (Contact Addition Technology, Des Plaines IL)* are now rarely used to treat myopia but have been applied for specific situations to treat post-LASIK ectasia[6] or keratoconus.[7] While the initial ICR FDA studies were promising[8], the procedure never gained widespread acceptance because of the inability to treat astigmatism, difficulty in duplicating the initial FDA results, competition from LASIK, and the high explantation rate.

Phakic intraocular lenses (IOLs) and *refractive lensectomy (RL)* remain the main options for the correction of extreme ametropias.

RL, also known as *clear lens exchange (CLE)* for myopia, has benefited from the availability of low diopter power IOLs; however, concerns about the increased risk of retinal detachment remain.[9] RL for hyperopia has used piggyback IOLs for eyes requiring heavy corrections;[10] however, high-power foldable IOLs (up to 40.0 D) may make this less necessary in the future.

Multifocal, accommodating, and diffractive IOLs such as the Rezoom, previously Array (AMO, Santa Ana, California), Crystalens, previously AT-45 (Eyeonics, Aliso Viejo, California) and the Restore IOL (Alcon Laboratories, Fort Worth, Texas) are currently being evaluated, which should expand the application of RL in the future to the treatment of presbyopia.

Radial keratotomy (RK) is no longer performed[11] as other refractive procedures offer a more predictable and stable outcome. For RK, a diamond knife was used to create radial incisions in the cornea.

LTK is no longer performed for low hyperopia, and the recent bankruptcy of the laser manufacturer officially ended its tenure. For LTK, peripheral thermal burns were applied to the peripheral cornea for the correction of small degrees of hyperopia.

LASIK, PRK, LASEK, and epi-LASIK are the main methods for the treatment of astigmatism. Astigmatic keratotomy (AK) and limbal relaxing incisions are now generally used in conjunction with other intraocular procedures to partially reduce astigmatism . The limits for the treatment of astigmatism by PRK, LASEK, or LASIK have been expanded by utilizing the cross-cylinder ablation or bitoric ablation technique originally proposed by Vinciguerra.[12] Toric pseudophakic and phakic IOLs have recently been introduced for the treatment of astigmatism associated with lens implantation.

U.S. Food and Drug Administration Studies: Advantages and Challenges

Apart from the Prospective Evaluation of Radial Keratotomy (PERK) Study of RK[13], there have been no large scale multicenter trials to evaluate the different techniques and technologies of refractive surgery as compared to the comprehensive studies performed for the other ophthalmic subspecialties. However, refractive procedures involve the use of new devices and therefore require the submission of detailed studies to the FDA, which are available on the FDA website shortly after approval (http://www.fda.gov). The FDA submission criteria requires that the data be submitted in a standardized format so that the results of different lasers, procedures, and devices can be compared.

While there are obvious advantages to using the FDA data for comparisons, in practice, there are some limitations also. First, excellent results in an FDA study do not always correlate with those in general practice. The most notable example of this discrepancy was with Intacs. The results of the FDA study for Intacs was outstanding; however, the results in the hands of most surgeons were disappointing, which led to the failure of Intacs as a viable option for the correction of myopia. Secondly, FDA studies are generally sponsored by the company seeking FDA approval and performed by physicians with close relationships with those companies so at least some degree of bias could be involved. Finally, in some cases, FDA studies have been submitted years apart so it is inappropriate to compare the results from one study submitted years before with another that used different and probably inferior technology. Despite these limitations, the FDA approval data provides an excellent comparison of the results of refractive procedures (see Table 4.1) as well as a good sample of the complications.

This chapter includes not only a detailed analysis and comparison of the FDA data but also other independent studies in the literature to provide a balanced and sometimes more updated view of the results of the procedures.

The Evaluation of Refractive Surgery Results

The results of refractive surgery are generally reported as the percentage of eyes achieving 20/20 and 20/40 vision (efficacy) and the percentage of eyes achieving within ±0.5 D of emmetropia and ±1.0 D of emmetropia (predictability). The overall reduction in the degree of myopia and the stability of this number over the length of follow-up in the study are also reported, as is the percentage of eyes with complications.

The indices of efficacy and safety may provide the best assessment of visual improvement using the standard methods of visual assessment.[14] The efficacy index is the ratio of the preoperative best-corrected visual acuity (BCVA) divided by the postoperative uncorrected visual acuity (UCVA), with both numbers in the decimal visual form. This value represents the result that patients truly wish to achieve—uncorrected vision at least as good as the corrected vision with their glasses or contact lenses. The safety index is the ratio of the preoperative BCVA divided by the postoperative BCVA with both numbers in the decimal visual form. This provides an overall assessment of the changes in BCVA that allows an excellent evaluation of safety using standard vision testing. Unfortunately, these reporting methods have not been widely accepted so the efficacy and predictability indices will not be reported in this chapter.

Photorefractive Keratectomy

Myopia

The efficacy and the predictability of the FDA results for the various excimer lasers for PRK are found in Table 4.1. After 2000, the FDA submissions were made for LASIK results rather than for PRK results. It can be seen that the early results for PRK were

TABLE 4.1 ■ FDA Data. FDA results of the various FDA studies reported on the FDA website. Since all new devices require an FDA study review, a tremendous amount of comparative data can be gathered

Device	Approval Range	Approval Number	Approval Date	Number of Eyes	≥20/20	≥20/40	0.5 D	1.0 D	Loss of two lines BCVA	Loss > two lines BCVA
Conventional Myopic PRK										
Alcon Apex Plus	1–6 D myopia, 1–4 D astigmatism	P930034/S9	3/11/98	151	48.3	84.1	49	73.5	n/a	3.4
Alcon LadarVision	1–10 D myopia	P970043	11/2/98	417	69.7	95.9	77.5	92.6	1	0.5
Alcon LadarVision	1–10 D myopia with 4 D astigmatism	P970043	11/2/98	177	59.3	93.2	74.3	92	2.1	0
Bausch and Lomb 116	1.5–7.0 D myopia (results 3–4 D spherical)	P970056	9/28/99	33	42.4	81.8	48.5	87.9	0	3
Bausch and Lomb 116	1.5–7.0 D myopia with astigmatism (results 3–4 D SE)	P970056	9/28/99	35	45.7	77.5	48.6	80	0	5.7
LaserSight LSX	1–6 D myopia	P980008	11/12/99	265	55.5	87.5	58.5	81.5	n/a	0
Nidek EC5000	0.75–7 D myopia	P970053	12/17/98	441	65.5	94.8	68.6	90.2	2.2	0.3
Nidek EC5000	7–13 D myopia	P970053	12/17/98	145	45.5	80.7	42.8	68.3	2.5	3
Nidek EC5000	1–8 D myopia with 4 D astigmatism	P970053/S1	9/29/99	631	64.3	93.5	62.3	86.1	1.1	0.5
VISX Star and Star2	0–12 D myopia with 4 D astigmatism	P930016/S5	3/27/96	156	50.7	79.5	45.9	70.9	n/a	7.5
Conventional Hyperopic PRK										
VISX Star and Star2	1–6 D hyperopia	P930016/S7	11/2/98	158	53.3	96	74.1	90.5	0	1
VISX Star and Star2	0.5–5 hyperopia with 4 D astigmatism	P930016/S10	10/18/00	231	50.2	95.4	69.5	91.2	5.1	1.5

62

Conventional Hyperopic LASIK

Device	Description	PMA	Date	N						
Alcon LadarVision (9 mo)	<6 D hyperia with up to 6 D myopia astigmatism	P970043/S7	9/22/00	66	57.6	95.2	70.2	91.5	5.8	0
Bausch and Lomb 116	1–4 D hyperia with 2 D astigmatism	P990027/S4	2/25/03	233	61.4	94.8	60	86.6	2.1	0.7
VISX S2 and S3	0.5–5 D hyopeopia with 3 D and astigmatism	P930016/S12	4/27/01	113	54	99.1	70.7	94.7	3.8	0
Wavelight Allegretto	Hyperopia up to 6 D with astigmatism up to 5 D	P30008	10/10/03	212	67.5	95.3	72.3	90.4	n/a	1.5

Conventional Mixed Astigmatism LASIK

Device	Description	PMA	Date	N						
Alcon LadarVision	Hyperopia <6 D with myopic astigmatism <6 D	P970043/S7	9/22/00	37	51.4	93.6	82	96	1.9	0
VISX S2 and S3	Mixed astigmatism up to 6 D (3 month data)	P930016/S14	11/16/01	115	58.3	98.3	79.1	97.4	0	0.9

Custom Myopic LASIK

Device	Description	PMA	Date	N						
Alcon LadarVision	myopia to 7 D with 0.5 D astigmatism	P970043/S10	10/18/02	139	79.9	91.4	74.8	95.7	0	0
Alcon LadarVision	Myopic astigmatism 0.5–4 D	P970043/S15	6/29/04	225	85.8	97.4	80.2	91.8	0	0
Bausch and Lomb 217Z	Myopia to 7 D with 3 D astigmatism	P990027/S6	10/10/03	117	90.1	99.1	71.3	92.4	0	0.4
VISX S4 Wavescan	Myopia to 6 D with 3 D astigmatism	P930016/S17	5/23/03	277	93.9	99.6	90.3	99.3	0	0

Custom Hyperopic LASIK

Device	Description	PMA	Date	N						
VISX S4 Wavescan	Hyperopia up to 3 D and astigmatism up to 2 D	P930016/S17	12/14/04	131	61.8	95.4	58	88.5	0	0

(continued)

TABLE 4.1 ■ (Continued)

Device	Approval Range	Approval Number	Approval Date	Number of Eyes	≥20/20	≥20/40	0.5 D	1.0 D	Loss two lines BCVA	Loss > two lines BCVA
Conductive Keratoplasty										
Keratec CK	Hyperopia from 0.75 to 3.25 D with <0.75 D astigmatism	P10018	4/11/02	205	63	96	70	96	4	1
Keratec CK	Presbyopia (16 spots)	P10018/S5	2/6/04	81	56(J1)	90(J3)	82	97	0	2
Intacs										
Keravision Intacs	1–3 D myopia with <0.5 D astigmatism	P980031	1/12/99	442	69	96	68	91	n/a	n/a
Phakic IOL										
Ophtec Verisyse	5–20 D of myopia with 2.5 D of astigmatism	P30028	2/5/04	581	33.2	86.7	72	94.5	n/a	0.344234079
Presbyopia										
AMO Array	Cataract–distance	P960028	9/5/97	400	39	91.5	n/a	n/a	n/a	n/a
AMO Array	Presbyopia–near	P960028	9/5/97	400	47.5	87.4	n/a	n/a	n/a	n/a
Alcon Restore	cataract–distance	P20040	3/21/05	110	29.2	92.7	n/a	n/a	n/a	n/a
Alcon Restore	presbyopia–near	P20040	3/21/05	110	30.9 (J1)	94.5 (J3)	n/a	n/a	n/a	n/a
Eyeonics Crystalens	cataract–distance	P30002	5/23/05	368	49.6	91.4	84.5	85.9	7.9	n/a
Eyeonics Crystalens	presbyopia–near	P30002	5/23/05	368	14.1 (J1)	89.1 (J3)	84.5	85.9	7.9	n/a

BCVA, best-corrected visual acuity; PRK, photorefractive keratectomy; LASIK, laser in situ keratomileusis modest, with only 40% to 60% of eyes achieving 20/20 UCVA. The high degree of loss of BCVA of two or more Snellen lines is of particular interest, ranging from 1% to 7%. There are few reports of the results of the use of modern excimer lasers and techniques for conventional PRK as most reports now focus on custom LASIK; however, the results have markedly improved, with 20/20 rates for conventional PRK as high as 92%.[15]

Hyperopia

Hyperopic PRK has received far less attention as compared to myopic PRK. This is because hyperopic patients make up a small proportion of the total number of refractive patients and are generally treated with LASIK rather than PRK because of concerns about regression of effect after hyperopic PRK. The FDA results for hyperopia on the VISX Star and Star2 are found in Table 4.1. An UCVA of 20/20 was achieved in about 50% of eyes, which is similar to the early myopic PRK results. Once again, there is a high loss of BCVA noted for the hyperopic PRK corrections. More recent reports on hyperopic PRK with conventional treatments have found modest results with an UCVA of 20/40 achieved in only 81% of eyes.[16]

Mixed Astigmatism

Most reports for the treatment of mixed astigmatism have been with LASIK because of the popularity of LASIK and the concern about regression of astigmatic treatments after PRK. There have been no FDA approvals for the treatment of mixed astigmatism with PRK. One independent PRK study with the MEL 60 excimer laser of 75 eyes with mixed astigmatism found that the mean preoperative −4.20 D cylinder and +3.00 D spherical equivalent refraction decreased to −0.50 D cylinder and −0.50 D spherical equivalent refraction. A UCVA of 20/40 or better was achieved in 83% (62/75 eyes); 20/20 or better in 32% (24/75 eyes); and 13.3% (10/75 eyes) lost two or more lines of BCVA.[17] More recently, cross-cylinder or bitoric ablations and custom ablations have been used for the treatment of mixed astigmatism, which has improved the results for LASIK and would presumably benefit PRK as well.

Photorefractive Keratectomy Complications

The complications of PRK are commonly related to the healing of the stroma and the epithelium after the procedure but can also be related to the placement and the type of excimer laser treatment. Common PRK complications reported in the FDA studies are found in Table 4.2.

Conventional Laser in situ Keratomileusis

Myopia

The results from conventional myopic LASIK from the FDA are reported in Table 4.3. The percentage of eyes achieving 20/20 can be seen to vary widely, depending on the excimer laser used, from a low of 46.4% to a high of 88.2%. The percentage of eyes achieving 20/20 can be seen to drop as the level of myopia increases.

Hyperopia

The results of conventional hyperopic LASIK are found in Table 4.1. The higher rates of loss of BCVA in this group, with a loss of two lines of BCVA ranging from 2.1% to 5.8%, are the biggest cause for concern. The 20/20 and 20/40 rates are similar to those reported for myopic LASIK. One independent study of 43 eyes at 3 months postoperatively has reported that the Alcon LadarVision achieves better results for primary hyperopic LASIK as compared to the VISX S3 with a UCVA 20/20 rate of 63% versus 24% and a UCVA 20/40 rate of 84% versus 100%.[18]

Mixed Astigmatism

Only two lasers have been approved from the treatment of mixed astigmatism with conventional LASIK, the VISX, and the Alcon LadarVision. The FDA results for mixed astigmatism (Table 4.1) are comparable to the results for myopic and hyperopic LASIK.

Adverse Events/Complications

The complications reported in the Alcon LadarVision LASIK study would be similar to the complications experienced with the other lasers at this time (see Table 4.4).

Custom Laser in situ Keratomileusis

Myopia

The FDA results for custom myopic LASIK show a vast improvement over those of conventional LASIK (Table 4.3). While there are slight differences among the results of the three systems, overall, they are

TABLE 4.2 □ The U.S. Food and Drug Administration (FDA) Study of Photorefractive Keratectomy (PRK) with the Bausch and Lomb 116 Reported a Number of Complications that were Typical of the PRK Experience at that Time.

PRK Complications with the Bausch and Lomb 116 ($n = 714$)	
Complications at 6 mo	(%)
Loss of $\geq$ two lines BCVA at 6 mo or later	7.4
BCVA worse than 20/40 at 6 mo or later	0.7
BCVA worse than 20/25 if 20/20 preoperatively	3.4
Haze $\geq$ trace with loss of >two lines BCVA	0.6
Increased manifest refractive astigmatism	0.5
Postoperative IOP increase >10 mm Hg	2.3
Postoperative IOP >25 mm Hg	3.2
Complications at any visit	
Blepharitis	0.3
Blurry vision	0.7
Burning	1.7
Conjunctivitis	1.0
Epithelial defect	0.4
Corneal scarring	1.0
Dry eye	1.0
Foreign body sensation	4.1
Ghosting/double image	2.1
Glare	11.3
Halos	4.8
Haze	1.1
Iritis	4.1
Light sensitivity	2.4
Night driving	4.5
Pain	0.6
Patient discomfort	3.2
Recurrent erosion	0.4
Redness	0.8
Tearing	0.7
Undercorrection	0.7

BCVA, best-corrected visual acuity; IOP, intraocular pressure.

remarkably similar. A UCVA of 20/20 was achieved in 79.9% to 93.9% of eyes. Another impressive result is the drop in the rate of loss of BCVA, with the highest level of 0.4% reported for a loss of > two lines of BCVA. These BCVA loss rates are much better than those of conventional LASIK. A study comparing the custom results of the Alcon CustomCornea and the VISX CustomVue in 93 eyes found that a UCVA of 20/15 or better was achieved by 32% of CustomCornea eyes and 23% of VISX CustomVue eyes while a UCVA of 20/20 or better was achieved by 98% of CustomCornea and 95% of CustomVue eyes.[19]

Hyperopia

At present, only the VISX laser has received FDA approval for custom hyperopic LASIK. The VISX custom hyperopic results demonstrate some improvement from the conventional hyperopic results; however, they do not achieve nearly the same efficacy and predictability of the custom myopic results (Table 4.1).

Mixed Astigmatism

While custom mixed astigmatism has recently been approved for the VISX S4 laser, this data has not been posted on the FDA website.

Adverse Events/Complications

Interestingly, complications were uncommon in the FDA custom LASIK studies; in fact, the VISX CustomVue LASIK report listed no complications out of 277 eyes at 6 months. The improved technology and techniques of LASIK are probably responsible for this dramatic improvement in safety.

Conductive Keratoplasty

CK has been approved by the FDA for both the treatment of low hyperopia and presbyopia (Table 4.1). While the results of CK for the correction of hyperopia and presbyopia are very similar to the results of conventional hyperopic LASIK, there has been concern regarding the regression of the thermal keratoplasty effect. Figure 4.2 demonstrates the regression reported in the FDA study, with extrapolation of the regression over 4 years. The only complication in the 146 eyes at 6 months reported in the FDA trial was a decrease in BCVA by more than ten letters due to irregular astigmatism. Most

TABLE 4.3 ■ The FDA Study Results for Myopic LASIK Demonstrate that Success of LASIK Decreases with Increasing Level of Myopia

Uncorrected Vision ≥20/20 at 6 mo Postoperative per Preoperative Manifest Refractive Spherical Equivalent

	1.00–1.99 D	2.00–2.99 D	3.00–3.99 D	4.00–4.99 D	5.00–5.99 D	6.00–6.99 D	7.00 D and above
Autonomous	68.8% (n = 11)	53.8% (n = 14)	35.3% (n = 6)	45.8% (n = 11)	30.0% (n = 6)	37.5% (n = 3)	34.4% (n = 11)
B + L Technolas (3 mo)	85.7% (n = 21)	90.4% (n = 73)	83.8% (n = 80)	84.0% (n = 81)	84.2% (n = 57)	77.5% (n = 40)	90.0% (n = 10)
LaserSight (12 mo)	55.6% (n = 9)	51.5% (n = 33)	67.9% (n = 53)	45.7% (n = 46)	41.7% (n = 36)	32.1% (n = 109)	
Nidek	88.2% (n = 17)	61.2% (n = 152)		54.3% (n = 164)		38.1% (n = 425)	
Summit	46.4% (n = 28)	54.7% (n = 53)	41.7% (n = 48)	47.7% (n = 44)	50.0% (n = 52)	37.8% (n = 37)	32.0% (n = 147)
VISX	59.0% (n = 39)	51.7% (n = 58)	65.2% (n = 89)	64.3% (n = 84)	45.1% (n = 82)	51.1% (n = 94)	43.0% (n = 200)

Uncorrected Vision ≥20/40 at 6 mo Postoperative per Preoperative Manifest Refractive Spherical Equivalent

	1.00–1.99 D	2.00–2.99 D	3.00–3.99 D	4.00–4.99 D	5.00–5.99 D	6.00–6.99 D	7.00 D and above
Autonomous	100% (n = 16)	88.5% (n = 23)	100% (n = 17)	87.5% (n = 21)	70.0% (n = 14)	87.5% (n = 7)	84.4% (n = 27)
B + L Technolas (3 mo)	100% (n = 21)	100% (n = 21)	100% (n = 80)	98.8% (n = 81)	100% (n = 57)	97.5% (n = 40)	100% (n = 10)
LaserSight (12 mo)	100% (n = 9)	87.9% (n = 33)	90.6% (n = 53)	80.4% (n = 46)	77.8% (n = 36)	32.1% (n = 114)	
Nidek	94.1% (n = 17)	86.2% (n = 152)		86.6% (n = 164)		82.6% (n = 425)	
Summit	92.9% (n = 28)	94.3% (n = 53)	91.7% (n = 48)	95.5% (n = 44)	98.1% (n = 52)	86.5% (n = 37)	88.4% (n = 147)
VISX	97.4% (n = 39)	96.6% (n = 58)	98.9% (n = 89)	95.2% (n = 84)	96.3% (n = 82)	94.7% (n = 94)	91.5% (n = 200)

(continued)

TABLE 4.3 ☐ (Continued)

Manifest Refractive Spherical Equivalent w/in ± 0.50 D of Intended at 6 mo Postoperative

	1.00–1.99 D	2.00–2.99 D	3.00–3.99 D	4.00–4.99 D	5.00–5.99 D	6.00–6.99 D	7.00 D and above
Autonomous	93.8% (n = 15)	65.4% (n = 17)	75.0% (n = 18)	75.9% (n = 22)	61.9% (n = 13)	77.8% (n = 7)	60.0% (n = 21)
B + L Technolas (3 mo)	76.2% (n = 21)	89.6% (n = 77)	83.5% (n = 85)	86.9% (n = 84)	76.3% (n = 59)	73.2% (n = 41)	50.0% (n = 10)
LaserSight (12 mo)	88.9% (n = 9)	75.8% (n = 33)	63.6% (n = 55)	39.1% (n = 46)	50.0% (n = 38)	32.5% (n = 114)	
Nidek	64.7% (n = 17)	80.7% (n = 150)			67.5% (n = 163)		52.5% (n = 425)
Summit	66.7% (n = 27)	78.8% (n = 52)	57.1% (n = 49)	76.5% (n = 51)	60.0% (n = 55)	66.7% (n = 39)	55.4% (n = 166)
VISX	87.9% (n = 33)	83.6% (n = 61)	86.8% (n = 91)	79.8% (n = 89)	65.9% (n = 91)	71.1% (n = 97)	61.8% (n = 212)

Source Document References: FDA "Summary of Safety and Effectiveness Data"

Autonomous	PMA# P970043/S5: Table #11
B + L Technolas	PMA # P990027: Table #19
LaserSight (12 mo)	PMA# P980008: Tables #12 and #13
Nidek	PMA# P970053/S002: Table #12
Summit	PMA# P930034/S13: Tables #20 and #22
VISX	PMA# P990010: Tables #22 and #24

FDA Web Site
www.fda.gov/cdrh/LASIK/lasers.htm

TABLE 4.4 ☐ The U.S. Food and Drug Administration (FDA) Study of the Alcon LadarVision Laser in situ Keratomileusis (LASIK) Complications at 6 Months (n = 324) Represents the Typical Complications for LASIK at that Time.

Alcon LadarVision LASIK Complications at 6 mo (n = 324)	
Clinical findings at 6 mo	(%)
Rolled flap edge with corneal melt	0.3
Corneal abrasion	0.3
Corneal folds/striae	0
Corneal opacities	0.3
Double/ghost images	1.5
Epithelial ingrowth	1.5
Foreign body sensation	0.3
Interface debris	1.5
Superficial punctate keratitis	3.1
Subjective symptoms worse at 6 mo	
Blurring of vision	15.3
Burning	8.0
Double vision	6.3
Dryness	17.7
Excessive tearing	1.8
Foreign body sensation	5.3
Fluctuation of vision	20.7
Glare	18.6
Halos	20.7
Headache	2.7
Light sensitivity	21.4
Night driving difficulty	14.2
Pain	4.5
Quality of vision	5.2
Redness	5.4

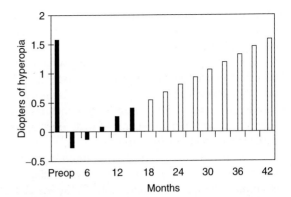

FIGURE 4.2 ☐ Extrapolation of the U.S. Food and Drug Administration (FDA) data on conductive keratoplasty found that the small amount of regression reported initially in the study (black bars) would result in complete elimination of the effect after 48 months if the regressive trend continues (white bars).

notably, there were no increases in astigmatism as were reported after FDA approval. A CK study of 38 eyes with an average of 30 months follow-up found that the UCVA was 20/20 or better in 52.5% and 20/40 or better in 89% of eyes and achieved within ±0.50 D of emmetropia in 68% and within ±1.00 D of emmetropia in 92%. No eye lost two or more Snellen lines or had an induced cylinder of 2.00 D or greater.[20] CK has now been largely abandoned as a refractive procedure because of regression although it is still sometimes used to correct presbyopia by the creation of "blended vision" in one eye.

Intacs

Intracorneal ring segments (Intacs) achieved good results in the FDA study that were better than those reported for conventional myopic LASIK (Table 4.1) but these results could not be duplicated by the average surgeon and the procedure has been abandoned except for the therapeutic use of Intacs for the treatment of keratoconus and post-LASIK ectasia.[21]

Phakic Intraocular Lenses

Phakic IOLs are generally reserved for the treatment of extreme myopia or hyperopia in the pre-presbyopic age-group (Fig. 4.1). While there are several phakic IOLs available worldwide, at present, only the Verisyse phakic IOL has received FDA approval, although approval for the Visian posterior chamber IOL is pending (Table 4.1). The results of efficacy and predictability for the spherical phakic IOLs are much poorer than those reported for both conventional and custom LASIK because of residual astigmatism and spherical error after implantation. Many of the eyes treated with phakic IOLs, required a secondary enhancement procedure or "bioptics" to achieve results similar to those of primary LASIK.[22,23] Toric phakic IOLs that allow the treatment of high levels of ametropia and astigmatism are now available internationally, which will reduce the need for secondary enhancement procedures.

Conversely, myopic phakic IOL implantation is usually associated with an improvement in the BCVA (and therefore a high safety index), which is probably because of the reduction of minification that has not been noted with the correction of high ametropias with the corneal refractive procedures.

The myopic results with the anterior chamber angle–supported phakic IOL (Vivarte, Bausch & Lomb Surgical, Claremont, CA)[24,25], the iris-claw phakic IOL (Verisyse, previously Artisan, OPHTEC USA, Boca Raton, FL),[26] and the posterior chamber implantable contact lens (Visian, previously Intraocular Contact Lens or ICL, Staar Surgical, Monrovia, CA)[27,28] have been reported in various studies (see Table 4.5). Results for the less common phakic

IOLs are scarce and are therefore not reported. The hyperopic phakic IOL results are also reported in Table 4.5 for each of the three main phakic IOLs.[29–31]

Phakic IOLs are associated with more risks than the corneal refractive procedures because phakic IOLs are intraocular procedures with greater surgical intervention in the eye (Table 4.5). The main risks of these procedures include pupil ovalization for angle-supported phakic IOLs[24], endothelial cell loss for iris-claw phakic IOLs[32], and anterior subcapsular cataracts for posterior chamber IOLs.[33] In the FDA study, the Verisyse IOL had an endothelial cell loss rate of 1.8% per year, which would lead to 39% of patients losing 50% of their corneal endothelial cells within 25 years of implantation.[34]

Clear Lens Extraction/Refractive Lensectomy

CLE is a procedure generally reserved for extreme myopia or hyperopia (Fig. 4.1). Because CLE makes use of the IOLs generally used for cataract surgery for a refractive purpose, there is no FDA approval required as CLE uses existing technology. There is a paucity of studies involving CLE, which may be due to the lower number of eyes requiring CLE.

There is considerable controversy about the use of this technique for myopia because of the high rate of retinal detachment reported in long-term follow-up studies of high myopes.[35] The results of CLE for the treatment of high degrees of hyperopia have been equally successful as those for high myopia; however, the risk of retinal detachment does not appear to be as significant.[36]

The studies of CLE do not report detailed results regarding the efficacy of the procedure. In terms of predictability, 1.0 D within emmetropia is achieved by 59% in myopic CLE[35] and 91.4% in hyperopic CLE.[36]

Presbyopia

Recently, several IOLs have been introduced for the treatment of cataracts and presbyopia. The FDA results for the AMO Array IOL, Alcon Restore IOL, and the Eyeonics Crystalens are found in Table 4.1. The AMO ReZoom IOL did not require a separate FDA study as it was a modification of the FDA approved ARRAY multifocal IOL. The results for the presbyopic IOLs show a UCVA of 20/20 rate in 39% to 49.6% and a UCVA of 20/40 in 91.4% to 92.7% of eyes. These results are worse than those for the corneal refractive procedures because of the residual

TABLE 4.5 ◻ The U.S. Food and Drug Administration (FDA) Study of the Crystalens Found a Number of Complications Not Uncommon for Intraocular Surgery

Complications with the Crystalens ($n = 324$)	(%)
Endophthalmitis	0.3
Hyphema	0.3
Cystoid macular edema	3.7
Secondary surgery	0.6
Intraocular lens dislocation	0
Papillary block	0
Retinal detachment	0
Night vision symptoms ($n = 130$)	
Night time glare	
Mild	23.8
Moderate	13.8
Severe	5.4
Night driving difficulty	
Mild	17.4
Moderate	11.6
Severe	3.3
Halos	
Mild	20
Moderate	12.3
Severe	6.2

astigmatism and sphere. The predictability data was only provided for the Eyeonics IOL.

The distance corrected near visual acuity (DCNVA) may be the best assessment of the ability of the presbyopic IOLs to simultaneously correct distance and near vision. The DCNVA with the ARRAY was 43.8% at J1 and 86.6% at J3, the Restore was 30.2% at J1 and 92.1% J3, and the Crystalens was 0.8% at J1 and 88.4% at J3.[37] The DCNVA results demonstrate that while presbyopic IOLs improve the near vision, they do not provide full simultaneous correction of distance and near vision.

References

1. Raviv T, Majmudar PA, Dennis RF, et al. Mytomycin-C for post-PRK corneal haze. *J Cataract Refract Surg*. 2000;26(8):1105–1106.
2. Anderson N, Beran R, Schneider T. Epi-LASEK for the correction of myopia and myopic astigmatism. *J Cataract Refract Surg*. 2002;28(8): 1343.
3. McDonald MB, Davidorf J, Maloney RK, et al. Conductive keratoplasty for the correction of low to moderate hyperopia: 1-year results on the first 54 eyes. *Ophthalmology*. 2002;109(4):637–649.
4. McDonald MB, Davidorf J, Maloney RK, et al. Conductive keratoplasty for the correction of low to moderate hyperopia: 1-year results on the first 54 eyes. *Ophthalmology*. 2002;109(4):637–649; discussion 649-50.
5. Pop M. Laser thermal keratoplasty for the treatment of photorefractive keratectomy overcorrections: A 1-year follow-up. *Ophthalmology*. 1998;105(5):926–931.
6. Alio J, Salem T, Artola A, et al. Intracorneal rings to correct corneal ectasia after laser in situ keratomileusis. *J Cataract Refract Surg*. 2002;28(9):1568.
7. Colin J, Velou S. Utilization of refractive surgery technology in keratoconus and corneal transplants. *Curr Opin Ophthalmol*. 2002;13(4): 230–234.
8. Rapuano CJ, Sugar A, Koch DD, et al. Intrastromal corneal ring segments for low myopia: A report by the American Academy of Ophthalmology. *Ophthalmology*. 2001;108(10): 1922–1928.
9. Colin J, Robinet A. Clear lensectomy and implantation of a low-power posterior chamber intraocular lens for correction of high myopia: A four-year follow-up. *Ophthalmology*. 1997;104(1):73–77; discussion 77-8.
10. Kolahdouz-Isfahani AH, Rostamian K, Wallace D, et al. Clear lens extraction with intraocular lens implantation for hyperopia. *J Refract Surg*. 1999;15(3):316–323.
11. Duffey RJ, Leaming D. U.S. trends in refractive surgery: 2001 International Society of Refractive Surgery Survey. *J Refract Surg*. 2002;18(2):185–188.
12. Vinciguerra P, Sborgia M, Epstein D, et al. Photorefractive keratectomy to correct myopic or hyperopic astigmatism with a cross-cylinder ablation. *J Refract Surg*. 1999;15 (2 Suppl):S183–S185.
13. Kemp JR, Martinez CE, Klyce SD, et al. Diurnal fluctuations in corneal topography 10 years after radial keratotomy in the Prospective Evaluation of Radial Keratotomy Study. *J Cataract Refract Surg*. 1999;25(7):904–910.
14. Koch DD, Kohnen T, Obstbaum SA, et al. Format for reporting refractive surgical data. *J Cataract Refract Surg*. 1998;24(3):285–287.
15. Serrao S, Lombardo M. One-year results of photorefractive keratectomy with and without surface smoothing using the technolas 217C laser. *J Refract Surg*. 2004;20(5):444–449.
16. Autrata R, Rehurek J. Laser-assisted subepithelial keratectomy and photorefractive keratectomy for the correction of hyperopia. Results of a 2-year follow-up. *J Cataract Refract Surg*. 2003;29(11):2105–2114.
17. Nagy ZZ, Krueger RR, Suveges I. Photorefractive keratectomy for astigmatism with the Meditec MEL 60 laser. *J Refract Surg*. 2001;17(4):441–453.
18. Seward MS, Oral D, Bowman RW, et al. Comparison of LADARVision and Visx Star S3 laser in situ keratomileusis outcomes in myopia and hyperopia. *J Cataract Refract Surg*. 2003;29: 2351–2357.
19. Awwad ST, El-Kateb M, Bowman RW, et al. Wavefront-guided laser in situ keratomileusis with the alcon CustomCornea and the VISX CustomVue: Three-month results. *J Refract Surg*. 2004;20:S636–S643.
20. Pallikaris IG, Naoumidi TL, Astyrakakis NI. Long-term results of conductive keratoplasty for low to moderate hyperopia. *J Cataract Refract Surg*. 2005;31(8):1520–1529.

21. Alio JL, Artola A, Hassanein A, et al. One or 2 Intacs segments for the correction of keratoconus. *J Cataract Refract Surg.* 2005;31(5): 943–953.

22. Guell JL, Vazquez M, Gris O. Adjustable refractive surgery: 6-mm Artisan lens plus laser in situ keratomileusis for the correction of high myopia. *Ophthalmology.* 2001;108(5):945–952.

23. Zaldivar R, Davidorf JM, Oscherow S, et al. Combined posterior chamber phakic intraocular lens and laser in situ keratomileusis: Bioptics for extreme myopia. *J Refract Surg.* 1999;15(3):299–308.

24. Allemann N, Chamon W, Tanaka HM, et al. Myopic angle-supported intraocular lenses: two-year follow- up. *Ophthalmology.* 2000;107(8): 1549–1554.

25. Munoz G, Alio JL, Montes-Mico R, et al. Angle-supported phakic intraocular lenses followed by laser-assisted in situ keratomileusis for the correction of high myopia. *Am J Ophthalmol.* 2003;136(3):490–499.

26. Maloney RK, Nguyen LH, John ME. Artisan phakic intraocular lens for myopia:short-term results of a prospective, multicenter study. *Ophthalmology.* 2002;109(9):1631–1641.

27. Uusitalo RJ, Aine E, Sen NH, et al. Implantable contact lens for high myopia. *J Cataract Refract Surg.* 2002;28(1):29–36.

28. Sanders DR, Doney K, Poco M, ICL in Treatment of Myopia Study Group. United States Food and Drug Administration clinical trial of the Implantable Collamer Lens (ICL) for moderate to high myopia: three-year follow-up. *Ophthalmology.* 2004;111(9):1683–1692.

29. Davidorf JM, Zaldivar R, Oscherow S. Posterior chamber phakic intraocular lens for hyperopia of +4 to +11 diopters. *J Refract Surg.* 1998;14(3):306–311.

30. Saxena R, Landesz M, Noordzij B, et al. Three-year follow-up of the Artisan phakic intraocular lens for hypermetropia. *Ophthalmology.* 2003;110(7):1391–1395.

31. Leccisotti A. Angle-supported phakic intraocular lenses in hyperopia. *J Cataract Refract Surg.* 2005;31(8):1598–1602.

32. Perez-Santonja JJ, Iradier MT, Sanz-Iglesias L, et al. Endothelial changes in phakic eyes with anterior chamber intraocular lenses to correct high myopia. *J Cataract Refract Surg.* 1996;22(8):1017–1022.

33. O'Brien TP, Awwad ST. Phakic intraocular lenses and refractory lensectomy for myopia. *Curr Opin Ophthalmol.* 2002;13(4):264–270.

34. (accessed /20/2005).

35. Colin J, Robinet A, Cochener B. Retinal detachment after clear lens extraction for high myopia: seven-year follow-up. *Ophthalmology.* 1999;106(12):2281–2284; discussion 2285.

36. Vicary D, Sun XY, Montgomery P. Refractive lensectomy to correct ametropia. *J Cataract Refract Surg.* 1999;25(7):943–948.

37. (accessed 9/21/2005).

SECTION III
GLAUCOMA

CHAPTER 5

Clinical Trials in Glaucoma

Paul E. Rafuse, PhD, MD, FRCS (C)

The association between intraocular pressure (IOP) and glaucomatous optic neuropathy has been appreciated for almost 150 years.[1] While it was long felt that IOP needed to be elevated, it has now been accepted that many people with glaucoma have IOPs consistently within the normal range.[2] Most recently, definitions of glaucoma describe an optic nerve pathology in which elevated IOP is a *risk factor* and not a defining feature of the disease.[3] As a risk factor for glaucoma, IOP is unique in that it is the only one modifiable; it is difficult to do anything about positive family history (i.e., genetic predisposition) and advanced age at this time.

All the current management strategies for glaucoma boil down to preventing, or at least minimizing, progression of the disease by lowering IOP adequately. The extent and means of IOP reduction have been the subjects of a number of quality studies in the last 20 years or so. This chapter will review some of the best studies. Some have corroborated what many have suspected for years, others have surprised us and several have changed the way we think about glaucoma and have altered our practice patterns.

The clinical trials reviewed here have been randomized, prospective, and comparison controlled. All reasonable efforts were made to mask the interventions from the patients and investigators. Since these are multicenter trials, large recruitments have given the studies statistical power. The questions addressed have been of pivotal importance. They are not presented in historical sequence but in the order of increasing severity of disease: (1) Ocular hypertension, (2) early to moderate open-angle glaucoma, and (3) advanced open-angle glaucoma.

A fourth section examines the therapeutic effectiveness of some of the more recent laser and incisional surgical methods. These procedures, which include selective laser trabeculoplasty (SLT), viscocanalostomy (VC), and deep sclerectomy (DS), have not yet been subjected to the same level of rigor as the preceding studies have been, but considerable experience is being obtained with them and they merit a discussion.

Ocular Hypertension

Veteran practitioners had observed that chronically elevated IOP could lead to glaucomatous optic disc and field damage after many years, but in most cases, modestly increased IOP was not associated with the development of glaucoma over significant follow-up periods.[4] It was therefore unclear as to when to initiate treatment and whether doing so was beneficial (halted or delayed the development of glaucoma with limited treatment side effects). Three previous studies were not in agreement, two showed a benefit[5,6], and one did not,[7] and it was felt that a large multicenter study with rigorous attention to end-point criteria was required. Two such studies will be reviewed—the Ocular Hypertension Treatment Study (OHTS),[8–14] and the European Glaucoma Prevention Study (EGPS).[15]

Ocular Hypertension Treatment Study

Recruitment period: February 1994 to October 1996.

Study Objectives

OHTS prospectively compared the conversion of ocular hypertension (OH) with primary open-angle glaucoma (POAG) in two groups of subjects: Those with medically lowered IOP and those observed without treatment.

Study Design, Treatment Groups, and Outcome Measures

Design. Prospective, multicenter, randomized, unmasked.

Sample Selection. Eligible subjects had to have normal eye examinations with visual acuities (VAs) of 20/40 or better in either eye. They needed to have an elevated IOP between 24 and 32 mm Hg in one eye and between 21 and 32 mm Hg in the fellow eye. The baseline IOP for all participants was 24.9 mm Hg. Two consecutive, normal visual fields (VFs) were obtained at screening. Normal clinical disc evaluations were documented by stereophotography. Patients were excluded if they had any sign of diabetic retinopathy. The mean age of the participants was 55 years. The prevalence rates (percentage of the number of patients [n]) of self-reported conditions are shown in Table 5.1.

Sample Size. A total of 1,636 subjects aged between 40 and 80 were recruited. Self-identification of race as white (1,132; 69.2%), black (389; 23.8%), and neither white nor black (87; 5.3%).

Intervention. At the discretion of the attending ophthalmologist; any combination of available topical glaucoma medications could be used in the treatment group to lower IOP to the required level.

Target Intraocular Pressure Reduction in the Treatment Group. <24 mm Hg and at least 20% less than the baseline.

Duration of Study. Minimum of 5 years, with follow-up intervals of 6 months.

Statistics. Comparisons between groups were on an intent-to-treat basis and based on univariate and multivariate analysis of risk factors.

Primary Outcome Measures. Reproducible (two) VF abnormality and/or verifiable optic disc deterioration determined by masked experts. Adverse local and systemic events.

TABLE 5.1 □ Prevalence Rates (%) of Self-Reported Conditions

Characteristic	Medication (*n* = 817)	Observation (*n* = 819)	Overall (*n* = 1636)
Previous use of ocular hypotensive agents	35.0	39.3	37.2
Systemic hypertension	37.5	38.1	37.8
Cardiovascular disease	5.8	6.5	6.1
History of diabetes	11.5	12.1	11.8
Positive family history for glaucoma	34.0	35.6	34.8

Secondary Outcome Measures. Baseline factors predictive of the onset of POAG.

Summary of Results

Impact on the Development of Primary Open-Angle Glaucoma.
Conversion to POAG at 60 months was 4.4% in the treated group as compared to 9.5% in the untreated group (hazard ratio 0.40; 95% confidence interval, 0.27 to 0.59; p <0.001). The Kaplan-Meier plot of the cumulative probability of developing glaucoma is reproduced in Figure 5.1.

Treatment conferred a protective effect of 54%; however, over 90% of the untreated subjects did not develop VF or disc changes consistent with POAG.

The end points for conversion to POAG were disc changes, 50% for treated and 57.3% for observed patients; VF changes, 41.7% for treated and 32.6% for observed patients; and both disc and VF changes, 8.3% for treated and 10.1% for observed patients.

A subgroup analysis showed that among black participants there was a higher rate of conversion to POAG in both arms of the study. In the treatment group, conversion occurred in 17/203 patients (8.4%); in the observation group conversion occurred in 33/205 patients (16.1%).

Of the 1,301 participants who had their central corneal thickness (CCT) measured, 549 received treatment. Regardless of the type of medication, the

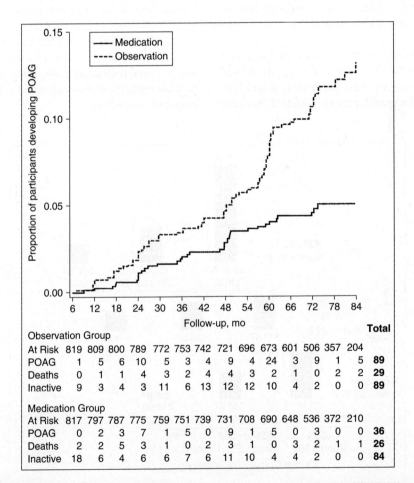

FIGURE 5.1 ☐ Kaplan-Meier plot of the cumulative probability of developing primary open-angle glaucoma (POAG) of the randomized group. The participants at risk were those who had not developed POAG at the beginning of each 6-month period. The number of participants classified as developing POAG is given for each interval. Participants who did not develop POAG and withdrew before the end of the study or who died are censored from the interval of their last completed visit. Reprinted with permission from *Arch Ophthalmol.* 2002;120:707.

effectiveness of topical treatment was found to be inversely related to the CCT.

Adverse Events. Cataracts were marginally more common in the treated group. Local side effects (e.g., stinging, blurring, and foreign body sensation) were more common in the treated group.

Baseline Factors Associated with the Onset of Primary Open-Angle Glaucoma. Advanced age and elevated IOP were risk factors as determined by both univariate and multivariate analyses. The strongest risk factor was a CCT thinner than the study mean. For every 40 μm less than the mean CCT, the hazard ratio for developing glaucoma was 1.71. Dividing the patients into three groups of CCT and examining the rates of POAG development at three levels of IOP shows a strikingly additive risk relationship between increasing IOP measurements and thinner CCTs (see Fig. 5.2).

Other baseline risk factors associated with conversion and assessed by multivariate analysis and were increased cup-to-disc ratio (both vertical and horizontal), and increased pattern standard deviation (PSD) on VF. These are summarized in Table 5.2 (Adapted with permission from *Arch Ophthalmol* 2002;120:717).

Black subjects had higher IOPs, larger cup/disc ratios and thinner CCT such that their race was not found to be an independent risk factor for the development of POAG by multivariate analysis.

Strengths of the Study

The study had sufficient enrollment and power to answer the question posed and there was a very low drop-out rate. Equally distributed in each arm, there were a total of 80 patients who violated the protocol (people taking drops in the observation group or not taking them in the treatment group), 173 who were lost to follow-up, and 56 who died.

Careful attention was paid to reproducing (i.e., VFs) and verifying (i.e., discs) the end points. There was minimal regression to the mean since adequate numbers of IOP measurements and reliable VFs were obtained at screening.

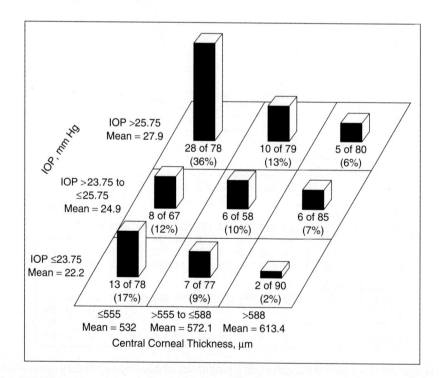

FIGURE 5.2 ☐ The percentage of participants in the observation group who developed primary open-angle glaucoma (median follow-up, 72 months) grouped by baseline intraocular pressure (IOP) of ≤23.75 mm Hg, >23.75 mm Hg to 25.75 mm Hg, and >25.75 mm Hg, and by CCT measurements of 555 μm, >555 μm to 588 μm, and >588 μm. These percentages are not adjusted for length of follow-up. (Reprinted with permission from *Arch Ophthalmol.* 2002;120:718.)

TABLE 5.2 □ The Baseline Factors Significantly[a] Associated with the Development of Primary Open-Angle Glaucoma

Putative Predictive Factor	Hazard Ratio (95% Confidence Interval) by Univariate Analysis	Hazard Ratio (95% Confidence Interval) by Multivariate Analysis[b]
Age (per decade)	1.43 (1.19−1.71)[a]	1.22 (1.01−1.49)[a]
African-American Origin	1.59 (1.09−2.32)[a]	0.98 (0.65−1.46)
Sex (male)	1.87 (1.31−2.67)[a]	1.42 (0.98−2.05)
Diabetes mellitus	0.40 (0.18−0.92)[a]	0.37 (0.15−0.90)[a]
Heart disease	2.11 (1.23−3.62)[a]	1.71 (0.95−3.09)
IOP (per mm Hg)	1.11 (1.04−1.18)[a]	1.10 (1.04−1.17)[a]
Corneal thickness (per 40 μm thinner)	1.88 (1.55−2.29)[a]	1.71 (1.40−2.09)[a]
Pattern standard deviation (per 0.3 dB greater)	1.36 (1.16−1.60)[a]	1.27 (1.06−1.52)[a]
Horizontal cup-disc ratio (per o.1 larger)[c]	1.25 (1.14−1.38)[a]	1.27 (1.14−1.40)[a]
Vertical cup-disc ratio (per 0.1 larger)	1.32 (1.19−1.46)[a]	1.32 (1.19−1.47)[a]

[a] $p < 0.05$
[b] Multivariate analysis adjusts for baseline age, IOP, pattern standard deviation, vertical cup-disc ratio, and corneal thickness, which were measured after randomization.
[c] Horizontal cup-disc ratio was not adjusted for vertical cup-disc ratio in the multivariate model
IOP, intraocular pressure.

This was the first study to establish a strong association between thinner than average CCTs and conversion from ocular hypertension to glaucoma.

Criticisms of the Study

CCT was not measured early in the recruitment period, and was never measured in one third of the participants. Owing to the effect of thicker corneas creating artifactually high Goldmann applanation IOP measurements, it is likely that the relatively thick CCTs noted in this study population reflect a sampling bias. If a correction factor were to be applied to this cohort, many would not have qualified as having ocular hypertension. At this time, however, there is no universally accepted or validated nomogram for adjusting measured applanation IOP readings for CCT.

Another sampling bias suspected is that there may have been subjects who had early manifestations of glaucoma. The baseline PSD correlated directly with the risk of conversion. Some would argue that an increased PSD alone, in the absence of the criteria for a focal glaucomatous VF defect, is suggestive of early glaucoma. Many subjects with increased cup-to-disc ratios but normal standard achromatic perimetry (SAP) might also be suspected of having early disease.

Surprisingly, diabetes was found to have a protective association with the development of POAG but it is likely that many of those that replied positively to the question of having this disease at screening did not have it but may have had a positive family history or had been warned that they had high blood sugar and were at risk of developing diabetes. In fact, any clinically apparent diabetic retinopathy was an exclusion criterion. Blood sugars were not taken.

There were an inordinately large number of participants (44%) stating that they had a positive family history for glaucoma. It is likely that many of these relatives were glaucoma suspects themselves without actually having the disease. The patient cohort was made up of healthy volunteers and not population based. There may have been a selection bias toward healthy people who were interested in enrolling in studies of this nature. They may have had a concern about glaucoma because of family members with the disease, hence the over-representation of people with a positive family history in the study. With such a high prevalence of patients with a stated positive family history, it might be difficult to statistically evaluate this as a risk factor.

Implications for Clinical Practice

A modest protective effect was determined for the medically treated group. However, to prevent one patient with ocular hypertension from developing glaucoma, 19 would need to be treated unnecessarily if risk factors were ignored.

The most important risk factor discovered was a CCT thinner than the median. For every 40 microns less than the median, there was a 40% increased risk of conversion to POAG.

The impact of lowering IOP in this cohort was a roughly 10% reduction in the risk for every 1 mm Hg.

The importance of carefully examining the optic disc is underlined by the fact that almost half of those individuals reaching an end point did so by developing a change in disc appearance. It may be acceptable not to treat those individuals with a few positive risk factors for conversion (i.e., thinner than average CCT, higher IOPs, greater cup-to-disc ratios, increased PSD) provided that detailed monitoring and close follow-up are assured.

With the end points measured in this study not being visually significant, it may be appropriate to take a conservative no-treatment approach in elderly patients with a limited life expectancy. Since only healthy volunteers were recruited, it would not be possible to predict the rate of visual deterioration, or protection with IOP-lowering medications, in patients with life-shortening illnesses.

European Glaucoma Prevention Study

Recruitment period: January 1997 to May 1999.

Study Objectives

This study examined the efficacy of a single IOP-lowering agent, dorzolamide, for the prevention of POAG.

Study Design, Treatment Groups, and Outcome Measures

Design. Prospective, multicenter, randomized, double-masked, placebo-controlled. Patients were randomized into two groups, medical treatment (dorzolamide) and placebo (the vehicle of the commercial dorzolamide preparation). The bottles in each group were identical in appearance so that both the patient and investigator were blind to the randomization.

Sample Selection. Patients were between 30 and 80 years and had at least one qualifying IOP recorded between 22 and 29 mm Hg in one eye without therapy or following a washout of 3 weeks, regardless of the prior treatment. Gonioscopy revealed open angles. Discs were determined to be normal clinically and by three independent evaluators at the Optic Disc Reading Center. Two normal and reliable VF tests were required. Patients were excluded if they had a VA worse than 20/40 in either eye, previous intraocular surgery, or any signs of diabetic retinopathy, or other diseases capable of causing VF loss or disc changes.

Sample Size. A total of 1,081 patients aged between 30 and 80 years were enrolled. No demographic information of gender, race, or concurrent diseases was provided in the initial publication. The sample size assured a statistical power of 80% to detect a difference of 5% between groups at 2.5 years, assuming a 10% drop-out rate over 2.5 years. The drop-out rate was greater than expected. It was calculated that a 5-year event rate of 20% in the placebo group and 12% in the treated group would have maintained the same power even with a drop-out rate of up to 36%.

Intervention. The treatment group was administered commercially prepared dorzolamide 2% t.i.d. The placebo group received the vehicle of only the commercially prepared dorzolamide, again at a t.i.d. schedule.

Target Intraocular Pressure in Treatment Group. A target IOP was not set for this study although the anticipated treatment effect with dorzolamide was in the published range of 18–22%.[15]

Duration of Study. While initially intending to have a minimum follow-up of 2.5 years, the lower than anticipated event rate led the Steering Committee to extend the observation time to allow the requisite number of end points to occur or until 5 years of follow-up was completed for each patient.

Statistics. Comparisons between groups were made on an intent-to-treat basis. All statistical tests were two-sided and performed at a 5% significance level. A "last observation carried forward" analysis was used to deal with the patients who withdrew from the study.

Primary Outcome Measures. The primary end points were the development of changes in the VF, optic disc, or both, consistent with glaucoma. The appearance of VF defects needed to be confirmed by two additional VFs and the disc changes required agreement between two of the three independent observers evaluating optic disc stereophotographs.

Secondary Outcome Measures. The safety end point for the study was an IOP of >35 mm Hg on two occasions. If this safety end point was met, the patient was withdrawn from the study.

Summary of Results

Impact on the Development of Primary Open-Angle Glaucoma.
Dorzolamide reduced the IOP by 15% at 6 months and 22% at 5 years. However, there was no statistically significant difference between the dorzolamide and placebo groups. There was an IOP reduction of 9% at 6 months and 19% at 5 years in the placebo group.

In terms of the cumulative probability of developing a VF and/or disc change consistent with glaucoma at 5 years, the percentage of patients reaching these end points was 13.4% for the dorzolamide group and 14.1% in the placebo group (hazard ratio, 0.86; 95% confidence interval. 0.58 to 1.26; $p = 0.45$). *Adverse Events.* Thirteen patients were withdrawn from the study because of safety end points. One out of the 536 patients (0.2%) in the dorzolamide group and 12 of the 541 (2.2%) in the placebo group had IOPs that recorded >35 mm Hg on two occasions. Adverse ocular reports related to the study groups were reported in 819 (22%) and 258 (6.5%) of visits in the dorzolamide and placebo groups, respectively. The most common complaint voiced in the dorzolamide group (12.9% of all patients in this group) was ocular burning or stinging on instillation of the drop. This complaint was heard from 2.7% of patients in the placebo group. Taste disorders were noted by 2.8% in the dorzolamide group and 0.1% in the placebo group. *Baseline Factors Associated with the Onset of Primary Open-Angle Glaucoma.* Baseline risk factors were not examined in their association with the development of glaucoma in the initial report of this study.

Strengths of the Study

In contrast to OHTS, this was a placebo-controlled study. Surprisingly, it demonstrated a very significant placebo effect, which in fact was statistically equivalent to the treated arm. The efficacy of a single glaucoma agent (i.e., dorzolamide) was carried out for 5 years and compared with placebo.

Criticisms of the Study

The 9.5% IOP reduction at 6 months in the placebo group likely reflects a regression to the mean. Patients could be recruited into the study with only two Goldmann applanation tonometer measurements of 22 mm Hg or greater, and they could occur within a few hours on the same day. Explaining the continued IOP-lowering effect of the placebo vehicle, let alone that of dorzolamide, over the duration of the study is more difficult. Most drugs gradually lose effectiveness over time.

There was a high rate of discontinuation by the patients in this study. While it was initially anticipated that the drop-out rate would be in the vicinity of 10% over 2.5 years, extension of the study to 5 years actually saw a drop-out rate of 35.6% for the dorzolamide group and 24.7% in the placebo group.

It could be inferred that the trend of lower IOPs over time in both groups could be due to patients with higher than mean IOPs preferentially dropping out or "self-selection bias." However, an analysis of the data using the "last observation carried forward" method reduced, but did not eliminate, this trend (see Figs. 5.3 and 5.4).

The efficacy of the placebo vehicle prompted a deliberate testing of the contents of the bottles to explore the possibility of contamination with the active ingredient. None was found.

Some reviewers might feel that if the objective of this study was to examine the impact of lowering the IOP medically on conversion from ocular hypertension to POAG, then a target IOP should have been set. It was the investigator's choice to examine the impact of an individual agent with few contraindications to its use instead of a specific level of IOP reduction. Dorzolamide was chosen because prostaglandins and α_2-agonists were not available at the beginning of the study and β-blockers would have excluded a large number of candidates.

Implications for Clinical Practice

It was shown by this study that dorzolamide does not provide better protection against the conversion of ocular hypertension to POAG over 5 years than the preparation vehicle for this drug. With the problems of the initial regression to the mean and the unexplained observation for both groups to show a continuing and parallel reduction in IOP, it is unclear how this study will impact clinical practice. More insight may be gained from a subgroup analysis of the contributing effects of baseline risk factors such as those examined in OHTS.

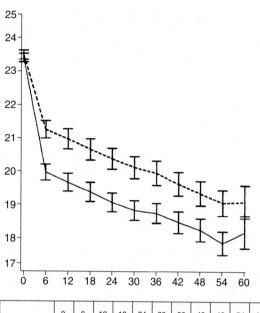

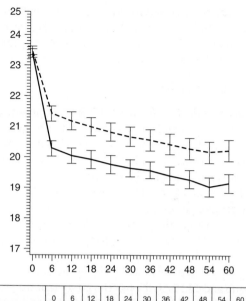

	0	6	12	18	24	30	36	42	48	54	60
Dorzolamid	536	484	453	415	391	365	356	333	311	290	192
Placebo	541	492	475	455	447	421	401	378	364	328	217

	0	6	12	18	24	30	36	42	48	54	60
Dorzolamid	536	484	453	415	391	365	356	333	311	290	192
Placebo	541	492	475	455	447	421	401	378	364	328	217

FIGURE 5.3 ◻ Mean intraocular pressure (IOP; 95% confidence intervals) at baseline and follow-up for the medication and placebo groups. Results for each participant's right and left eye were averaged to calculate a mean. The numbers of participants completing each follow-up visit are shown at the bottom. The solid line represents the dorzolamide group and the dotted line the placebo group. X-axis = months from randomization; y-axis = IOP. Reprinted with permission from *Ophthalmol* 2005;112:371.

FIGURE 5.4 ◻ Mean intraocular pressure (IOP; 95% confidence intervals) at baseline and follow-up fro the medication and placebo groups using the last observation carried forward analysis. Each participant's right and left eye was averaged to calculate the mean. The solid line corresponds to the dorzolamide group, and the dotted line to the placebo group. X-axis = months from randomization; y-axis = IOP. Reprinted with permission from *Ophthalmol* 2005;112:371.

More people progressed to glaucoma in this study compared to the treatment arm of OHTS, presumably because the IOP reduction was greater in OHTS. It would be useful to have similar studies conducted with prostaglandins and other single agents compared to their vehicles for placebo-control.

More research needs to done on the IOP-lowering effect of the buffered vehicle in this and other commercial preparations.

Early to Moderate Open-Angle Glaucoma

The long established relationship between IOP and glaucoma has been strengthened in the past few decades. Compelling epidemiologic evidence has been published demonstrating a direct relationship between IOP and glaucoma prevalence in a general population.[16] Persuasive testimonials have been made regarding the long-term outcomes of glaucoma at different starting points; the likelihood of blindness increases with the severity of the disease at baseline.[17] Some retrospective[18,19] and uncontrolled prospective[20,21] treatment trials have suggested a protective effect of therapy. However, until very recently, there were no rigorous prospective clinical trials to quantitatively examine the effects of lowering IOP by various means.

In this chapter, four such studies will be critiqued. Two studies, the Early Manifest Glaucoma Trial Study (EMGT study)[22–28] and the Collaborative Normal-Tension Glaucoma Study (CNTGS)[29–34] look at the basic question of whether or not lowering IOP by a specified level prevents progression, compared with no intervention. The Collaborative Initial Glaucoma Treatment Study (CIGTS)[35-41] compares an individualized level of IOP lowering by two different means—medications first as compared to incisional surgery first. The Glaucoma Laser Trial (GLT)[42-48] examines the outcomes between initiating treatment with medications first rather than laser first.

Early Manifest Glaucoma Treatment Study

Recruitment period: October 1992 to January 1997.

Study Objectives

To evaluate the safety and effectiveness of lowering IOP by a specified level in patients with open-angle glaucoma.

Study Design, Treatment Groups, and Outcome Measures

Design. Prospective, multicenter, randomized, unmasked.

Sample Selection. Candidates were screened from the general population (44,243 people). Subjects were between the ages of 50 and 80 and had newly diagnosed open-angle glaucoma, which included POAG, exfoliation glaucoma, and normal-tension glaucoma. The diagnosis of glaucoma required reproducible defects on the Humphrey 24-2 in at least one eye. Patients were predominantly white and were residents of Sweden. Exclusion criteria included advanced VF damage (mean deviation [MD] >-16 dB) or threat to fixation, mean IOP >30 mm Hg (or any IOP >35 mm Hg) in either eye or VA in either eye of $<20/40$.

Sample Size. A total of 255 patients were recruited; 129 in the treatment arm, and 126 in the control arm.

Intervention. The group randomized to treatment underwent argon laser trabeculoplasty (ALT) (360°) and were placed on betaxolol 0.5% b.i.d. The control group received no treatment. All patients were examined every 3 months. Visits included a recent medical and ophthalmologic history with questioning about adverse events and compliance. The examinations included VA testing, subjective refraction, Goldmann tonometry, full threshold Humphrey 30-2, ophthalmoscopy, and inspection with a slit lamp. Lens opacification (nuclear sclerosis, cortical and posterior subcapsular opacification) was graded according to the Lens Opacities Classification System (LOCS) II as described in the initial publication.[22]

Target Intraocular Pressure Reduction in Treatment Group. Minimum 25% reduction in IOP with an absolute maximum of 25 mm Hg.

Duration of Study. Patients were examined every 3 months for a minimum of 4 years.

Statistics. Intent-to-treat analysis, univariate and multivariate analyses.

Primary Outcome Measures. Progression of the glaucoma due to the worsening of the VF and/or increased cupping of the optic disc, each according to specific criteria, were the primary end points. VF progression was defined as 3 points showing significant progression, as compared with baseline, at the same location on three consecutive tests. Optic disc progression was determined by masked graders comparing baseline and follow-up disc photographs using side-by-side photograding and flicker chronoscopy. (This technique detects differences in discs by superimposing two aligned photographs taken at different times and rapidly alternating the images. Differences in topography, or cupping, will be revealed as flickering of the images).

Secondary Outcome Measures. Subgroup analysis examined selected baseline characteristics for responsiveness to treatment. Baseline characteristics examined included IOP level, presence of exfoliation syndrome, severity of glaucomatous VF damage (as measured by MD), and age. The development of cataract was monitored for each group.

Summary of Results

Impact on Progression of Glaucoma. Patient retention for 4-year minimum follow-up was excellent. Only 22 patients died (15 in the treatment group and seven controls) and three patients in each group were lost to follow-up for reasons other than death. The median follow-up periods were 66 months for the treatment group and 69 months for the control group.

Many of the patients in this study would likely have been classified as POAG at normal pressures, or normal-tension glaucoma, if diurnal tension curves had been observed. Approximately half the patients in each group had baseline IOPs <21 mm Hg.

The mean IOP in the treatment group was reduced from 20.6 mm Hg at baseline to 15.5 mm Hg at 3 months (25% reduction) and this was maintained throughout the observation period. The IOP reduction was more pronounced (29%) in eyes with baseline IOP of 21 mm Hg or greater than in eyes starting at <21 mm Hg (18%).

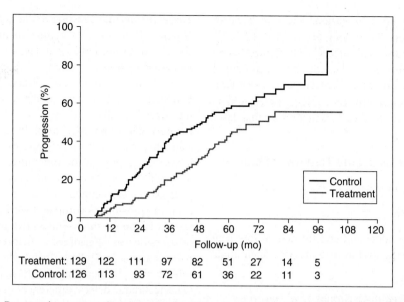

FIGURE 5.5 ◻ Progression across time in patients of the study group. The cumulative probability of patients with progression was larger in the control group than in the treatment group (*p* = 0.007). The number of patients at risk for progression of glaucoma in the treatment group and control group is shown below the x-axis. Reprinted with permission from *Arch Ophthalmol.* 2002;120:1272.

At 4 years, the proportion of patients demonstrating definite progression of their optic disc cupping or VF defects was 78/126 (62%) in the control group and 58/129 (45%) in the treatment group (*p* = 0.007). This represented a reduced risk of progression of approximately 50% with treatment. Progression in all patients over time is shown in Figure 5.5.

The rate of progression was highly variable among individual patients with the same IOP reduction. The mean rate of progression, by change in MD, was −0.03 ± 0.05 dB per month with treatment versus −0.05 ± 0.07 without treatment (*p* = 0.008). All the end points for progression were established by the study protocol for VF deterioration, with or without a disc change, except for one patient who showed only a disc change.

For the range of IOPs in this study (13.0 to 31.0 mm Hg), the protective effect of lowering IOP was approximately 10% for every 1 mm Hg.

Adverse Events. There were no patients in the control group who needed to be started on treatment because their IOPs reached 35 mm Hg. Adverse events and self-reported conditions were marginally more often recorded in the treatment group. Twice as many patients in the treatment group died as compared to the control group (15 versus 7), but this was not statistically significant. The development of lens opacification as measured by LOCS II scoring was significantly greater in the treatment group only for nuclear sclerosis (see Fig. 5.6). Eight patients underwent cataract surgery, 6 of whom were in the treatment arm.

Factors Associated with Progression. The baseline factors associated with progression that were obtained by multivariate analysis were age >67 years, IOP >20 mm Hg, PSD ≥4, presence of exfoliation, and bilateral eligibility for the study.

Postbaseline factors associated with progression, which were also obtained by multivariate analysis, included less change in IOP at the 3-month visit, higher IOP at the first follow-up visit, higher mean IOP at all follow-up visits and higher percentage of visits with a disc hemorrhage.

Strengths of the Study

A racially homogeneous cohort of patients with definite open-angle glaucoma was drawn from a general population using a massive screening program. As a result, there is no selection bias as is often seen when volunteers step in because they have a strong motivation to participate in a particular study. For example, in OHTS there were a disproportionate number of people claiming a positive family history of glaucoma.[8]

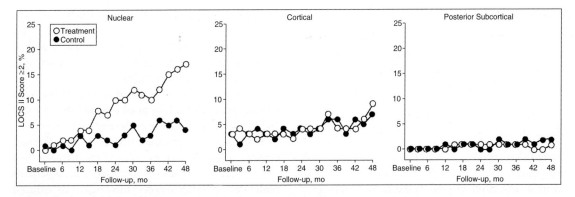

FIGURE 5.6 ☐ Lens Opacities Classification System (LOCS) II scores of 2 and higher for the study group during the first 48 months of follow-up. Reprinted with permission from *Arch Ophthalmol.* 2002;120:1275.

The treatment and monitoring protocol was standardized. All treated patients received a single medication and the same laser procedure. The follow-up schedule was rigorously applied with a very low attrition rate. The end point for VF progression was highly sensitive and clinically useful to the practicing clinician. Some studies, such as CIGTS and Advanced Glaucoma Intervention Study (AGIS) use VF scores, which are more difficult for practicing ophthalmologists to use.

While this study did not enroll very large numbers of subjects, the initial power calculations based on expected rates of progression gave it the statistical ability to answer the main question.

Criticisms of the Study

The study population was racially homogeneous and provided no direct information to guide the treatment of open-angle glaucoma in groups other than northern European Caucasians.

The IOP range studied was narrow but it was also a mixture of POAG at normal and elevated pressures. The subgroup analysis for baseline IOPs (IOP > and <21 mm Hg) lacked the power to compare and quantify the protective effect of a set amount of IOP lowering. Despite lowering the IOP by 29% instead of 18%, the VF progression was greater in the treated subgroup starting at the higher IOPs.

There were surprisingly few patients with exfoliation glaucoma (23/255, 9%). It might have been expected that this population would have yielded larger numbers of this aggressive glaucoma. How exfoliation glaucoma, the most common secondary glaucoma in the world, differs in natural history and treatment goals/effects from POAG will be useful information.

The restricted treatment protocol limited the IOP reduction to 25%. The fact that 45% of treated subjects progressed might suggest that a more vigorous IOP lowering would have led to a lower progression rate.

The fact that only one patient reached a progression end point solely on the basis of disc changes renders the examiners' abilities to detect change with this protocol questionable. Alternatively, it could mean that the VF protocol was too sensitive and that some of the VF progression end points might have been false positives.

Implications for Clinical Practice

This is a very important study. It is the first, and may be the last, study to compare the treatment of manifest glaucoma (where the untreated IOPs were often above the normal range) with the natural course of the disease. Future studies may, and should, be done to compare different target pressures, but this study shows unequivocally that lowering the IOP immediately by 25% is better than doing nothing initially.

Regardless of the reasons for almost all of the progression events being VF events (and not disc events), it is clear that careful follow-up of the VFs is the most important way to detect worsening of the disease, once an early VF defect is present.

Collaborative Normal-Tension Glaucoma Study

Recruitment period: April 1987 to September 1998.

Study Objectives

To examine whether lowering the IOP significantly, by medical or surgical means, would influence the course of the disease in open-angle glaucoma occurring at normal pressures.

Study Design, Treatment Groups, and Outcome Measures

Design. Prospective, multicenter, randomized, unmasked.

Sample Selection. Eligible subjects had glaucomatous optic disc damage and VF abnormalities based on three reliable Octopus 32 or Humphrey 30-2 tests. VAs needed to be at least 20/30. Untreated IOPs or IOPs following a 1-month washout period needed to average 20 mm Hg or less, with no measurements >24 mm Hg. Ten baseline IOP readings were taken to confirm that this criterion was fulfilled.

Patients were excluded if they had had previous laser treatments or intraocular surgery. They could not be taking a systemic β-blocker or clonidine. Their eye examination could not uncover other reasons for a VF defect such as a vascular occlusion. The angles needed to be open.

Sample Size. Two hundred and thirty patients from 24 institutions were enrolled. From this cohort, 145 eyes in 145 patients demonstrated progression, or had a VF defect that threatened fixation at recruitment, and were randomized to either the treatment or control groups. Five patients withdrew from the treatment group before the target IOP was achieved. These five eyes were nonetheless included in the intent-to-treat analysis. Of the 140 patients followed up, 116 were white, 12 Asian, 7 black and 3 Hispanic. Ninety-three of them were female and 47 were male.

Intervention. Randomization to either the treatment or control groups was made following a progressive event defined as a documented change in the VF, a change in the optic disc or the development of a disc hemorrhage. Randomization occurred immediately if the selected eye had a VF defect that threatened fixation or the reading committee was provided with past VF tests that indicated recent progression.

Patients randomized to treatment were prescribed medications and/or received laser and/or incisional surgery. The objective was to reach the IOP target within 6 months but it often took longer. Topical β-blockers and adrenergic agonists were not permitted because of their potential cardiovascular effects.

After randomization, the patients in both groups were followed every 3 months for the first year and every 6 months thereafter. If an end point was reached for a control patient, the protocol was lifted and treatment was offered promptly.

Investigators were asked to report all instances when Snellen acuities dropped by two lines or more and to ascertain the cause of the reduced acuity.

Target Intraocular Pressure Reduction in Treatment Group. Medical, laser, or surgical means were used to lower the IOP by 30% from the baseline. If patients underwent filtering surgery, the target was reduced to 20% in order to limit second and third surgeries.

Duration of Study. 5 to 7 years.

Statistics. Per protocol, and intent-to-treat analysis, multivariate analysis.

Primary Outcome Measures. The end point of VF change consisted of deepening of an existing scotoma, its expansion, a new or expanded threat to fixation, or a newly appearing scotoma in an area which had been previously normal. As per protocol, VF progression had to be verified by two of three VFs done within 1 month and again by two of three VFs done 3 months later. A second VF analysis was developed, which considered progression to have occurred when four of five consecutive follow-up VFs showed worsening, relative to the baseline. This was referred to as the four-of-five (4/5) criterion.

A suspected optic disc change was photographed and the images submitted to a reading committee of two experts who had to agree independently that the new stereophotograph was different from the baseline photographs.

It should be noted that disc hemorrhages were used only as a criterion to allow randomization. After randomization, a disc hemorrhage prompted new photography and review by the reading center for glaucomatous disc changes, but the hemorrhage did not in itself constitute a progressive end point.

If an end point for progression (i.e., disc of VF change) was confirmed, all protocol constraints were lifted and the patient was treated according to the individual physician's judgment.

Secondary Outcome Measures. Baseline characteristics were examined by multivariate analysis as possible risk factors for progression. Attention was given to a number of continuous variables consisting of age, various cardiovascular parameters (e.g., blood pressure, pulse, refraction), various optic disc parameters (e.g., disc size, cup-to-disc ratios), IOP, MD of the VF and VA. Gender and race were also considered.

A large number of discrete variables were similarly examined and these included a constellation of medical conditions, family history for glaucoma, diabetes, and stroke as well as the finding of a disc hemorrhage on follow-up examinations.

Summary of Results

Impact on Progression of Glaucoma. In the control group at randomization, the IOP was 16.9 mm Hg, and at follow-up it was 16.0 mm Hg. In the treatment group, the corresponding IOPs were 16.1 mm Hg at randomization and 10.6 mm Hg at follow-up.

Using the end points outlined in the protocol, 28/79 (35%) of the control group reached an end point with 3 of the 28 eyes progressing solely on the basis of a disc change. In contrast, only 7/61 (12%) eyes in the treated group progressed, with only one eye in this group progressing on the basis of a disc change ($p <0.0001$).

Using the four-of-five criterion for VF progression, 24/79 (30%) progressed in the control group and 11/61 (18%) in the treatment group ($9 = 0.0116$).

It should be appreciated that until the VF data was censored for cataract effect, which was more significant in the treatment arm, there was no apparent protective effect of lowering IOP by 30% in this study by an intent-to-treat analysis. Of the 145 eyes randomized to the study, there was an indistinguishable rate of subsequent progression between the treated 22/66 (33%) eyes and untreated 31/79 (39%) eyes.

After the foveal thresholds were adjusted to account for the two lines of reduced acuity caused by the cataracts, VF progression became significantly more common in the untreated group 21/79 (27%) as compared to the treated group 8/66 (12%). Figures 5.7 and 5.8 show the differences in survival curves and p values before and after censoring for cataract.

In the treatment arm, 28/61 eyes achieved a 30% reduction in IOP by laser (argon laser trabeculoplasty, ALT) and/or medications.

There was a wide individual variability in progression rates in both arms of this study. During the 5 to 7 years of careful follow-up, 20% of eyes progressed despite a 30% reduction in IOP. Furthermore, over 50% of those who were not treated showed no progression.

Adverse Events. The development of cataract was the principle adverse event followed and analyzed in this study. Cataracts were noted in 23/61 (38%) treated eyes; 16/33 (48%) were treated with filtering surgery and 7/28 (25%) were treated medically and/or with laser. There were 11/79 (14%) cataracts in the control group.

Baseline Factors Associated with Progression. A multitude of characteristics potentially associated with VF progression were carefully analyzed in the 160 patients enrolled in this study who had not received IOP-lowering treatment.[33] None of the continuous variables examined were positively associated with VF progression. Strikingly, advanced age and increased IOP at baseline were not found to be risk

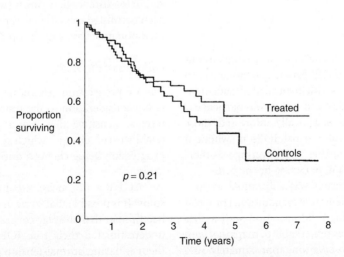

FIGURE 5.7 ☐ Survival curves of end points in untreated control subjects and treated patients from visual field baselines obtained at randomization using 4/5 defined end points. Reprinted with permission from *Am J Ophthalmol.* 1998;126:502.

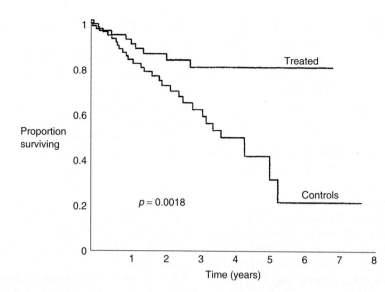

FIGURE 5.8 □ Survival curves of end points in untreated control subjects and treated patients from visual field baselines obtained at randomization using 4/5 defined end points with data on eyes developing cataracts, censored at the time of the diagnosis of the cataract. Reprinted with permission from *Am J Ophthalmol.* 1998;128:503.

factors for progression. The risk ratios for the discrete variables that were positively associated with VF progression were migraine (2.58) and disc hemorrhage (2.72). The risk ratio for the female gender was 1.85. Asian ancestry appeared to be associated with a slower rate of progression and, while the number of patients was small, African ancestry was associated with a faster rate of progression. A self-declared family history did not have an effect on the rate of VF progression.

Strengths of the Study

This was the first prospective, randomly assigned clinical trial that compared IOP-lowering treatment with no treatment in patients with documented glaucomatous damage to their disc and VFs. It was particularly important because it specifically addressed those patients with POAG at normal IOPs in whom it was unclear whether further IOP lowering was therapeutic. This was shown, in fact, to be the case.

The follow-up period was substantial (5 to 7 years), allowing sufficient time for additional progression to occur following randomization with a 30% reduction of IOP. It was remarkable perhaps that with this long period of observation, approximately 50% of the untreated eyes did not show any progression.

The impact of cataract development with treatment was carefully examined. In fact, it was shown

to be so important a factor that the treatment effect, evaluated by an intent-to-treat analysis, was entirely concealed until it was dealt with.

At the conception of the study, it was felt that most patients would require filtering surgery in order to achieve an IOP reduction of 30%. It is important to recognize that the target IOP was reached in almost 50% of the time with medications and/or laser, and without prostaglandins (which were not available yet) or α_2-adrenergic agonists (which would not have been permitted even if they were available because of their potential vasoactive properties).

Criticisms of the Study

The VF progression criteria were very sensitive as a safety consideration to the untreated patients. They were so sensitive that it was perhaps difficult to establish true change, which led to the criteria for progression being changed during the course of the study.

CCT was not measured at any time during the study. It is possible that some of the patients enrolled had thinner than average corneas, which would have underestimated their true IOPs, falsely classifying them as having normal-tension glaucoma.

There appeared to be some ambivalence about the significance of optic disc hemorrhages. They were regarded as a progressive event for randomization but not as an end point for progression thereafter. They were found to be a risk factor for VF progression.

Implications for Clinical Practice

This study supports the practice of lowering IOP in patients with POAG at normal IOPs. Many had regarded this entity as a subgroup of POAG,[2,49] or a separate condition altogether,[50,51] which was IOP-independent in terms of pathogenesis or treatment potential. This study showed that there was a role for IOP and its reduction in this condition.

The development, or progression, of cataract with the treatment of glaucoma was shown to be a major confounder in the interpretation of the value of the glaucoma treatment.

There was tremendous individual variability in the response to treatment and observation. Many people progressed despite a 30% reduction in baseline IOP while others showed no progression over 5 to 7 years without treatment. This study was able to elucidate several important risk factors for VF progression in untreated subjects—female gender, disc hemorrhages, and migraine headache sufferers. Special attention should be afforded to patients with these risk factors in terms of surveillance and the aggressiveness of IOP-lowering therapy.

It was also shown here that there is a dissociation of risk factors associated with prevalence as opposed to progression of glaucoma. A positive family history, advanced age, and elevated IOP are recognized risk factors for glaucoma, but not for its progression, according to this study.

Collaborative Initial Glaucoma Treatment Study

Recruitment period: October 1993 to April 1997.

Evidence has been published recently in the British literature demonstrating better long-term IOP control and VF preservation in eyes that had had immediate filtering surgery as compared with eyes that had received topical antiglaucoma medications.[52–54] These were prospective studies with relatively small numbers of subjects from a few surgeons. It was felt that a large multicenter trial involving several surgeons would further address the efficacy, safety, patient acceptance, and advisability of bypassing the traditional practice of initiating glaucoma treatment with medications and going directly to surgery.

Study Objectives

This study was designed to compare the long-term efficacy, safety, and patient acceptance of initiating treatment for POAG with topical medications against treatment with incisional surgery.

Study Design, Treatment Groups, and Outcome Measures

Design. Prospective, multicenter, randomized, unmasked.
Sample Selection. Volunteers were recruited at 14 clinical centers. There was a slight predominance of males (55%) among the enrollees. Most patients were diagnosed with POAG (90.6%), while a few had exfoliation glaucoma (4.8%) and pigmentary glaucoma (4.6%). Thirty-eight percent of the participants were black. The mean ages at entry were 56 and 61 years for black and white patients respectively. Approximately one third of all participants stated they had a positive family history for glaucoma and 17% said they had diabetes.
Sample Size. Between October 1993 and April 1997, a total of 607 newly diagnosed patients with open-angle glaucoma were recruited.
Intervention. Random assignment placed 307 patients in the medication-first group and 300 in the surgery-first group. If intervention failure occurred in either group, the next step would be an ALT. If ALT did not provide adequate control, then the third step for the medication-first group would be a trabeculectomy, and for the surgery group, the third step would be adjuvant medications (see Table 5.3).

An intervention failure was defined as a failure to achieve or maintain target IOP or the worsening of CIGTS VF score by three units from the baseline. Trabeculectomy was accomplished by a technique that was familiar to the individual surgeon who was free to use intraoperative or perioperative antimetabolites as deemed necessary. Mitomycin C

TABLE 5.3 ◻ Steps Involved in Glaucoma Treatment

Medication-First Group	Medications → ALT → Trabeculectomy
Surgery-First Group	Trabeculectomy→ ALT → Medications

ALT, argon laser trabeculoplasty.

was not permitted for initial trabeculectomies, but could be used for reoperations.

To address quality of life measures, a custom-designed questionnaire for telephone use was created. It queried several areas of interest including 16 questions on health perceptions, 4 questions about adaptations and social supports, a 33-item visual activity questionnaire, a 43-item symptom and health problem list, an 8-item questionnaire about depression and a 136-item sickness impact profile. This telephone interview was carried out every 6 months. The interview took an average of 48 minutes to conduct.

Target Intraocular Pressure Reduction in the Treatment Group. A unique CIGTS target IOP was determined for each eye on the basis of a preintervention (reference) IOP score a and preintervention VF score. The following formula was used:

$$(1 - [\text{reference IOP} + \text{VF score}]/100)$$
$$\times \text{reference IOP}$$

Example: if reference IOP = 28 mm Hg and VF score is 5,

$$(1 - [28 + 5]/100) \times 28 = 0.67(28)$$
$$= 18.76 \text{ or } 19 \text{ mm Hg}$$

Duration of Study. Results at 5 years have been published for clinical outcomes and quality of life measures.[38,39] Immediate perioperative (within the first month) complications have also been analyzed and reported more recently.[41]

Primary Outcome Measures. A sustained VF progression was defined by an increase of 3 units in VF score on a scale from 0 to 20 from 2 baseline Humphrey 24-2 full threshold tests. The VF scale was a global VF deficit from 0 (no defects) to 20 (end stage; all 52 points of the Humphrey 24-2 field test had a defect at $p < 0.005$). It is similar, but not identical, to the AGIS VF scale.

Secondary Outcome Measures. The impact of the intervention on the patients' well being and quality of life was evaluated. Other secondary outcome measures were VA (using a modified Early Treatment Diabetic Retinopathy Scale [ETDRS] scale) and IOP (by Goldmann tonometry).

Summary of Results

Impact on the Progression of Primary Open-Angle Glaucoma. Over 60 months of follow-up, there was no significant change in CIGTS VF score for either the medicine-first or the surgery-first group. The eyes undergoing trabeculectomy experienced a greater drop in IOP throughout the study period than those receiving topical medication (see Fig. 5.9). VA loss was greater in the surgical group initially

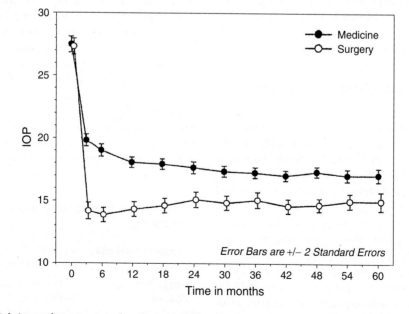

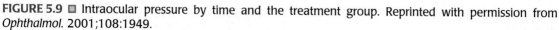

FIGURE 5.9 ☐ Intraocular pressure by time and the treatment group. Reprinted with permission from *Ophthalmol.* 2001;108:1949.

but this difference disappeared after 4 years. Much of the VA decrease was due to cataract formation and the rate of cataract surgery was substantially increased in the surgery-first group, resulting in the acuities coming together later in the study (see Fig. 5.10).

The Total Symptom Impact Glaucoma Score, a composite measure of 43 possible symptoms or health problems related to the glaucoma or its treatment scored from 1 to 5 (for a total score up to 215) decreased slightly in parallel between the two groups. Likewise, the percentage of patients worried about blindness dropped in both groups from about 50% at the outset of the observation period to approximately 25% from 6 months until 5 years. Initially, patients receiving a trabeculectomy were more satisfied with their treatment than those receiving eye drops (95% satisfied versus 75% satisfied), but this difference disappeared over time with patients in both groups being 95% satisfied with their treatment (see Fig. 5.11).

There was no difference between the groups in terms of VA perception on questioning during the interviews.

Adverse Events. Most of the adverse events encountered were related to perioperative complications of the trabeculectomies. There were a total of 465 trabeculectomies performed on the 300 patients randomized to the initial surgery group.[41]

Intraoperative complications occurred in 55 eyes or 12% of all cases. The two most commonly noted problems were anterior chamber bleeding (37 eyes, 8%) and conjunctival buttonhole formation (5 eyes, 1%).

Complications occurred within 1 month of surgery in half the cases (232 eyes). The most frequent complications consisted of shallow or flat anterior chamber (62 eyes, 13%), encapsulated blebs (56 eyes, 12%), ptosis (55 eyes, 12%), serous choroidal detachment (52 eyes, 11%), and anterior chamber bleeding or hyphema (48 eyes, 10%). There were three small suprachoroidal hemorrhages and no cases of endophthalmitis. Subgroup analysis showed that older patients were more likely to experience serous choroidal detachment, new anterior or posterior synechiae, and wound leaks. Blacks had less anterior chamber bleeding but more ptosis than whites. In cases of patients requiring bilateral surgery, there was a tendency for fellow eyes to experience a greater rate of complications than due to chance alone.

On perioperative complication evaluation, the authors noted that it was unlikely that any of the problems encountered in the first month would have caused any sustained vision loss.

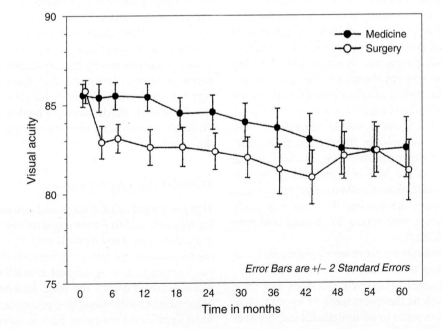

FIGURE 5.10 ◻ Visual acuity by time and the treatment group. Reprinted with permission from *Ophthalmol.* 2001;108:1947.

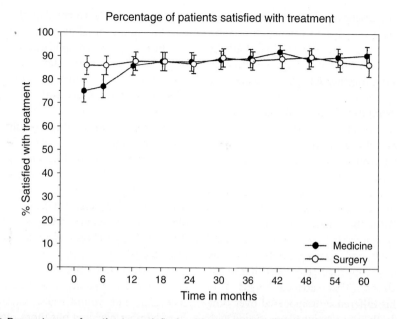

Percentage of patients satisfied with treatment

FIGURE 5.11 ▢ Percentage of patients satisfied with treatment (single item): Percent of respondents indicating that their glaucoma treatment has been "moderately" or "very successful". Reprinted with permission from *Ophthalmol.* 2001;108:1964.

Strengths of the Study

This is the first study of this nature to carefully examine quality of life issues surrounding two very different treatment routes. The questioning was comprehensive and exhaustive, covering most of the concerns regarding perception of disease, the likelihood of going blind and the real and perceived disabilities.

This study gives serious attention and credibility to the modern concept of setting a target pressure as a treatment objective. A unique formula for calculating target pressure, requiring a VF score, was presented, which may not make it readily adoptable by the practicing ophthalmologist. Nonetheless, the formula could be modified to use other more accessible global indices such as the MD of a Humphrey field. A simple treatment plan of reducing IOP by a certain percentage from the baseline does not adequately treat the patient with severe VF damage and very high initial IOPs.

Since the target pressures were significantly lower (by as much as 45% on average in the surgical arm) than the preintervention levels, this study may serve as a testament to the importance of lowering IOP substantially in order to achieve clinical stability over 5 years, regardless of the means used to achieve that target.

Criticisms of the Study

The absence of any significant outcome differences between the surgically and medically treated groups might suggest one of two possibilities. Firstly, open-angle glaucoma is usually a slow and indolent disease; maybe the follow-up was not long enough to show a difference. Perhaps five years is long enough to show the differences with this enrollment size but the reason none was shown was that there were many very early stage disease subjects (i.e., those with very low VF scores), which may have rendered the study incapable of providing the dynamic range to show differences.

Implications for Clinical Practice

This study validated the safety and efficacy of choosing medications first for the initial treatment of open-angle glaucoma. The average IOP of 38% achieved in the medication-first group was substantial, it avoided the immediate risk of surgical complications, and it was achieved despite the nonavailability of many of the newest medications (i.e., prostaglandins). The most significant implication for our current clinical practice patterns is that we need not change them if substantial target pressures are achieved.

Glaucoma Laser Trial and Glaucoma Laser Trial Follow-Up Studies

Recruitment period: February 1984 to April 1987.

ALT was quickly adopted for patients inadequately responsive to medical therapy and it gained acceptance as a safer alternative or next step, to incisional filtering surgery.[55] It was soon questioned whether this treatment modality might be a safe and efficacious way to initiate treatment in patients with open-angle glaucomas. Supporters of this approach espoused the benefits of avoiding the side effects of medication, sidestepping the issue of drug compliance, reducing costs to the patient in the long-term, and potentially improving quality of life. To address some of these issues the GLT Research Group was formed and GLT was carried out,[42−46] and was subsequently reported in the GLT Follow-up Study.[47,48]

Study Objectives

To examine the differences in safety, IOP-lowering capacity, and optic disc and VF protection in patients with open-angle glaucomas treated with medication (i.e., timolol 0.5%) or ALT first.

Study Design, Treatment Groups, and Outcome Measures

Design. Prospective, multicenter, randomized, unmasked clinical trial comparing two treatments.
Sample Selection. Patients enrolled in this study were newly diagnosed with POAG. They were 35 years or older, with an IOP of 22 mm Hg or more in both eyes and a glaucomatous VF defect in at least one eye, or higher IOP with various combinations of increased cup-to-disc ratios or asymmetry of the discs without definite VF defects.

Patients with glaucoma other than POAG, severe VF defects that threatened fixation, or contraindications to the use of any of the study medications, were excluded.
Sample Size. A total of 271 patients were included in the Glaucoma Laser Trial Studies (GLTS). Of these original subjects, 203 were followed up in the companion study, GLT Follow-up Study. Of the 271 patients enrolled, 125 identified themselves as white, 120 as black, and 26 as Hispanic. There were 152 females and 119 males.
Intervention. One eye of each patient was randomly assigned to the medication-first or ALT-first group.

ALT was performed in two sessions of 180° separated by four weeks. The argon blue–green laser was used with settings of 0.1 seconds, 50-μm spot size, and power adjusted between 600 and 1,200 mW to achieve a threshold bubble for 45 to 50 burns per session. Efforts were made to place the burns at the junction of the pigmented and nonpigmented trabecular meshwork. Patients were examined 1 and 4 hours after each ALT. Pretreatment with an IOP-lowering agent was not done, but the attending ophthalmologist could use medication to lower IOP postlaser if it was felt that an IOP spike could be harmful. An anti-inflammatory drug was used four times a day for 6 days following treatment.

Medication-first eyes were administered topical agents according to the following stepwise protocol (see Table 5.4).

After a few visits immediately following initiation of treatment, patients in both arms of the study were followed up every 3 months. VA and IOP were measured at each visit. VFs were performed at set intervals using either the Octopus 201 or 2000 perimeter with Program 32. Strict VF criteria for enrollment and progression were adhered to. Progression was deemed to have occurred if scotomas arose in locations which were previously normal (11 dB or more below the age-adjusted normal level), deepened (7 dB or more below baseline level), or expanded (test location adjacent to baseline scotoma deteriorated by 9 dB from its baseline level). One confirmatory VF was required to establish progression. Conversely, the criteria for VF improvement were the changes for VF progression, inverted.

TABLE 5.4 □ Step-wise Protocol for Administering Topical Agents

---

Step 1—Timolol 0.5% b.i.d.

Step 2—Dipivefrin 0.1% b.i.d.

Step 3—Low-dose pilocarpine q.i.d.

Step 4—High-dose pilocarpine q.i.d.

Step 5—Timolol 0.5% b.i.d. plus high-dose pilocarpine q.i.d.

Step 6—Dipivefrin 0.1% b.i.d. with high-dose pilocarpine

Step 7—Release from stepped regimen/treatment as per the GLT ophthalmologist

---

GLT, glaucoma laser trial.

Disc stereophotographs were evaluated at a reading center using a customized cup-to-disc measurement grid.

Target Intraocular Pressure Reduction in the Treatment Group. A successfully treated IOP was considered to be <22 mm Hg or 80% or less of the baseline reference IOP. The reference IOP could be changed by the GLT ophthalmologist if there was VF deterioration.

Duration of Study. Median follow-up of 7 years with a maximum of 9 years for the GLT Follow-up Study.

Primary Outcome Measures. The primary outcome measure for the GLT Study was the number of medications needed to control IOP.

Secondary Outcome Measures. Secondary measures were IOP control, VA change, VF progression, and optic disc deterioration. Adverse events were recorded with special attention to immediate IOP spikes.

Summary of Results

Primary and Secondary Outcome Measures. At 2 years' follow-up, 44% of the eyes were controlled by ALT first (achieved target IOP), 70% were controlled by ALT or ALT plus timolol and 89% were controlled within the stepped medical protocol. The ALT-first group maintained an average IOP, which was slightly lower (1 to 2 mm Hg) than the medication-first group and this was statistically significant (p <0.001). However, there were no major differences between the treatment arms in terms of VAs or fields.

At 42 months' follow-up, differences in outcomes between the treatment arms started to emerge. The mean VF threshold for the ALT-first eyes was 0.3 dB better than for the medication-first eyes. More eyes in the medication-first group 82/261 (31%) than in the ALT-first group 61/261 (23%) had confirmed localized VF deterioration. However, in both treatment arms there were twice as many VFs showing improvement than deterioration, which was suggestive of some regression to the mean and possibly an extended learning effect. Most experts are reluctant to acknowledge that glaucomatous VFs improve, especially when the IOP treatment effect is less than dramatic.

At final follow-up (median of 7 years), eyes initially treated with ALT had a 1.2 mm Hg greater reduction in IOP (p <0.001) than those eyes receiving medication first. The ALT-first eyes had 0.6 dB greater improvement in VF (p <0.001) compared to entry into the study. In terms of optic disc changes, there was a tiny but statistically significant (p = 0.005) difference in cup-to-disc areas in favor of the ALT-first eyes.

Adverse Events. Acute elevations in IOP were commonly observed at 1 and 4 hours after ALT treatments. Spikes of >5 mm Hg occurred in 34% of eyes and those >10 mm Hg were seen in 12% of eyes. The only risk factor for an IOP spike that was noted after a first treatment, was increased pigmentation of the trabecular meshwork. IOP spikes were more likely for the second treatment, if there had been a spike with the first treatment. Peripheral anterior synechiae (PAS) formation was more common in brown-colored irides. Forty-six percent of eyes developed >1 degree of PAS.

Strengths of the Study

This was the first study to prospectively evaluate the efficacy and safety of ALT first, instead of the traditional use of medications, over a long observation period and with a large enrollment. It was rigorously carried out, with many checks and balances. It employed highly sensitive criteria for VF and disc changes and it was one of the first major studies to define a treatment objective for IOP, or target pressure.

Criticisms of the Study

The observation that ALT-first eyes had a net improvement in VF of 0.6 dB over 7 years, and that the medication-first eyes showed no change in either direction, may reflect a biased enrollment. It is possible that there was a significant learning effect in both groups with many of the subjects normalizing, or nearly normalizing, their VFs. Many of the patients may not have had glaucoma. This might also explain the very minor changes in optic cup-to-disc areas in both groups.

It is also likely that the VF end points were too sensitive to detect true deterioration. With the criteria for VF improvement being the inverse of those for progression and with twice as many patients showing improvement than progression, it is probable that the criteria were at too high a resolution and much of what was noted at 42 months could have been long-term fluctuation. Some net VF progression should have been expected with this long follow-up (up to 9 years) even with IOP reductions of 23 to 29%.

Fewer medications were required to reach the pressure target when ALT was the initial treatment, therefore ALT was a drug-sparing intervention. However, if ALT was considered an equivalent intervention to a drug, there would have been no difference in the number of interventions in the two groups.

The medication protocol in this study was unwieldy and it must have been difficult to get patients to adhere to it. Multiple medication changes must have been necessary. Since the actual medication algorithm was not an outcome of the study, it might have been less cumbersome to simply allow the attending physicians the latitude to choose what they felt would be best tolerated and provide the best effect, as was done in the OHTS.

There were significant baseline differences between the groups in terms of race, gender, age, and cardiovascular history. Compared to the eyes of whites, those of blacks had more damaged VFs and larger cup-to-disc ratios on enrollment. Unlike the AGIS, these racial differences were not examined for their influences on the results.

Each patient had one eye entered in one of the two arms of the study. It was shown in one analysis that the cross-over effect of the timolol was only 0.5 mm Hg, despite previous reports that the cross-over effect could be as much as 30%.[56] The effect of the use of ALT on one eye on the fellow eye is unclear. If there was an effect, it could influence the perceived cross-over effect of timolol in this study. Also, the ALT effect in the eye of a patient receiving topical medications in the contralateral eye might be different from that in the eye of a patient not receiving any treatment in the other eye. These confounding possibilities would have been eliminated if only one eye of a patient had been randomized.

Implications for Clinical Practice

This study showed that ALT applied as initial therapy was safe and at least as effective as starting with topical medications. Patients unable, or unwilling, to start with topical medications for reasons of adverse drug effects, lack of response, poor compliance, excessive cost, or a philosophical objection to the use of drugs now have an alternative treatment route in ALT.

ALT has not replaced topical medications as the first modality of treatment in POAG. The use of medications is reversible whereas the use of ALT

is not. ALT causes permanent structural changes to the trabecular meshwork. Even with the use of perioperative IOP-lowering agents, there remains a small but real possibility of a pressure spike and, as such, ALT is not recommended for use in patients with advanced VF damage splitting fixation.

Trabeculoplasty has been performed with other lasers. While the diode laser[57] did not gain wide popularity for this purpose, the SLT using a Q-switched, frequency-doubled Nd:YAG laser has shown promise.[58] The final section of this chapter explores the evidence to date that supports this new laser method, as well as a few of the newer incisional procedures (i.e., the nonpenetrating filtering procedures), for effective and sustained IOP reduction.

Advanced Open-Angle Glaucoma

Advanced Glaucoma Intervention Study

Recruitment period: April 1988 to November 1992.

AGIS was designed and carried out to answer questions about the best way to proceed with those patients with significant glaucomatous damage who had failed to improve with (i.e., condition progressed under) maximum medical management.

Until about 1980, filtering surgery would have been the next step. By this time the trabeculectomy[59,60] had largely supplanted full-thickness techniques[61,62] as the initial surgical choice. Also, around this time a new nonincisional laser procedure[55], ALT, was being used as an intermediate step, positioned between medical and incisional surgical treatments. This chapter will review the peer-reviewed publications of AGIS to evaluate the role of modern surgical methods in the treatment of advanced open-angle glaucoma.

Study Objectives

To assess the long-range outcomes of different sequences involving trabeculectomy and ALT following failed medical management. In particular, is it worthwhile to do ALT or should we proceed directly to trabeculectomy?

Study Design, Treatment Groups, and Outcome Measures

Design. Prospective, multicenter (11 US centers), randomized, unmasked.

Sample Selection. Candidates for recruitment were aged between 35 and 80 years and were deemed to

TABLE 5.5 ◻ **Criteria for Advanced Open-angle Glaucoma**

Criterion[a]	IOP Consistently Elevated (mm Hg)[b]	Visual Field Score	Documented Disc Rim Deterioration[c]
A	≥18[d]	Increase of ≥3 ("visual field deterioration")[c]	Not required
B	≥18[d]	≥2	Required
C	≥21	≥6, with at least one of four paracentral points depressed 20 dB or more from normal	Not required
D	≥21	≥11	Not required
E	≥22	≥7	Not required
F	≥23	≥4	Not required
G	≥24	≥3	Not required
H	≥26	≥2	Not required
I	≥30	≥1	Not required

[a] When an eye meets more than one of the eligibility or failure criteria, it is classified according to the criteria whose letter designation appears last in the alphabet (e.g., an eye meeting criteria G and H is classified H).
[b] IOP is consistently elevated at or above a specified pressure when two IOP determinations made on separate days not more than 30 days apart while the eye is on maximum tolerated and effective medical therapy are both at, or above, that pressure.
[c] Visual field (VF) deterioration and disc rim deterioration must be ascertained while the eye has been on maximum tolerated and effective medications.
[d] For eligibility, the eye must have had at least one previous measurement, with or without medicines, of IOP ≥21 mm Hg by applanation or indentation tonometry.
IOP; intraocular pressure.

have "advanced" open-angle glaucoma. This degree of glaucoma was established by fulfilling at least one of nine criteria, consisting of various combinations of IOP, VF defect, and disc damage (see Table 5.5; modified with permission from *Control Clin Trials* 1994;15:302). Eyes with previous incisional surgery or laser trabeculoplasty were excluded.

There were more blacks than whites in this study. Some of their baseline characteristics differed[63] and these included age (blacks were younger than whites), self-reported systemic disease (there were more blacks than whites with systemic hypertension, diabetes, and coronary artery disease), and ocular characteristics (blacks were more hyperopic and had fewer disc hemorrhages than whites). The VFs of blacks were more severely damaged than those of whites. IOPs and VA scores were not significantly different between the two groups (see Table 5.6).

Sample Size. A total of 591 patients (789 eyes) were enrolled. Of these participants, 332 identified themselves as black, 249 as white and 10 as neither black nor white.

Intervention. Eyes were randomly assigned to undergo one of two sequences of surgical treatments.

One group started with ALT, which, if unsuccessful would be followed by a trabeculectomy, and if necessary a second trabeculectomy. This sequence/group was referred to as the argon laser trabeculoplasty-trabeculotomy-trabeculotomy (ATT) sequence/group. The other arm of the study involved the eyes initially receiving a trabeculectomy, which, if failure occurred was followed by an ALT and if this failed a second trabeculectomy. This sequence/group was referred to as the trabeculotomy-argon laser trabeculoplasty-trabeculotomy (TAT) sequence/group (see Table 5.7; Adapted from *Control Clin Trials* 1995;15:303).

Target Intraocular Pressure Reduction in Treatment Group. There was no target IOP set at the beginning of this study although an IOP measured above 18 mm Hg was considered to be enough grounds to step-up treatment at the discretion of the attending ophthalmologist.

Duration of Study. Patients were recruited between 1988 and 1992 with the initial reports made after a follow-up of 4 to 7 years. Follow-up has been ongoing since then, allowing for multiple subgroup analyses.

TABLE 5.6 ☐ Racial Distribution of Baseline Characteristics

Baseline Patient and Ocular Characteristic	Blacks	Whites	Adjusted p Value[a]
Total enrollment (n)	332	249	
Mean age (y)	67.0	68.0	
Systemic hypertension (%)	59.6	39.0	
Diabetes (%)	26.5	12.4	
Vascular or coronary disease (%)	17.2	23.7	
Mean spherical equivalent	+0.3	−0.4	<0.001
Presence of disc hemorrhages (%)	0.9	3.7	0.008
Visual acuity score[b]	79.1	79.8	0.188
Visual field score	9.2	7.5	<0.001
Intraocular pressures (mm Hg)	23.7	24.5	0.077

[a] p value adjusted for correlation between eyes within patient, and for age and gender.
[b] Approximate Snellen equivalents of visual acuity scores: 85 = 20/20, 80 = 20/25, 70 = 20/40, 55 = 20/80.

Primary Outcome Measure. Percentage of eyes with a decrease in visual function (VF and VA) in the two treatment arms. VA was measured using the ETDRS chart where a maximum score of 100 letters, corresponding to Snellen acuity of 20/10, was possible. The end point for a decrease in VA was defined as a decrease of 15 letters (3 lines) on the ETDRS chart.

VFs were recorded using the Humphrey Visual Field 24-2 full threshold test algorithm. The VF was considered abnormal if three or more contiguous test locations in the total deviation plot were depressed to dB levels equal to or greater than the dB levels shown in Figure 5.12. Also, the VF would be considered abnormal if two contiguous points, excluding the six in the nasal area, were depressed to values equal to or greater than the dB levels shown in Figure 5.12, and at least one of these sites was reduced by 12 dB or more. A nonlinear scale from 0 to 20 was developed, with 0 indicating no VF damage, 1–5 indicating mild damage, 6–11 indicating moderate damage, 12–17

indicating severe damage and 18–20 indicating the end stage. The end point for VF progression was an increase in score of 4 or more.[64,65]

Secondary Outcome Measures. The effect of IOP on visual function, complications of surgery, time to treatment failure, and the requirement for additional medical therapy were some of the secondary measures examined. Separate publications have addressed the rate of cataract formation with surgery, the effect of cataract on the VF, the risk of bleb encapsulation, risk factors for filtration failure and VF progression, and racial differences to treatment between blacks and whites.

Late intervention failure was based on maximum tolerated medical management being reestablished and the IOP being greater than the preintervention level after 6 weeks postop. Alternatively, if at any IOP, the VF score criteria were met or clinical disc progression as determined by the attending ophthalmologist was noted, then failure was declared.

Summary of Results

Impact on the Progression of Primary Open-Angle Glaucoma. The most often quoted results of this study relate to the positive impact that IOP lowering had on VF preservation.[66] Two analyses for evaluating the relationship between IOP and VF stability were performed. The outcome measure for both was the change from baseline in follow-up VF defect score (0 to 20 units).

TABLE 5.7 ☐ Sequences of Three Assigned Glaucoma Operations

Operation	Sequence 1 (TAT)	Sequence 2 (ATT)
First	Trabeculectomy	Argon laser trabeculoplasty
Second (after failure of first)	Argon laser trabeculoplasty	Trabeculectomy
Third (after failure of second)	Trabeculectomy	Trabeculectomy

TAT, trabeculotomy-argon laser trabeculoplasty-trabeculotomy; ATT, argon laser trabeculoplasty-trabeculotomy-trabeculotomy.

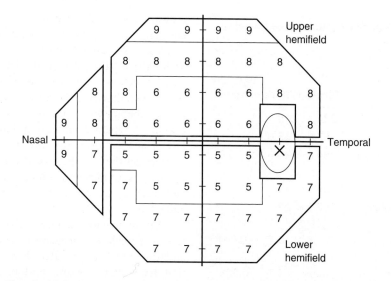

FIGURE 5.12 ☐ Threshold decibel values in the three sectors of the C-24-2 field Statpac total deviation plot. Depressions equal to or greater than the threshold values in contiguous locations indicate abnormality. Reprinted with permission from *Control Clin Trials.* 1994;15:306.

The first, designated *Predictive Analysis,* categorized 738 eyes into three groups on the basis of the IOPs measured over the first three 6-month visits. By this analysis, there was a direct correlation between the initial IOP measurements and worsening of the VF over 7 years (see Fig. 5.13).

The second analysis was referred to as the *Associative Analysis* and it categorized 586 eyes into four groups based on the percentage of the 6 monthly visits over 6 years with IOP measurements of <18 mm Hg. One of the most reproduced figures in the recent ophthalmologic literature (see Fig. 5.14) shows that in Group A, where the IOP was <18 mm Hg for 100% of the visits (with a mean IOP recorded of 12.3 mm Hg), there was no net change in the VF score.

As there were large enrollments of both blacks and whites in AGIS, three publications[67-69] were devoted to comparisons in outcomes between these two groups. At ten years follow-up, visual function outcomes were better for blacks than for whites in the ATT sequence and better for whites than for blacks in the TAT sequence. While initial ALT was marginally more effective in the black patients, the failure rate with initial trabeculectomy (almost all cases were done without antimetabolites) was significantly lower and the surgery was less complicated in whites.

Adverse Events. Cataracts occurred at a higher rate following trabeculectomy than ALT.[70] At 7 years, the cumulative occurrence of cataract was 56% for

eyes in the TAT sequence and 47% for eyes in the ATT sequence. At 7 years, a first trabeculectomy increased the cataract extraction rate by 78% while a second trabeculectomy nearly tripled the odds of cataract surgery.[71] Vision diminished by cataracts and vision diminished by cataract surgery were not directly related. Presumably, surgery was undertaken electively when the patients' perception of their disability outweighed the risk of the surgery.

While there has long been a concern that ALT predisposes one to the formation of encapsulated blebs after trabeculectomy,[72,73] this was not supported by AGIS.[74] Male gender, however, was shown to be a risk factor for bleb encapsulation in both white and black patients.[75]

Late surgical failure was defined as returning to preintervention IOP, with or without a change in VF score, or progressive disc changes. Often failure was simply a return to the situation that had qualified the patient for entry to the study. For both blacks and whites, ALT failure was associated with younger age and higher preintervention IOP. In the case of trabeculectomy failure, the risk factors were younger age, high preintervention IOP, diabetes, and one or more postoperative complications, most notably an increase in IOP or inflammation.

Baseline Factors Associated with Progression[76].
Sustained VF progression, defined as a change in baseline VF score by at least four units over three

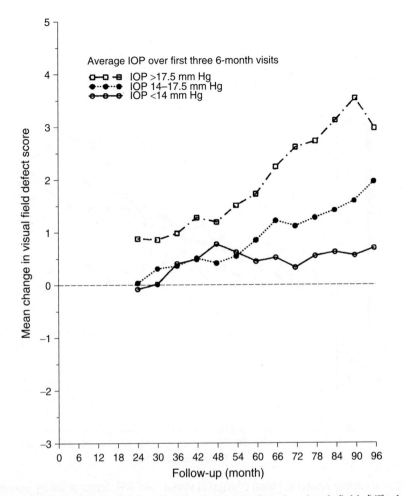

FIGURE 5.13 ◻ Predictive Analysis. Mean change from baseline in visual field (VF) defect score by intraocular pressure classified according to average value over the first three 6-month visits. Reprinted with permission from *Am J Ophthalmol.* 2000;130:434.

consecutive 6 month follow-up visits, was most likely to occur in older patients and all patients demonstrating >3 mm Hg IOP fluctuations between visits. The odds of VF progression increased by 30% for every 5-year increment in age and 1 mm Hg at enrolment.[77] The risk of VF progression was greater for fluctuating IOP than for mean IOP by most statistical analyses.

Strengths of the Study

This was a large enrollment study with the longest follow-up yet (between 7 and 11 years) for a prospective treatment trial. It was multiracial with enough power to make it relevant to black patients, a population at increased risk of suffering vision loss from glaucoma. The criteria for VF progression were conservative so that the false positive rate for progression would be low. The subgroup analyses have been exhaustive, resulting in 14 AGIS Investigator publications with a variety of clinically useful inferences being made.

Criticisms of the Study

The criteria for intervention failure were not very rigorous. In other words, unless the IOP did not return to the preintervention level with maximal medical therapy having been reestablished, the intervention (ALT or trabeculectomy) was considered a success. This is subject to the attending ophthalmologist not detecting a change in the disc or the VF score not

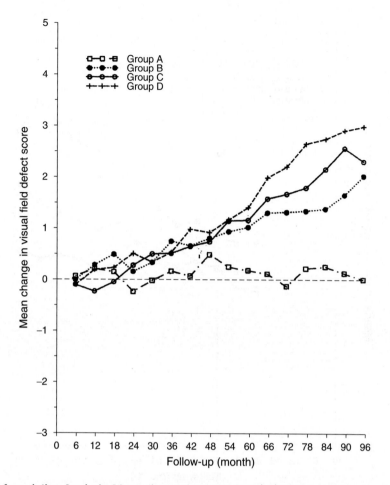

FIGURE 5.14 □ Associative Analysis. Mean change in visual field (VF) defect score by percent of visits over 6 years at which an eye presented with intraocular pressure <18 mm Hg (group A is 100%, group B is 75% to <100%, group C is 50% to <75%, and group D is 0% to <50%.). Reprinted with permission from *Am J Ophthalmol.* 2000;130:437.

worsening by at least four units. Many would argue that unless a preset target IOP was achieved, an intervention should not be considered successful.

While the ALT technique would not have changed substantially during the study, the trabeculectomy technique and the use of adjuvant antimetabolites (i.e., 5-fluorouracil and MMC) would have undergone some evolution. It also would have varied between surgeons and by the same surgeon depending on the stage of the intervention sequence. Antimetabolites were virtually never used in first trabeculectomies but were used to varying degrees in the second surgeries. For example, an antifibrotic agent was used in only 6% (4/63) of white patients and 39% (30/77) of black patients at the time of the second trabeculectomy.

Although there is valuable intrarace information provided in this study, it is difficult to compare outcomes between whites and blacks. The black patients were younger, had more systemic hypertension and diabetes, had worse baseline VF scores, and were more likely to receive antimetabolites at the time of trabeculectomy than the white patients. It therefore becomes impossible to make direct comparisons of treatment.

Implications for Clinical Practice

The Predictive and Associative Analyses for IOP and VF stability have guided the development of target pressures for treatment in advanced open-angle glaucoma. Perhaps even more importantly,

IOP measurements at each visit should not fluctuate by more than 3 mm Hg. The Associative Analysis confirmed that on average the VF score did not change if all IOP measurements were <18 mm Hg with a mean of about 12.3 mm Hg.

It should be recognized, however, that keeping the IOP consistently below 18 mm Hg does not guarantee that the VF will not progress in a person with advanced open-angle glaucoma. In fact, while the Associative Analysis showed that the net effect of having all visit IOPs under 18 mm Hg was no average change in VF score over 7 years, 13.1% of eyes had a worse VF score at 2 years, 13.9% were worse at 5 years, and 14.4% were worse at 7 years. The net effect was zero because roughly equal numbers of patients had VF scores that were 4 or more units better than baseline at the same time periods. Since this data represents a mean trend for a study population, it can not be assumed that an individual patient would follow the same trend.

This study reaffirms the importance of considering ALT in the postmedication management of patients with advanced open-angle glaucoma. Black patients, in particular, may benefit from postponing their exposure to the risk of complications associated with trabeculectomy. It was also shown that the risk of cataract formation was less with ALT and that the rate of bleb encapsulation was not significantly greater for trabeculectomy following ALT.

New Laser And Incisional Surgical Methods

Fluorouracil Filtering Surgery Study

Recruitment period: September 1985 to June 1988.

As a rule, new surgical procedures are not validated for their safety and effectiveness by prospective, randomized controlled trials (RCT) before they are widely adopted. For the past 35 years or more, trabeculectomy has been the gold standard incisional procedure for medically controlled glaucoma..[59,60] It became the accepted standard within a very short time, and without an RCT, because of its superior safety profile when compared to the full-thickness procedures. However, enhanced safety was traded for effectiveness ; the older full-thickness procedures seemed to lower IOP more, albeit with a higher complication rate.[78] As a result, interest in chemically inhibiting wound healing emerged. The Fluorouracil Filtering Surgery Study (FFSS) Group embarked on a multi-center trial to properly examine the safety and effectiveness of adjuvant subconjunctival 5-fluorouracil (5-FU) following trabeculectomy.[79–83]

Design, Treatment Groups, and Outcome Measures

This was a prospective, randomized, masked trial involving seven centers in the United States. Patients were selected if they were considered at higher risk of surgical failure on the basis of having had previous cataract extraction or previous failed filtering surgery in a phakic eye. One eye each of 213 patients was randomized to trabeculectomy alone (108 patients) or trabeculectomy with adjuvant postop 5-FU injections (105 patients). A standardized surgical technique was employed in all cases. Those patients in the 5-FU arm were given subconjunctival injections of 5 mg 5-FU 180 degrees from the trabeculectomy site twice daily on days 1–7 and once daily on days 8–14. Non-5-FU patients did not receive sham injections. Daily clinical examinations were made and both groups used frequent topical corticosteroids and atropine sulfate 1% in the immediate postop period.

Treatment failure was defined as either reoperation to decrease IOP, or an IOP >21 mm Hg with or without adjuvant IOP-lowering medications. VAs, VFs, and complications were also monitored.

Summary of Results

The results of the study were reported at 1,[79] 3[81] and 5 years.[82] The failure rates as reported in the abstracts are summarized in Table 5.8.

The major complications reported were related to the toxicity of 5-FU and its impact on wound healing. Corneal epithelial erosions were common in the 5-FU group, which resulted in more discomfort and transiently reduced VAs. Suprachoroidal hemorrhages were reported in 10 of the 162 eyes (6.2%) that had undergone previous cataract extraction,[80] but they were not statistically associated with the eyes

TABLE 5.8 □ Treatment Failure Rates

Year of Follow-up	With 5-FU	Without 5-FU
1	28/105 (27%)	54/108 (50%)
2	49/100	73/99
3	54/105 (51%)	80/108 (74%)

receiving postop 5-FU. Early wound leaks were associated with failure and they were more common in the 5-FU group.[83] Figure 5.15 shows the cumulative proportion of patients with successful surgery in the two groups with and without wound leaks.

After 5 years, a greater proportion of the patients receiving 5-FU had controlled IOPs and avoided further surgery. Risk factors for failure in both groups were high preop IOPs, a short time interval after the last procedure involving a conjunctival incision, the number of procedures with conjunctival incisions, and Hispanic ethnicity. Lower IOPs in both groups were associated with better maintenance of VA.

Implications for Clinical Practice

This study is perhaps the best example of a clinical trial to compare two surgical techniques. It was compelling in its evidence to show that adjuvant 5-FU can enhance surgical success, but at a potential cost. The toxicity of 5-FU to the external eye was troublesome to many and contraindicated in patients with severe dry eye syndromes, and wound leaks and infection were more of a worry. It was recommended by the study group that 5-FU only be used in patients at high risk for failure.

As the results of AGIS, the CNTGS, and others started to appear in the literature, lower target IOPs were sought and this validated the emerging preference for MMC applied once intraoperatively over postop 5-FU injections.[84,85] The frequent 5-FU injections were not popular with either the patients or the surgeons. The antibiotic alkylating agent MMC was found in the laboratory to be several-folds more potent than 5-FU in its inhibition of fibroblast proliferation. Despite a number of comparison studies with 5-FU, albeit with shorter follow-up than the FFSS, it has been difficult to show a large difference in treatment effect between the two antimetabolites.[86,87] Most glaucoma surgeons believe that there are clear advantages to MMC over 5-FU in terms of efficacy, safety, and patient acceptance. A large meta-analysis has recently been published, which slightly favors MMC over 5-FU in combined cataract and glaucoma surgery.[88]

Nonpenetrating Procedures. The past 10 to 15 years have seen renewed interest in IOP-lowering surgery, which does not require a direct communication between the anterior chamber and the suprascleral surface, VC and DS (with or without an implant). These nonpenetrating methods potentially avoid

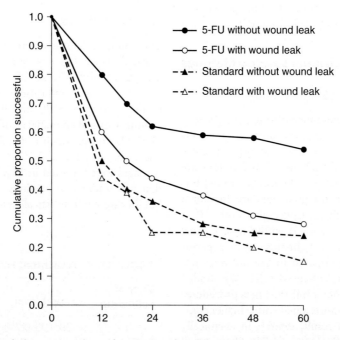

FIGURE 5.15 ◻ Cumulative proportion of patients who did not undergo a reoperation and who did not have an intraocular pressure >21 mm Hg in months after trabeculectomy, by treatment group and wound leak status. Reprinted with permission from *Am J Ophthalmol.* 2001;132:636.

many of the risks and hazards of the trabeculectomy, particularly in an era of antimetabolite use. Intraoperatively, nonpenetrating approaches decompress the eye less abruptly and may pose less risk of hypotony, flat anterior chamber, and suprachoroidal hemorrhage. Peripheral iridectomies are only required with fistulizing surgery, and without the formation of a conjunctival bleb, a number of unwanted possibilities are averted. Blebs can be uncomfortable, can cause astigmatism and leak, and become infected. Endophthalmitis becomes a lifelong concern when an avascular bleb is present. It is claimed by the proponents of these techniques that visual recovery from surgery is more rapid and subsequent cataract formation less likely.

Deep Sclerectomy (with or Without and Implant). This procedure bears some similarities to a number of "unroofing" procedures, the best remembered being the sinusotomy of Krasnov.[89] It was modified to serve as the basis for a number of subsequent variations.[90] After a large (5 × 5 mm) one-third thickness scleral flap is turned on the limbus, a rectangle of deeper sclera is excised, which exposes the Schlemm's canal and creates an intrascleral cavity (which will later fill with aqueous). An important objective is to fashion a Descemet's window without perforation. An egress of aqueous should be apparent and the scleral flap is loosely closed. An implant can be inserted under the flap to act as a spacer and/or aqueous wick. A popular implant is one that is processed from lyophilized porcine scleral collagen (Aquaflow™, Staar Surgical, Monrovia, California).

As DS is undergoing rapid development, with many modifications emerging, long-term, comparative, prospective studies have been few. One nonrandomized, noncomparative, prospective series of 105 patients has been presented with a mean follow-up of 64 months.[90] For the patients followed up to 78 months, the mean IOP was 12 ± 3 mm Hg (preop IOP was 26.8 ± 7.7 mm Hg). The number of glaucoma medications used dropped from 2.3 ± 0.7 to 0.5 ± 0.7. YAG laser goniopuncture was used in 51% of cases and 23% were given postop 5-FU injections. No flat chambers, endophthalmitis, or surgery-induced cataracts were noted.

In comparing DS with trabeculectomy, a prospective RCT was reported.[91] Out of 65 patients (eyes), 32 underwent DS—17 as single procedures and 15 combined with phacoemulsification—and 33 patients underwent trabeculectomy—18 alone and 15 combined with phacoemulsification. No

goniopuncture, laser suturlysis, or antimetabolites were allowed. The mean follow-up period was 22.5 months. Substantial IOP reductions were noted in all groups with the only statistically significant intergroup difference being that trabeculectomy alone lowered IOP more than DS alone.

Viscocanalostomy. VC starts out with a deep scleral flap dissection and exposure of a Descemet's window as does DS, but instead of an aqueous wick being placed under the flap, a high-density viscoelastic is injected into both exposed ends of the Schlemm's canal.[92] This technique by Stegmann had the scleral flap closed tightly with little to no external filtration developing (i.e., bleb formation). It is believed that the IOP-lowering effect of the resulting intrascleral lake and dilated Schlemm's canal occur through intrascleral filtration and enhanced conventional outflow.[93]

Five-year results of VC have been presented on 57 eyes in 57 patients with a mean follow-up of 34.1 months.[94] This was a prospective, nonrandomized, consecutive case series. The mean preop IOP was 24.6 mm Hg and at 36 months, it was 13.9 mm Hg. Sixty percent of those patients who had made it to 60 months had the IOP controlled to <21 mm Hg without medications. YAG laser goniopuncture was required for 37% of the study patients and the mean time for this treatment was 9.4 months. In these patients, goniopuncture further reduced the IOP from a mean of 20.4 mm Hg to 12.6 mm Hg ($p < 0.001$).

VC and DS were directly compared in a prospective, nonrandomized, consecutive series between two centers involving 192 eyes.[95] A mixture of VC, DS, and VC with phacoemulsification and DS with phacoemulsification cases were included. The mean follow-up was 36 months (9 to 60 months). At this time period, there were no statistically significant differences between the mean postop IOPs in the four groups. Large or cystic drainage blebs were observed only in the DS eyes.

Implications for Clinical Practice

The nonpenetrating group of procedures is in a rapid state of evolution, with a number of variables being reported for their relative safety and efficacy. Interventions such as the use of implants (of variable materials), perioperative antimetabolites, postop goniopuncture and bleb-enhancing maneuvers such as laser suturlysis need to find their proper indications. The logic is that this type of surgery should be safer than trabeculectomy with or without antimetabolites. The option that is best for a given indication, alone or in combination with cataract surgery, will be made clear once the technical developments stabilize somewhat and the results of RCTs comparing them to trabeculectomy become available. These studies will need to compare surgical techniques for common indications that consider the type of glaucoma, risk factors for surgical failure, level of glaucomatous VF, disc damage and target pressure.

Selective Laser Trabeculoplasty. The GLT and vast individual experience have highlighted the virtues and shortcomings of ALT. The mechanical effect of the thermal energy delivered to the trabecular meshwork likely contributes both to the IOP-lowering effect itself and its self-limiting effectiveness.[96] Owing to the thermally induced coagulation of the trabecular meshwork, ALT is a somewhat destructive procedure. Overtreatment can cause synechiae formation or persistent IOP elevation[97,98] which has been corroborated histopathologically.[99] Aggressive treatment of the primate angle has given us an animal model for high-pressure glaucoma.[100]

As recently as 1995, Latina et al. reported that the frequency-doubled Nd:YAG laser emitting at a wavelength of 532 nm with a 3-nanosecond pulse width and low fluency could selectively photolyze pigmented trabecular meshwork cells without significant collateral damage.[101] Selective Laser Trabeculoplasty (SLT), as it was called, was quickly introduced clinically with the first comparative series published by Latina in 1998.[102] Six month follow-up was reported for 53 eyes in 53 patients with medically uncontrolled open-angle glaucoma. Thirty eyes received 50 applications of laser over 180 degrees while 23 patients received the same number of treatment applications of ALT over 180 degrees. This small series showed no major differences in terms of effectiveness or safety between the two groups.

The next year Damji et al. followed with a more rigorously controlled prospective, comparative series with 18 patients in each group.[103] Again there was no statistically significant difference in the IOP effect between ALT and SLT after 6 months. This same group has recently published longer follow-up results on 72 patients receiving SLT with at least 1-year follow-up.[104] At 1 year, 43/72 (59.8%) had an IOP reduction of >20%. An analysis of baseline characteristics showed that only preop IOP level predicted IOP reduction; the magnitude of IOP reduction was positively correlated with the height of the pretreatment IOP. Patient age, type of open-angle glaucoma, degree of angle pigmentation, and previous ALT showed no predictive value. The lack of significance of whether the patient had received previous ALT could be indirect support for repeatability of SLT. Generally, repeat ALT shows a diminished effect compared to primary treatment and the risk of IOP spikes increase.[97,98]

Among a number of smaller studies with limited follow-up periods, three more substantial studies provide information regarding the relative efficacy and safety of SLT. Jurych et al. assembled retrospective data on 195 eyes of 195 patients, 154 of whom underwent ALT while 41 underwent SLT.[105] Both treatments were given over 180 degrees of the angle. With a mean follow-up of 37.4 months in the SLT group and 33.6 months in the ALT group, there was no statistically significant difference in the IOP-lowering effectiveness between the groups up to 5 years.

The most impressive IOP-lowering results have been shown in a non-comparative, consecutive series where SLT was used in open-angle glaucomas (POAG, exfoliation, pigment dispersion, and normal-tension glaucomas) and ocular hypertensive patients as the primary therapy.[106] Melamed et al. reported on 45 eyes of 31 patients with a follow-up of 18 months. Mean IOP reductions of 30% were recorded for all eyes and the best effect of a 41% mean reduction was seen in five eyes with exfoliation syndrome. Only two eyes did not have even a 20% reduction in IOP. No significant complications were encountered.

The first RCT comparing SLT to latanoprost has been published at 10.3 months mean follow-up.[107] Latanoprost 0.5% given once each evening was compared to SLT delivered to 90, 180 and 360 degrees of the angle. Postoperative ocular pain, uveitis, and pressure spikes were noted in a dose-dependent manner as more of the angle was treated. Success rates were higher with latanoprost than with 90 or 180-degree treatments of SLT. There was no statistically significant difference in the effect of 360 degrees of SLT treatment and latanoprost with 60% of the eyes receiving laser, achieving an IOP reduction of 30% or more.

Implications for Clinical Practice

It would appear that the available evidence supports that ALT and SLT are, on the whole, equivalent in terms of effectiveness. Comparisons of safety issues in the short-term have also not uncovered any major differences. Anecdotal reports have suggested that pressure spikes may be seen in highly pigmented angles with SLT but these have been seen with ALT as well. The more important issues are whether SLT is so benign in its effects on the trabecular meshwork that it can be safely repeated once, twice, or more. Is it wise to use SLT in the place of medications first in patients with ocular hypertension? Do the medications work as well after SLT as before? What are the best treatment parameters in terms of energy, spot size, and duration? Can SLT be safely used in eyes not ideal for ALT (e.g., partially closed angles, pseudophakia, glaucomas with inflammatory etiologies)? These are a few of the questions that will be partly answered with personal experience being reported in the literature, but also by rigorous RCTs such as the GLT.

Concluding Comments And Future Directions

In the late 1980s, when most of the studies in the first three sections were conceived, some health care policy analysts were saying that there was inadequate scientific evidence to support the belief that lowering IOP was therapeutic in glaucoma.[108] The implications of this doubt were protean. It called into question the vocation of ophthalmologists practicing the accepted standards of care for managing glaucoma patients. Were patients accepting the risk of therapies with no true benefit and what exactly were ophthalmologists being paid for in terms of deliverables? The policy makers and health care economists demanded RCTs to validate the practice of lowering IOP with medications, lasers, and surgery.

Several of these studies have answered the basic question of the therapeutic value of IOP-lowering treatments in at least open-angle glaucoma and ocular hypertension in Europeans and North Americans. The effectiveness of lowering IOP appears to be dose dependent and a number of risk factors for conversion to, and progression of, glaucoma have been identified. Some of the relative risks and benefits of the different treatment options have been elucidated but many questions remain to be answered. This chapter concludes with an incomplete list of some of the most important questions.

The protective effect of IOP lowering is dose dependent for ocular hypertension and POAG in the populations studied. Several risk factors have been identified. How can we use this information to develop relative risk calculations and target IOP determinations for individual patients?

For ocular hypertension and POAG, there are several options within each of the three traditional modalities of IOP-lowering therapy: Medications, lasers, and surgery.

- Which is the best initial drug?
- Which is the best initial laser treatment?
- Which is the best initial surgery?
- How do we expeditiously evaluate new therapies against the current "gold standards?"

There are many varieties of glaucoma. How effective are IOP-lowering treatments in closed-angle glaucomas and in secondary glaucomas with angles, which are both open and closed?

Cataract and glaucoma often coexist. The cataract can influence the pathogenesis and management of the glaucoma. Treating the glaucoma can cause or exacerbate the cataract. What are the best strategies, from a risk-benefit standpoint, for the management of glaucoma and coincident cataract?

An IOP that is too high for a particular optic nerve is the only accepted risk factor studied to date. Are there other modifiable risk factors amenable to RCTs?

Each of the aforementioned questions spawns a multitude of other questions and further studies. For the results of these studies to be weighty enough to change the way we manage glaucoma, the studies will need to be prospective, randomized, sufficiently powered, and properly controlled. The outcome measures will need to be as quantitative and reliable as possible. The studies reviewed here were plagued with reliability issues for the VFs and quantification issues for the optic disc assessments. New objective and functional tests will need to be developed and validated for any future studies. Greater emphasis will need to be placed on quality of life issues.

References

1. Mueller H. Anatomische beirtrage zur ophthalmologie: Ueber nervean-veranderungen an der eintrittsstelle des schnerven. *Arch Ophthalmol.* 1858;4:1.

2. Drance SM, Sweeney VP, Morgan RW, et al. Studies of factors involved in the production

of low tension glaucoma. *Arch Ophthalmol.* 1973;89:457.

3. Stamper RL, Leiberman MF, Drake MV, eds. *Becker and Shaffer's: Diagnosis and Therapy of the Glaucomas.* 7th ed. St. Louis: Mosby; 1999.

4. Chandler PA. Long term results in glaucoma therapy. *Am J Ophthalmol.* 1960;49:221–246.

5. Kass MA, Gordon MO, Hoff MR, et al. Topical timolol administration reduces the incidence of glaucomatous damage in ocular hypertensive individuals. A randomized, double masked, long term study. *Arch Ophthalmol.* 1989;107:1590–1598.

6. Epstein DL, Krug JH Jr, Hertzmark E, et al. A long term clinical trial of clinical therapy versus no treatment in the management of glaucoma suspects. *Ophthalmology.* 1989;96:1460–1476.

7. Schulzer M, Drance SM, Douglas GR. A comparison of treated and untreated glaucoma suspects. *Ophthalmology.* 1991;98:301–307.

8. Gordon MO, Kass MA. The ocular hypertension treatment study: design and baseline description of the participants. *Arch Ophthalmol.* 1999;117:573–583.

9. Johnson CA, Keltner JL, Cello KE, et al. Baseline visual field characteristics in the ocular hypertension treatment study. *Ophthalmology.* 2002;109:432–437.

10. Kass MA, Heuer DK, Higginbotham EJ, et al. The Ocular Hypertension Treatment Study: A randomized trial determines that topical ocular hypotensive medication delays or prevents the onset of primary open-angle glaucoma. *Arch Ophthalmol.* 2002;120:701–713.

11. Gordon MO, Beiser JA, Brandt JD, et al. The Ocular Hypertension Treatment Study: Baseline factors that predict the onset of primary open-angle glaucoma. *Arch Ophthalmol.* 2002;120:714–720.

12. Brandt JD, Beiser JA, Gordon MO, et al. Central corneal thickness and measured IOP response to topical ocular hypotensive medication in the Ocular Hypertension Treatment Study. *Am J Ophthalmol.* 2004;138:717–722.

13. Higginbotham EJ, Gordon MO, Beiser JA, et al. The Ocular Hypertension Treatment Study: Topical medication delays or prevents primary open-angle glaucoma in African American individuals. *Arch Ophthalmol.* 2004;122: 813–820.

14. Keltner JL, Johnson CA, Levine RA, et al. Normal visual field results following glaucomatous visual field end points in the Ocular Hypertension Treatment Study. *Arch Ophthalmol.* 2005;123:1201–1206.

15. The European Glaucoma Prevention Study (EGPS) Group. Results of the European Glaucoma Prevention Study. *Ophthalmology.* 2005; 112:366–375.

16. Sommer A, Tielsch JM, Katz J, et al. Relationship between intraocular pressure and primary open-angle glaucoma among white and black Americans. *Arch Ophthalmol.* 1991; 109:1090–1095.

17. Grant WM, Burk JF Jr. Why do some people go blind from glaucoma? *Ophthalmology.* 1982;89:991–998.

18. Odberg T. Visual field prognosis in advanced glaucoma. *Acta Ophthalmol (Copenh).* 1987;65: 27–29.

19. Mao LK, Stewart WC, Shields MB. Correlation between intraocular pressure control and progressive glaucomatous damage in primary open angle glaucoma. *Am J Ophthalmol.* 1991;111:51–55.

20. Jay JL, Allan D. The benefit of early trabeculectomy versus conventional management in primary open angle glaucoma relative to severity of disease. *Eye.* 1989;3:528–535.

21. Crick RP, Newson RB, Shipley MJ, et al. The prognosis of the visual field in chronic simple glaucoma and ocular hypertension treated topically with pilocarpine or with timolol. *Eye.* 1990;4:563–571.

22. Leske MC, Heijl A, Hyman L, et al. Early manifest glaucoma trial: Design and baseline data. *Ophthalmology.* 1999;106:2144–2153.

23. Heijl A, Leske MC, Bengtsson B, et al. Reduction of intraocular pressure and glaucoma progression: Results from the Early Manifest Glaucoma Trial. *Arch Ophthalmol.* 2002;120:1268–1279.

24. Lichter PR. Expectations from clinical trials: Results of the early manifest glaucoma trial. *Arch Ophthalmol.* 2002;120:1371–1372.

25. Leske MC, Heijl A, Hussein M, et al. Factors for glaucoma progression and the effect of treatment: The early manifest glaucoma trial. *Arch Ophthalmol.* 2003;121:48–56.

26. Heijl A, Leske MC, Bengtsson B, et al. Measuring visual field progression in the early

manifest glaucoma trial. *Acta Ophthalmol Scand.* 2003;81:286–293.

27. Leske MC, Heijl A, Hyman L, et al. Factors for progression and glaucoma treatment: The early manifest glaucoma trial. *Curr Opin Ophthalmol.* 2004;15:102–106.

28. Hyman LG, Komaroff E, Heijl A, et al. Treatment and vision related quality of life in the early manifest glaucoma trial. *Ophthalmology.* 2005;112:1505–1513.

29. Schulzer M, The Normal Tension Glaucoma Study Group. Intraocular pressure reduction in normal-tension glaucoma patients. *Ophthalmology.* 1992;99:1468–1470.

30. Collaborative Normal-Tension Glaucoma Study Group. Comparison of glaucomatous progression between untreated patients with normal-tension glaucoma and patients with therapeutically reduced intraocular pressures. *Am J Ophthalmol.* 1998;126:487–497.

31. Collaborative Normal-Tension Glaucoma Study Group. The effectiveness of intraocular pressure reduction in the treatment of normal-tension glaucoma. *Am J Ophthalmol.* 1998;126:498–505.

32. Drance SM. The Collaborative Normal-Tension Glaucoma Study and some of its lessons. *Can J Ophthalmol.* 1999;34:1–6.

33. Drance SM, Anderson DR, Schulzer M, et al. Risk factors for progression of visual field abnormalities in normal-tension glaucoma. *Am J Ophthalmol.* 2001;131:699–708.

34. Anderson DR. Collaborative normal tension glaucoma study. *Curr Opin Ophthalmol.* 2003;14:86–90.

35. Musch DC, Lichter PR, Guire KE, et al. The Collaborative Initial Glaucoma Treatment Study: Study design, methods, and baseline characteristics of enrolled patients. *Ophthalmology.* 1999;106:653–662.

36. Janz NK, Wren PA, Lichter PR, et al. Quality of life in newly diagnosed glaucoma patients: The Collaborative Initial Glaucoma Treatment Study. *Ophthalmology.* 2001;108:887–897.

37. Mills RP, Janz NK, Wren PA, et al. Correlation of visual field with quality-of-life measures at diagnosis in the Collaborative Initial Glaucoma Treatment Study (CIGTS). *J Glaucoma.* 2001;10:192–198.

38. Lichter PR, Musch DC, Gillespie BW, et al. Interim clinical outcomes in the Collaborative Initial Glaucoma Treatment Study comparing initial treatment randomized to medications or surgery. *Ophthalmology.* 2001;108:1943–1953.

39. Janz NK, Wren PA, Lichter PR, et al. The Collaborative Initial Glaucoma Treatment Study: Interim quality of life findings after initial medical or surgical treatment of glaucoma. *Ophthalmology.* 2001;108:1954–1965.

40. Gillespie BW, Musch DC, Guire KE, et al. The collaborative initial glaucoma treatment study: Baseline visual field and test-retest variability. *Invest Ophthalmol Vis Sci.* 2003;44:2613–2620.

41. Jampel HD, Musch DC, Gillespie BW, et al. Perioperative complications of trabeculectomy in the collaborative initial glaucoma treatment study (CIGTS). *Am J Ophthalmol.* 2005;140:16–22.

42. Glaucoma Laser Trial Research Group. The Glaucoma Laser Trial. 1. Acute effects of argon laser trabeculoplasty on intraocular pressure. *Arch Ophthalmol.* 1989;107:1135–1142.

43. Glaucoma Laser Trial Research Group. The Glaucoma Laser Trial (GLT). 2. Results of argon laser trabeculoplasty versus topical medicines. *Ophthalmology.* 1990;97:1403–1413.

44. Glaucoma Laser Trial Research Group. The Glaucoma Laser Trial (GLT): 3. Design and methods. *Control Clin Trials.* 1991;12:504–524.

45. GLT Research Group. The Glaucoma Laser Trial: 4. Contralateral effects of timolol on the intraocular pressure of eyes treated with ALT. *Ophthalmic Surg.* 1991;22:324–329.

46. Glaucoma Laser Trial Research Group (GLT): 5. Subgroup differences at enrollment. *Ophthalmic Surg.* 1993;24:232–240.

47. Glaucoma Laser Trial Research Group. The Glaucoma Laser Trial (GLT): 6. Treatment group differences in visual field changes. *Am J Ophthalmol.* 1995;120:10–22.

48. Glaucoma Laser Trial Research Group. The Glaucoma Laser Trial (GLT) and glaucoma laser trial follow-up study: 7. Results. *Am J Ophthalmol.* 1995;120:718–731.

49. Lewis RA, Hayreh SS, Phelps CD. Optic disk and visual field correlations in primary open-angle and low-tension glaucoma. *Am J Ophthalmol.* 1983;96:148–152.

50. Chumbley LC, Brubaker RF. Low-tension glaucoma. *Am J Ophthalmol.* 1976;81:761–767.

51. Caprioli J, Spaeth GL. Comparison of visual field defects in the low-tension glaucomas with

those in the high-tension glaucomas. *Am J Ophthalmol.* 1984;97:730–737.

52. Migdal C, Hitchings R. Control of chronic simple glaucoma with primary medical, surgical and laser treatment. *Trans Ophthalmol Soc U K.* 1986;105:653–656.

53. Jay JL, Murray SB. Early trabeculectomy versus conventional management in primary open angle glaucoma. *Br J Ophthalmol.* 1988; 72:881–889.

54. Migdal C, Gregory W, Hitchings R. Long-term functional outcome after early surgery compared with laser and medicine in open-angle glaucoma. *Ophthalmology.* 1994;101: 1651–1656.

55. Wise JB, Witter SL. Argon laser therapy for open-angle glaucoma: A Pilot Study. *Arch Ophthalmol.* 1979;79:319–322.

56. Zimmerman TJ, Kass MA, Yablonski ME, et al. Timolol maleate: Efficacy and safety. *Arch Ophthalmol.* 1979;97:656–658.

57. Chung PY, Schuman JS, Netland PA, et al. Five-year results of a randomized, prospective, clinical trial of diode vs argon laser trabeculoplasty for open-angle glaucoma. *Am J Ophthalmol.* 1998;126:185–190.

58. Latina MA, Tumbocon JA. Selective laser trabeculoplasty: A new treatment option for open angle glaucoma. *Curr Opin Ophthalmol.* 2002;13:94–96.

59. Sugar HD. Experimental trabeculectomy in glaucoma. *Am J Ophthalmol.* 1961;51:623.

60. Cairns JE. Trabeculectomy: Preliminary report of a new method. *Am J Ophthalmol.* 1968;66: 672–679.

61. Sugar HS. Limboscleral trepanation: Eleven year's experience. *Arch Ophthalmol.* 1971;85: 703–708.

62. Viswanathan B, Brown IAR. Peripheral iridectomy with scleral cautery for glaucoma. *Arch Ophthalmol.* 1975;93:34–35.

63. The AGIS Investigators. The Advanced Glaucoma Intervention Study (AGIS): 3. Baseline characteristics of black and white patients. *Ophthalmology.* 1998;105:1137–1145.

64. The AGIS Investigators. The Advanced Intervention Study (AGIS): 1. Study design and methods and baseline characteristics of study patients. *Control Clin Trials.* 1994;15:299–325.

65. The AGIS Investigators. Advanced Glaucoma Intervention Study. 2. Visual field scoring and reliability. *Ophthalmology.* 1994;101:1445–1455.

66. The AGIS Investigators. The Advanced Glaucoma Intervention Study (AGIS): 7. The relationship between control of intraocular pressure and visual field deterioration. *Am J Ophthalmol.* 2000;130:429–440.

67. The AGIS Investigators. The Advanced Glaucoma Intervention Study (AGIS): 4. Comparison of treatment outcomes within race. Seven-year results. *Ophthalmology.* 1998;105:1146–1164.

68. AGIS Investigators. The Advanced Glaucoma Intervention Study (AGIS): 9. Comparison of glaucoma outcomes in black and white patients within treatment groups. *Am J Ophthalmol.* 2001;132:311–320.

69. Ederer F, Gaasterland DA, Dally LG, et al. The Advanced Glaucoma Intervention Study (AGIS): 13. Comparison of treatment outcomes within race: 10-year results. *Ophthalmology.* 2004;111:651–664.

70. The AGIS Investigators. The advanced glaucoma intervention study, 6: Effect of cataract on visual field and visual acuity. *Arch Ophthalmol.* 2000;118:1639–1659.

71. AGIS (Advanced Glaucoma Intervention Study) Investigators. The Advanced Glaucoma Intervention Study: 8. Risk of cataract formation after trabeculectomy. *Arch Ophthalmol.* 2001;119:1771–1779.

72. Richter CU, Shingleton BJ, Bellows AR, et al. The development of encapsulated filtering blebs. *Ophthalmology.* 1988;95:1163–1168.

73. Feldman RM, Gross RL, Spaeth GL, et al. Risk factors for the development of Tenon's capsule cysts after trabeculectomy. *Ophthalmology.* 1989;96:336–334.

74. AGIS Investigators. The Advanced Glaucoma Intervention Study (AGIS): 11. Risk factors for failure of trabeculectomy and argon laser trabeculoplasty. *Am J Ophthalmol.* 2002; 134:481–498.

75. Schwartz AL, Van Veldhuisen PC, Gaasterland DE, et al. The Advanced Glaucoma Intervention Study (AGIS): 5. Encapsulated bleb after initial trabeculectomy. *Am J Ophthalmol.* 1999;127:8–19.

76. AGIS Investigators. The Advanced Glaucoma Intervention Study (AGIS): 12. Baseline risk factors for sustained loss of visual field and

visual acuity in patients with advanced glaucoma. *Am J Ophthalmol.* 2002;134:499–512.

77. Nouri-Mahdavi K, Hoffman D, Coleman AL, et al. Predictive factors for glaucomatous visual field progression in the Advanced Glaucoma Intervention Study. *Ophthalmology.* 2004;111:1627–1635.

78. Lamping KA, Bellows AR, Hutchinson BT, Afran SI. Long-term evaluation of initial filtration surgery. *Ophthalmology.* 1986;93:91–101.

79. The Fluorouracil Filtering Surgery Group. Fluorouracil Filtering Surgery Study one-year follow-up. *Am J Ophthalmol.* 1989;108:625–635.

80. The Fluorouracil Filtering Surgery Study Group. Risk factors for suprachoroidal hemorrhage after filtering surgery. *Am J Ophthalmol.* 1992;113:501–507.

81. The Fluorouracil Filtering Surgery Study Group. Three-year follow-up of the Fluorouracil Filtering Surgery Study. *Am J Ophthalmol.* 1993;115:82–92.

82. The Fluorouracil Filtering Surgery Study Group. Five-year follow-up of the Fluorouracil Filtering Surgery Study. *Am J Ophthalmol.* 1996;121:349–366.

83. Parrish II RK, Schiffman JC, Feuer WJ, et al. Prognosis and risk factors for early postoperative wound leaks after trabeculectomy with and without 5-fluorouracil. *Am J Ophthalmol.* 2001;132:633–640.

84. Chen CW, Huang HTBair JS, et al. Trabeculectomy with simultaneous topical application of mitomycin-C in refractory glaucoma. *J Ocul Pharmacol.* 1990;6:175–182.

85. Palmer SS. Mitomycin as adjunctive chemotherapy with trabeculectomy. *Ophthalmology.* 1991;98:317–321.

86. Singh K, Mehta K, Shaikh NM, et al. Trabeculectomy with Intraoperative mitomycin C versus 5-fluorouracil. Prospective randomized clinical trial. *Ophthalmology.* 2000;107:2305–2309.

87. WuDunn D, Cantor LB, Palanca-Capistrano AM, et al. A prospective randomized trial comparing Intraoperative 5-fluorouracil vs mitomycin C in primary trabeculectomy. *Am J Ophthalmol.* 2002;143:521–528.

88. Jampel HD, Friedman DS, Lubomski LH, et al. Effect of technique on intraocular pressure after combined cataract and glaucoma surgery: An evidenced-based review. *Ophthalmology.* 2002;109:2215–2224.

89. Krasnov MM. Externalization of Schlemm's canal (sinusotomy) in glaucoma. *Br J Ophthalmol.* 1968;52:157–161.

90. Shaarawy T, Mansouri K, Schnyder C, et al. Long-term results of deep sclerectomy with collagen implant. *J Cataract Refract Surg.* 2004;30:1225–1231.

91. Cillino S, Di Pace F, Casuccio A, et al. Deep sclerectomy versus punch trabeculectomy with or without phacoemeulsification. A randomized clinical trial. *J Glaucoma.* 2004;13:500–506.

92. Stegmann R, Pienaar A, Miller D. Viscocanalostomy for open-angle glaucoma in black African patients. *J Cataract Refract Surg.* 1999;25:316–322.

93. Smit BA, Johnstone MD. Effects of viscoelastic injection into Schlemm's canal in primate and human eyes. Potential relevance to viscocanalostomy. *Ophthalmology.* 2002;109:786–792.

94. Shaarawy T, Nguyen C, Schnyder C, et al. Five year results of viscocanalostomy. *Br J Ophthalmol.* 2003;87:441–445.

95. Wishart PK, Wishart MS, Porooshani H. Viscocanalostomy and deep sclerectomy for the surgical treatment of glaucoma: A longterm follow-up. *Acta Ophthalmol Scand.* 2003;81:343–348.

96. Van Buskirk EM, Pond V, Rosenquist RC, et al. Argon laser trabeculoplasty. Studies of mechanism of action. *Ophthalmology.* 1984;91:1005–1010.

97. Thomas JV, Simmons RJ, Belcher CD III. Argon laser trabeculoplasty in the pre-surgical glaucoma patient. *Ophthalmology.* 1982;89:187–197.

98. Hoskins HD Jr, Hetherington J Jr, Minckler DS, et al. Complications of laser trabeculoplasty. *Ophthalmology.* 1983;90:796–769.

99. Greenidge KC, Rodrigues MM, Spaeth GL, et al. Acute intraocular pressure elevation after argon laser trabeculoplasty and iridectomy: A Clinicopathologic Study. *Ophthalmic Surg.* 1984;15:105–110.

100. Gasaterland D, Kupfer B. Experimental glaucoma in the rhesus monkey. *Invest Ophthalmol.* 1974;13:455–457.

101. Latina MA, Park C. Selective targeting of trabecular meshwork cells: in vitro studies of

pulsed and CW laser interactions. *Exp Eye Res.* 1995;60:359–371.

102. Latina MA, Sibayan SA, Shin DH, et al. Q-switched 532-nm Nd:YAG laser trabeculoplasty (selective laser trabeculoplasty): A Multicenter, Pilot, Clinical Study. *Ophthalmology.* 1998;105:2082–2090.

103. Damji KF, Shah KC, Rock WJ, et al. Selective laser trabeculoplasty v argon laser trabeculoplasty: a prospective randomized clinical trial. *Br J Ophthalmol.* 1999;83:718–722.

104. Hodge WG, Damji KF, Rock W, et al. Baseline IOP predicts selective laser trabeculoplasty success at 1 year post-treatment: Results from a randomized clinical trial. *Br J Ophthalmol.* 2005;89:1157–1160.

105. Juzych MS, Chopra V, Banitt MR, et al. Comparison of long-term outcomes of selective laser trabeculoplasty versus argon laser trabeculoplasty in open-angle glaucoma. *Ophthalmology.* 2004;111:1853–1859.

106. Melamed S, Ben Simon G, Levkovitch-Verbin H. Selective laser trabeculoplasty as primary treatment for open-angle glaucoma. A prospective, nonrandomized Pilot Study. *Arch Ophthalmol.* 2003;121:957–960.

107. Nagar M, Ogunyomade A, O'Brart DPS, et al. A randomized, prospective study comparing selective laser trabeculoplasty with latanoprost for the control of intraocular pressure in ocular hypertension and open angle glaucoma. *Br J Ophthalmol.* 2005;89:1413–1417.

108. Eddy DM, Billings J. The quality of medical evidence: implications for quality of care. *Health Aff (Millwood).* 1988;7:19–32.

SECTION IV
RETINA

CHAPTER **6A**

Diabetic Retinopathy: Prevention and Screening

Dean Eliott, MD

Clinical Trials and Epidemologic Studies

Diabetes Control and Complications Trial

Introduction

Long-term microvascular and neurologic complications cause considerable morbidity and mortality in patients with insulin-dependent diabetes mellitus. These complications develop over a period of years, and in the 1960s, there was evidence to suggest that the underlying cause is chronic elevation of blood glucose. Subsequently, there was controversy as to whether improved control of blood glucose would reduce the chronic complications of diabetes, including diabetic retinopathy.[1-7] If such a relationship existed, and if improved control of blood glucose could be achieved, then there would be potential benefit in pursuing effective treatment strategies to reduce blood glucose levels. However, the effects of such intervention might not become apparent for years, and maintaining blood glucose concentrations as close to the normal range as possible (normoglycemia) has associated costs and potential complications. To address these questions of considerable public health importance, a prospective, multicenter, randomized, controlled clinical trial was needed.

Background and Study Questions

The Diabetes Control and Complications Trial (DCCT) was established in the 1980s to determine whether improved control of blood glucose levels would reduce the frequency and severity of diabetic retinopathy and other chronic complications of diabetes.[8] Improved control of blood glucose was termed *intensive control*, with the goal of achieving normoglycemia.

Patients Included in the Study

A total of 1,441 patients with type 1 diabetes, aged between 13 and 39, with no retinopathy and a duration of diabetes of 1 to 5 years (the primary-prevention cohort, 726 patients) or mild to moderate nonproliferative retinopathy and a duration of diabetes of 1 to 15 years (the secondary-intervention cohort, 715 patients) were enrolled.

Intervention and Outcome Measures

Patients were randomly assigned to intensive or conventional insulin therapy. Intensive therapy consisted of the use of an external insulin pump (continuous subcutaneous insulin infusion) or three or more daily insulin injections, and was guided by four or more blood glucose tests daily (doses adjusted on the basis of self-monitoring). Conventional therapy involved one or two daily insulin injections and once-daily monitoring. Outcome measures included

the appearance and progression of retinopathy using the Early Treatment Diabetic Retinopathy Study (ETDRS) retinopathy severity scale (see Tables 6A.1 and 6A.2) and systemic findings related to nephropathy and neuropathy.

Major Findings

At a mean follow-up of 6.5 years (range 3.5 to 9 years) in the primary-prevention cohort, intensive therapy reduced the risk of developing retinopathy by 76% as compared with conventional therapy. In the secondary-intervention cohort, intensive therapy slowed the progression of retinopathy by 54% and reduced the development of severe nonproliferative or proliferative retinopathy by 47%. In both cohorts, intensive therapy reduced the occurrence of microalbuminuria and albuminuria, and clinical neuropathy.[9-11]

Cumulative 8.5-year rates of progression of retinopathy by three or more steps at two consecutive visits were 12% with intensive treatment as compared to 54% with conventional treatment in the primary-prevention cohort and 17% as compared to 49% in the secondary-intervention cohort (see Fig. 6A.1). Once progression occurred, subsequent recovery was

TABLE 6A.1 ◻ Abbreviated Summary of the Final Version of the Early Treatment Diabetic Retinopathy Study Scale of Diabetic Retinopathy Severity for Individual Eyes

Level	Severity	Definition
10	No retinopathy	Diabetic retinopathy absent
20	Very mild NPDR	Microaneurysms only
35	Mild NPDR	Microaneurysm plus hard exudates, soft exudates (cotton-wool spots) and/or mild retinal hemorrhages
43	Moderate NPDR	Microaneurysms plus mild IRMA or moderate retinal hemorrhages
47	Moderate NPDR	More extensive IRMA, severe retinal hemorrhages, or venous beading in one quadrant only
53	Severe NPDR	Severe retinal hemorrhages in 4 quadrants, or venous beading in at least 2 quadrants, or moderately severe IRMA in at least 1 quadrant
61	Mild PDR	NVE <1/2 disc area in 1 or more quadrants
65	Moderate PDR	NVE ≥1/2 disc area in 1 or more quadrants, or NVD <1/4−1/3 disc area
71−75	High-risk PDR	NVD ≥1/4−1/3 disc area and/or vitreous hemorrhage
81−85	Advanced PDR	Fundus partially obscured

NPDR, nonproliferative diabetic retinopathy; PDR, proliferative diabetic retinopathy; IRMA, intraretinal microvascular abnormalities; NVE, neovascularization elsewhere; NVD, new vessels on or within 1 disc diameter of optic disc. From Diabetes Control and Complications Trial Research Group. The effect of intensive diabetes treatment on the progression of diabetic retinopathy in insulin-dependent diabetes mellitus. *Arch Ophthalmol.* 1995;113:36−51.

TABLE 6A.2 ☐ Abbreviated Final Version of the Early Treatment Diabetic Retinopathy Study Scale of Diabetic Retinopathy Severity for Individual Patients

Step	Level (worse eye/ better eye)
1	10/10
2	20/<20
3	20/20
4	35/<35
5	35/35
6	43/<43
7	43/43
8	47/<47
9	47/47
10	53/<53
11	53/53
12–23	61/<61 or greater

From Diabetes Control and Complications Trial Research Group. The effect of intensive diabetes treatment on the progression of diabetic retinopathy in insulin-dependent diabetes mellitus. *Arch Ophthalmol.* 1995;113:36–51.

at least two times more likely with intensive treatment than with conventional treatment.[12]

The level of glycemic exposure (HbA_{1c}) measured at eligibility screening and the duration of insulin-dependent diabetes were the dominant baseline predictors of the risk of progression.[13] The intensive treatment group achieved a median HbA_{1c} of 7.2% as compared to 9.1% in the conventional treatment group. Mean blood glucose was 155 mg per dL in the intensive treatment group and 230 mg per dL in the conventional group.

The major adverse event associated with intensive therapy was a two- to three-fold increase in severe hypoglycemia.[9] At the 6- and 12-month visits, a small adverse effect of intensive treatment occurred, termed *early worsening of retinopathy*. Worsening was defined as any of the following: Progression of retinopathy >3 steps, the development of soft exudates and/or intraretinal microvascular abnormalities, or the development of clinically important retinopathy (clinically significant diabetic macular edema [CSDME], severe nonproliferative diabetic retinopathy [NPDR], retinal neovascularization elsewhere [NVE], or neovascularization of the optic disc [NVD]). Worsening was considered early if it

occurred between baseline and the 12-month follow-up visit. Early worsening was noted in 13% of patients undergoing intensive treatment and in 8% undergoing conventional treatment. Risk factors were higher HbA_{1c} level at screening, and reduction in this level during the first 6 months of the study (but not related to the rate of reduction).[14] Early worsening was followed by a beneficial effect that increased with follow-up duration,[12] and the long-term benefits of intensive treatment greatly outweighed the risks of early worsening.

Implications for Clinical Practice

The DCCT demonstrated the powerful impact of glycemic control on the microvascular complications of diabetes mellitus. In patients with insulin-dependent diabetes who met the inclusion criteria, intensive insulin therapy as administered in this trial delayed the onset effectively and slowed the progression of diabetic retinopathy, nephropathy, and neuropathy.

The DCCT concluded that the beneficial effect of intensive treatment in slowing the progression of retinopathy was very substantial, increased with time, was consistent across all outcome measures assessed, and was present across the spectrum of retinopathy severity included in the study.

However, intensive therapy did not prevent retinopathy completely, and it was associated with early worsening in some patients with long-standing poor glycemic control (elevated HbA_{1c}), especially if retinopathy was at or beyond the moderate nonproliferative stage. In such patients, examination before initiation of intensive treatment and at frequent (3- to 4-month) intervals for the first year was recommended. In patients with elevated HbA_{1c} whose retinopathy approached high risk, prompt photocoagulation was recommended if intensive treatment was to be initiated.[14] The magnitude, but not the rapidity, of the reduction in HbA_{1c} during the first 6 months of intensive treatment was an important risk factor for early worsening.

Despite this, intensive treatment had a remarkable beneficial effect that began after 3 years of therapy on all levels of retinopathy that were studied.[15] The reduction in risk observed in the DCCT translated into a reduced need for laser treatment and reduced risk of visual loss, and the DCCT recommendation was to implement intensive treatment as early as possible in as many patients with insulin-dependent diabetes as is safely possible.

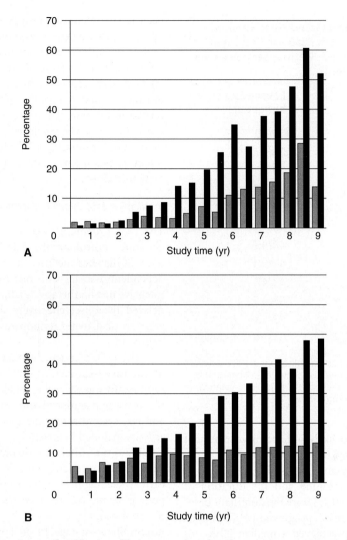

FIGURE 6A.1 ☐ Percentage of patients with progression by three or more steps at each semiannual follow-up visit for the intensive (shaded bars) and conventional (solid bars) treatment groups in the primary-prevention **(A)** and secondary-intervention **(B)** cohorts. (From Diabetes Control and Complications Trial Research Group. The effect of intensive diabetes treatment on the progression of diabetic retinopathy in insulin-dependent diabetes mellitus. *Arch Ophthalmol.* 1995;113:36–51.)

The Epidemiology of Diabetes Interventions and Complications (EDIC) study assessed whether the benefits demonstrated in the DCCT persisted after the end of the DCCT. This study concluded that the benefits associated with intensive treatment extended well beyond the period of intensive implementation. The recommendation was that once intensive treatment was initiated in patients with insulin-dependent diabetes, it should be maintained thereafter, aiming for a target HbA_{1c} level of 7.0% or less (normal 3.0% to 6.0%) and a fasting blood glucose level of 110 mg per dL or less.[16]

Unanswered Questions

The DCCT demonstrated a substantial beneficial effect of intensive insulin therapy in slowing down the progression of retinopathy. Although this treatment effect increased during the follow-up period, its relation to long-term functional outcome can be only estimated.

Inclusion criteria for the DCCT were the absence of retinopathy or the presence of mild to moderate nonproliferative retinopathy, while patients with more advanced levels of retinopathy were excluded from the study. When early worsening occurred in the study patients, it was not associated with any cases of serious visual loss. It is possible, however, that patients with severe nonproliferative or proliferative diabetic retinopathy may experience early worsening that is clinically relevant when intensive treatment is initiated. Although increased surveillance and a lower threshold for photocoagulation are recommended for these patients when intensive treatment is initiated, the early effects of intensive treatment are unknown.[12]

Furthermore, the disease process appears to have considerable momentum, as evidenced by the number of years of intensive therapy required before a treatment effect becomes manifest. In patients with advanced retinopathy, although the long-term effects are unknown, it is unlikely that intensive treatment alone can halt the progression.[15]

Wisconsin Epidemiologic Study of Diabetic Retinopathy

Introduction

In the 1970s, there was limited data concerning the epidemiology of diabetic retinopathy. Information on the prevalence and severity of retinopathy in a large cohort of patients with diabetes was needed to plan a well-coordinated approach to this important public health problem. To recommend the guidelines for ophthalmologic care, patients with a broad distribution of retinopathy severity needed to be examined and followed up, and patients with risk factors for developing visual loss from diabetic retinopathy needed to be identified. Such data would also be helpful in planning future clinical trials to better define etiologic relationships and to assess the effects of new treatments.

The Wisconsin Epidemiologic Study of Diabetic Retinopathy (WESDR) was established to address these issues. The WESDR was a cross-sectional and longitudinal study designed to provide data on the prevalence, severity, incidence, and progression of diabetic retinopathy in a geographically defined population of patients with diabetes. It was the largest and the most comprehensive epidemiologic study of diabetic retinopathy.

Background and Study Questions

Established in the late 1970s, the WESDR sought (a) to describe the prevalence and severity of diabetic retinopathy and its component lesions, and to determine the frequency of visual impairment in a total population of patients with diabetes who were under physicians' care in a defined geographic region, and (b) to determine the relationships between risk factors, prevalence, and severity of diabetic retinopathy in these patients.

Patients Included in the Study

The patient population described in the WESDR was obtained in the following manner. In an 11-county area in southern Wisconsin, 452 primary care physicians (99% of total) provided charts of all the patients with diabetes they had seen over a 1-year period. Approximately 10,000 charts were identified and reviewed, and a sample of approximately 3,000 patients was selected for examination.

Intervention and Outcome Measures

Patients were examined in the early 1980s to determine the prevalence and severity of diabetic retinopathy and associated risk variables. The WESDR cohort was reexamined periodically thereafter to determine the incidence and progression of visual impairment and retinopathy. Both the younger- and older-onset groups were reexamined 4 and 10 years later, but only the younger-onset group was reexamined at the 14-year follow-up due to the high death rate among older-onset patients.

Outcome measures included visual acuity using the ETDRS protocol: Visual impairment, grouped into four levels (no impairment: >20/40, mild impairment: 20/40 to 20/63, moderate impairment: 20/80 to 20/160, blind: <20/200); the relative contribution of diabetic retinopathy in eyes with impaired vision; the severity and progression of diabetic retinopathy using a modification of the Airlie House classification scheme that specifies nine levels;[17] the presence of macular edema; and metabolic control as determined by glycosylated hemoglobin and protein levels in the urine.

Major Findings

Fifteen percent of patients were diagnosed with diabetes before 30 years of age and were taking insulin (younger-onset group), while 85% were diagnosed at 30 years of age or older (older-onset group). The older-onset patients had their diagnosis confirmed by a random or postprandial serum glucose level of at least 200 mg per dL or a fasting level of at least 140 mg per dL, and approximately 50% of these patients were taking insulin.

Visual impairment (visual acuity in the better eye <20/40) increased with increasing age. Legal blindness (visual acuity in the better eye <20/200) was related to the duration of diabetes in both the younger- and the older-onset groups. In the younger-onset group, legal blindness was present in 3.6% of patients, and diabetes was at least partly responsible in 86% of such patients. In the older-onset group, legal blindness was present in 1.6%, and diabetes was a cause in 33%.[18]

In the younger-onset group, the prevalence of diabetic retinopathy was 17% in patients with diabetes for <5 years and 98% for those with diabetes for >15 years. Proliferative retinopathy was present in 23%. Retinopathy severity was related to longer duration of diabetes and higher levels of glycosylated hemoglobin (see Fig. 6A.2).[19] In the older-onset group, the prevalence of retinopathy was 29% in patients with diabetes for <5 years and 78% in those with diabetes for >15 years. Proliferative disease was present in 9%. Retinopathy severity was related to longer duration of diabetes, younger age at diagnosis, higher glycosylated hemoglobin levels, higher systolic blood pressure, and the use of insulin (see Fig. 6A.3).[20]

In the younger-onset group, the prevalence of macular edema varied from 0% in those with diabetes for <5 years to 29% in those with diabetes for >20 years. In the older-onset group, prevalence rates of

macular edema varied from 3% in those with diabetes for <5 years to 28% in those with diabetes for >20 years. Macular edema was associated with a longer duration of diabetes, higher glycosylated hemoglobin level, and the presence of proteinuria.[21]

In the younger-onset group, the prevalence rate was 14% for panretinal photocoagulation and 4% for focal laser, and in the older-onset group, the rates were 4% and 3%, respectively. At the time of the WESDR, focal treatment for macular edema had not been proved to be efficacious.[22]

At the 4-year follow-up examination, the rates of blindness were 1.5% in the younger-onset patients, 3.2% in the older-onset insulin users, and 2.7% in the older-onset nonusers of insulin. The rate of blindness increased with increasing age, increasing retinopathy severity, and lower baseline visual acuity in all three groups.[23] The 4-year incidence of retinopathy (59%, 47%, and 34%) and the progression to proliferative disease (11%, 7%, and 2%) were highest in the younger-onset group, intermediate in the older-onset insulin user group, and lowest in the older-onset insulin nonuser group, respectively (see Table 6A.3).[24,25]

At the 10-year follow-up examination, the incidence of blindness was 1.8% in the younger-onset patients, 4.0% in the older-onset insulin users, and 4.8% in the older-onset nonusers of insulin.[26] The 10-year incidence of retinopathy (89%, 79%, and 67%) and the progression to proliferative disease (30%, 24%, and 10%) were highest in the younger-onset group, intermediate in the older-onset insulin

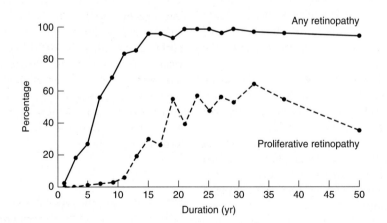

FIGURE 6A.2 ◻ Frequency of retinopathy or proliferative retinopathy for patients with younger-onset diabetes by duration of diabetes (in years). (From Klein R, Klein BEK, Moss SE, et al. The Wisconsin Epidemiologic Study of Diabetic Retinopathy II: Prevalence and risk of diabetic retinopathy when age at diagnosis is less than 30 years. *Arch Ophthalmol.* 1984;102:520–526.)

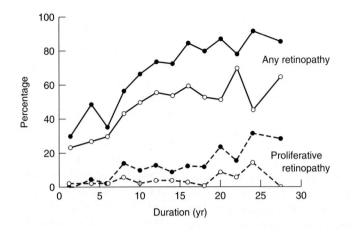

FIGURE 6A.3 ☐ Frequency of retinopathy or proliferative retinopathy for patients with older-onset diabetes by duration of diabetes (in years) for insulin users (black circles or black squares) and nonusers of insulin (white circles or white squares). (From Klein R, Klein BEK, Moss SE, et al. The Wisconsin Epidemiologic Study of Diabetic Retinopathy III: Prevalence and risk of diabetic retinopathy when age at diagnosis is 30 or more years. *Arch Ophthalmol.* 1984;102:527–532.)

user group, and lowest in the older-onset insulin nonuser group, respectively (Table 6A.3).[27]

At the 14-year follow-up examination, the incidence of blindness was 2.4%, the rate of progression to proliferative disease was 37%, and the incidence of macular edema was 26%. Visual loss (doubling of the visual angle) was associated with older age, longer duration of diabetes, higher glycosylated hemoglobin, higher systolic and diastolic blood pressure, the presence of proteinuria, more pack-years smoked, the presence of macular edema, and more severe retinopathy.[28,29]

There was a strong association between glycosylated hemoglobin levels and multiple outcomes. At both the 4- and 10-year follow-up visits, for all three groups (younger-onset, older-onset insulin users, older-onset nonusers of insulin), there was a statistically significant relationship between glycosylated

TABLE 6A.3 ☐ **Rate of blindness, incidence of retinopathy, and progression to proliferative disease at the 4- and 10-year follow-up examinations for younger-onset patients, older-onset insulin users, and older-onset nonusers of insulin in the Wisconsin Epidemiologic Study of Diabetic Retinopathy**

	4-y Follow-up Examination			10-y Follow-up Examination		
	Younger-onset Patients	Older-onset Patients Taking Insulin	Older-onset Patients Not Taking Insulin	Younger-onset Patients	Older-onset Patients Taking Insulin	Older-onset Patients Not Taking Insulin
Rate of blindness	1.5%	3.2%	2.7%	1.8%	4.0%	4.8%
Incidence of retinopathy	59%	47%	34%	89%	79%	67%
Progression to proliferative disease	11%	7%	2%	30%	24%	10%

hemoglobin and the incidence of retinopathy, progression of retinopathy, and progression to proliferative retinopathy. At the 10-year follow-up visit, this relationship existed for macular edema also in the younger- and older-onset groups and for visual loss in the younger-onset group and the older-onset insulin user group.[30,31] At the 14-year follow-up visit, glycosylated hemoglobin level was associated with doubling of the visual angle.[28]

An important relationship also existed between hypertension and the incidence and progression of diabetic retinopathy. Elevation of both systolic and diastolic blood pressure was associated with an increased risk of developing proliferative retinopathy in the younger-onset and older-onset insulin user groups.[32]

Dyslipidemia, particularly in patients with diabetes with poor glycemic control, is characterized by increased levels of cholesterol, low-density lipoproteins (LDLs), and triglycerides, and by decreased levels of high-density lipoproteins (HDLs). In patients who used insulin, there was a significant trend of increasing severity of retinopathy and retinal hard exudates with increasing cholesterol levels.[33]

Nephropathy is a common microvascular complication of diabetes, and proteinuria was measured in the WESDR. Gross proteinuria was found to be a risk factor for proliferative retinopathy in younger-onset patients.[34]

All-cause and cause-specific mortality was determined from death certificates in the WESDR. The presence of more severe retinopathy or visual impairment in patients with diabetes was a risk indicator for all-cause, stroke, and ischemic heart disease mortality.[35]

Implications for Clinical Practice

The WESDR provided data on the prevalence and severity of diabetic retinopathy, the frequency of visual impairment, and the relationships of risk factors in a geographically defined population of patients with diabetes. Before the WESDR, most information about the prevalence, severity, incidence, and progression of diabetic retinopathy had been derived from specific groups of patients presenting to specific clinics, where patients with severe disease may be overrepresented. This study was unique in that a large cohort with a broad distribution of retinopathy severity was examined at baseline and reexamined 4, 10, and 14 years later.

Longitudinal data from the WESDR has proved valuable in the design of clinical trials that evaluate interventions to prevent incidence of new events or progression of existing lesions. Reliable incidence rates of visual impairment have had important public health uses, such as projecting the need for services and costs, defining etiologic relationships, and assessing the effect of treatment. In addition, information obtained in the WESDR has helped define current guidelines for care in patients with diabetes. For example, ophthalmologic evaluation for the detection of vision-threatening retinopathy is not indicated in patients who are younger than 12 years since proliferative disease is rare in that age group. Thereafter, patients should be under ophthalmologic observation depending on the duration of diabetes and the severity of retinopathy detected. Although the progression from no retinopathy to proliferative disease is low in the first few years after diagnosis in younger-onset patients, the disease shows continued progression with increasing duration. In older-onset patients, proliferative disease is observed after a shorter duration of diabetes, and continued progression occurs with increasing duration. Periodic, lifelong ophthalmologic care is therefore absolutely essential for all patients with diabetes.

In addition to providing data of considerable importance from a public health standpoint, the WESDR has provided clinically useful information for individuals with diabetes. The WESDR demonstrated that several modifiable risk factors are associated with diabetic retinopathy and visual loss. The need for improved glycemic control, at any level of hyperglycemia and at any time during the course of diabetes, and improved control of blood pressure cannot be overemphasized, while control of cholesterol and cessation of smoking are additional recommendations. For patients with diabetes, risk factor modification can have a substantial impact on the vision-threatening complications.

Unanswered Questions

In the WESDR, almost all patients with diabetes in an 11-county area in southern Wisconsin who were seen by their primary care physician during a 1-year period were identified. A sample of these patients was available for ophthalmologic examination. These patients, by definition, demonstrated a level of compliance that may not be representative of the entire diabetic population. In addition, the racial composition of this group may not reflect the demographics of the population as a whole. Since the manifestations of diabetes are related to many factors including compliance and race, the findings of the WESDR may be applicable only to certain patient populations.

Patients were initially examined in the early 1980s, a time when many of the currently accepted treatments for diabetic retinopathy had not yet been proved effective. Some of the findings of the WESDR, therefore, may not be applicable today because of the 25-year evolution of the standard of care. Ironically, it was the WESDR that helped establish the current standard of care by substantially increasing the available epidemiologic data and by identifying modifiable risk factors for diabetic retinopathy.

The WESDR remains one of the most valuable epidemiologic studies ever conducted, as data obtained in the WESDR helped define screening guidelines for ophthalmologic care and helped identify risk factors for retinopathy and visual loss. This study has provided important public health data and clinically useful information for individuals with diabetes.

Beaver Dam Eye Study

Background and Study Questions

In adult individuals, the majority of newly diagnosed cases of diabetes are noninsulin-dependent (type 2). In the 1980s, there were conflicting data regarding the prevalence of diabetic retinopathy at the time of diagnosis of noninsulin-dependent diabetes mellitus (NIDDM), with some studies suggesting that retinopathy is relatively rare, whereas others suggested that retinopathy may appear at or shortly after the time of diagnosis.

To address this and other issues related to diabetic eye disease, the Beaver Dam Eye Study was established. It sought to evaluate the prevalence of diabetic retinopathy in people aged between 43 and 86 with previously diagnosed and newly discovered NIDDM who lived in a defined geographic area. It also sought to determine if relationships existed between older-onset diabetes and cataract, glaucoma, and age-related macular degeneration.

Patients Included in the Study

The patient population described in the Beaver Dam Eye Study was obtained in the following manner. A census of the residents of Beaver Dam, Wisconsin,

was performed in the late 1980s to identify individuals aged between 43 and 84. Almost 6,000 people were identified, and 4,926 (83%) of them were examined. Some people (4.5%) permitted only an interview.

Patients whose diabetes was diagnosed before 30 years of age were excluded from analysis because of the small sample size and because they were typically insulin dependent.

The remaining NIDDM patients ($n = 416$) were divided into one group with newly discovered NIDDM ($n = 49$) and three groups with previously diagnosed diabetes at 30 years of age or after: Insulin users ($n = 79$), those using oral hypoglycemic agents and/or diet ($n = 271$), and those using a combination of oral hypoglycemic agents and insulin ($n = 17$).

Intervention and Outcome Measures

Patients were examined over a 30-month period in the late 1980s to determine the prevalence and severity of diabetic retinopathy in adults with newly discovered and previously diagnosed diabetes.[36] Additional data obtained included standardized grading of lens opacities to determine the prevalence of cataract in the older-onset patients with diabetes;[37] standardized grading of optic discs and cups, measurement of intraocular pressure, and visual field testing to evaluate the relationship of open-angle glaucoma to older-onset diabetes;[38] and standardized grading for lesions associated with age-related maculopathy to examine the association among hyperglycemia, diabetes status, and age-related maculopathy in older-onset patients with diabetes.[39]

The Beaver Dam Eye Study cohort was reexamined 5 and 10 years later to evaluate the change in visual acuity over this period. Of the surviving patients who had participated in the baseline examination, 81% participated in the 5-year follow-up examination,[40] and of these, 83% participated in the 10-year follow-up.[41] Since the longitudinal data did not specifically address changes in patients with diabetes, the results are not covered in this review.

Major Findings

The prevalence of retinopathy was lowest in people with newly discovered NIDDM (10%), intermediate in those who were using oral hypoglycemic agents and/or diet (30%) or oral hypoglycemic agents combined with insulin (35%), and highest in insulin users (70%). Proliferative retinopathy was present in <1%

of nonusers of insulin and in 6% of insulin users. In the newly diagnosed group, none had proliferative retinopathy and 2% had macular edema.[36]

Older-onset diabetes was associated with increased frequency of a specific age-related lens change, cortical opacity, and increased frequency of cataract surgery.[37]

Rates of persons meeting optic disc, visual field, and intraocular pressure criteria for definite glaucoma were more common in the older-onset diabetes group than in the group without diabetes.[38]

The data also suggested that diabetes was not related to early age-related maculopathy or geographic atrophy.[39]

Implications for Clinical Practice

These data suggest that asymptomatic individuals discovered to have NIDDM during epidemiologic studies may not need immediate ophthalmoscopic examination at the time of their diagnosis because they have a relatively low risk of visual loss from diabetic retinopathy at that time. In the Beaver Dam Eye Study, it was unusual to discover either proliferative retinopathy or macular edema in the newly diagnosed group. However, the initial ophthalmoscopic examination may represent an opportunity to educate newly diagnosed patients about the importance of controlling modifiable risk factors and the importance of periodic ophthalmologic examination.

Since the presence of cataract and open-angle glaucoma was found to be increased in older-onset diabetes, patients should be educated and periodically followed up for these conditions as well.

Unanswered Questions

Differences in the reported prevalence of diabetic retinopathy in people with newly discovered NIDDM may be due to variations in the time between onset and detection of diabetes. Because the prevalence of retinopathy increases with increasing duration of hyperglycemia, retinopathy is more likely to be found in patients who have a longer interval between the onset of diabetes and its discovery. This interval may depend on a variety of factors including the availability of and access to medical care, and the health care–seeking behavior of the specific group. The patient population studied in the Beaver Dam Eye Study was, by definition, relatively compliant and this may not represent the behavior patterns of other groups.

Blue Mountains Eye Study

Background and Study Questions

To better understand visual impairment and ocular disease among a representative older community in a geographically defined area, the Blue Mountains Eye Study was established. It sought (a) to estimate the prevalence and severity of diabetic retinopathy among persons with both previously diagnosed and undiagnosed diabetes and (b) to examine systemic and ocular associations (cataract and glaucoma) with diabetic retinopathy.

Patients Included in the Study

The patient population described in the Blue Mountains Eye Study was obtained in the following manner. A census of the residents of an urban area west of Sydney, Australia was performed in the early 1990s to identify individuals born before 1943 (aged 49 years or older). Approximately 4,000 people were identified, and 3,654 (88%) of them were examined. Some patients permitted only an interview.

The population examined included 6% ($n = 217$) with a history of diabetes, including 21% ($n = 46$) who were treated with insulin, 46% ($n = 99$) treated with oral hypoglycemic agents, and 33% ($n = 72$) treated with diet only. An additional 1% ($n = 39$) were found to have undiagnosed diabetes, with a fasting blood glucose of 7.8 mmol/L or more.

Intervention and Outcome Measures

Patients were examined over a 2-year period in the early 1990s to determine the prevalence and severity of diabetic retinopathy in those with newly discovered and previously diagnosed diabetes.[42] Additional data obtained included standardized grading of lens opacities to determine the prevalence of cataract in a defined older diabetic population[43] and standardized grading of optic discs, applanation tonometry, and automated perimetry to evaluate the relationship of open-angle glaucoma to diabetes.[44]

The Blue Mountains Eye Study cohort was reexamined 5 years later to evaluate the change in visual acuity over this period. Of the surviving patients who had participated in the baseline examination, 75% participated in the 5-year follow-up examination. Since the longitudinal data did not specifically address changes in patients with diabetes, the results are not covered in this review.

Major Findings

Diabetes was present in 7% of the population. Signs of diabetic retinopathy were found in 2.3% of the overall study population (32% of those with known or newly diagnosed diabetes). The prevalence was 1.7% in patients younger than 60 years, 2.4% in patients aged between 60 and 69 years, 2.7% in patients aged between 70 and 79 years, and 2.3% in patients 80 years of age or older. Higher blood glucose was related to the finding of moderate-to-severe retinopathy compared to milder retinopathy.[42]

Both the presence and severity of diabetic retinopathy were strongly related to the known duration of diabetes. Retinopathy was found in 21% of those with diabetes diagnosed for <1 year versus 68% in patients with a history of diabetes for 20 years or longer.[42]

In the newly diagnosed cases, retinopathy was prevalent in 16%. No cases of proliferative retinopathy or macular edema were found in this group.[42]

In the Blue Mountains Eye Study, the presence of posterior subcapsular cataract and past cataract surgery were associated with diabetes.[43]

In addition, the prevalence of glaucoma and ocular hypertension were increased in patients with diabetes compared with those without diabetes. In many cases, glaucoma was diagnosed before diabetes.[44]

Implications for Clinical Practice

The Blue Mountains Eye Study provided an estimate of diabetic retinopathy prevalence in a representative Australian population aged 49 years or more. Systemic and ocular associations were also explored.

This study estimated the prevalence and severity of diabetic retinopathy in people with undiagnosed noninsulin-dependent diabetes, detected from fasting blood glucose levels. The failure to find any cases of vision-threatening retinopathy among the newly diagnosed group suggests that for such patients, ophthalmologic examinations can be scheduled on a routine basis, unless visual symptoms are present. However, the clinical diagnosis of diabetes provides an opportunity to emphasize the importance of blood glucose control and the need for periodic ophthalmologic examinations.[42]

For patients with known diabetes, the results of the Blue Mountains Eye Study and the Beaver Dam Eye Study are similar. A slightly lower rate for the prevalence of any retinopathy was found in the current study (32%) as compared with the Beaver Dam study (37%), but the rates for signs of proliferative retinopathy (1.6% in Blue Mountains vs. 1.8% for Beaver Dam) and macular edema (4.3% in Blue Mountains vs. 3.9% in Beaver Dam) were very similar.[36,42]

Since the presence of cataract and open-angle glaucoma was found to be increased in patients with diabetes, patients should be educated and periodically followed up for these conditions as well.

Unanswered Questions

The Blue Mountains Eye Study found a higher overall retinopathy prevalence for patients with newly diagnosed diabetes (16%) as compared with the Beaver Dam Eye Study (10%). This difference could reflect the different criterion used to detect undiagnosed diabetes (elevated fasting blood glucose in the Blue Mountains Study vs. nonfasting glycosylated hemoglobin in the Beaver Dam Study), differences in access to health care, and the different probabilities of early diagnosis between the two communities.[36,42]

Los Angeles Latino Eye Study

Background and Study Questions

The Latino population is the largest minority group in the United States, comprising 12.5% of the US population in the 2000 census. Latinos are individuals who are born into or have descended from a Spanish-speaking community, regardless of the race. In the United States, they are a heterogeneous group, with most of them with Mexican ancestry (66%). Latinos are a racial/ethnic population with unique ocular disease characteristics, yet there have been relatively few epidemiologic studies in the Latino population.[45]

To study the prevalence of eye disease and to determine both modifiable and nonmodifiable risk indicators that may be associated with these ocular diseases among Latinos, the Los Angeles Latino Eye Study (LALES) was established. It had five specific aims: (a) to determine the age-specific prevalence of blindness, visual impairment, and ocular disease among Latinos 40 years or older; (b) to determine what proportion of the prevalence of blindness and visual impairment can be attributed to refractive error, lens opacities, glaucoma, diabetic retinopathy, and age-related maculopathy; (c) to evaluate the importance of suggested risk factors and the degree to which these factors may be associated with visual impairment and the prevalence of each ocular disease; (d) to determine the impact of blindness, visual impairment, and presence of ocular disease and comorbid medical conditions on self-reported visual impairment and health-related quality of life; and (e) to evaluate utilization of eye care and general health care services.[45]

Patients Included in the Study

The patient population described in the LALES was obtained in the following manner. A census of the residents of an area of Los Angeles County, California was used to identify Latino individuals age 40 years or older. Almost 8,000 people were identified, and 6,357 (82%) of these were examined. Some patients (7%) permitted only an interview.[45]

Intervention and Outcome Measures

Patients were examined from 2000 to 2003 to determine the prevalence and severity of diabetic retinopathy in those with newly discovered and previously diagnosed diabetes. Additional data obtained included standardized grading of lens opacities, evaluation for open-angle glaucoma, and measurements of quality of life and health care utilization.[45]

Primary outcome variables included prevalence of visual impairment, blindness, cataract, glaucoma, diabetic retinopathy, and age-related macular degeneration. Secondary outcomes included risk factors associated with eye disease, health-related quality of life, and vision-related quality of life.[45]

Major Findings

Diabetes was present in 20% of the population. Retinopathy was present in 47% of patients with diabetes, and proliferative retinopathy was present in 6%. Macular edema was observed in 10% of patients; of these, 60% (6% of total diabetic population) had clinically significant macular edema. Eight percent of patients with diabetes had either proliferative diabetic retinopathy with high-risk characteristics or clinically significant macular edema requiring laser treatment.[46]

Twenty percent of the patients with diabetes were newly diagnosed, and retinopathy was noted in 23% of these. Proliferative retinopathy was present in <1% and macular edema was present in 2.4% of newly diagnosed patients.[46]

The rate of visual impairment was 6% in those with diabetes as compared with 2% in those without diabetes.[46]

Implications for Clinical Practice

Data from the LALES suggests that the prevalence of diabetic retinopathy is high among Latinos of primarily Mexican ancestry. The increase in prevalence of retinopathy with longer duration of diabetes emphasizes the importance of early diagnosis and management in Latinos. Since Latinos are the largest minority group and the fastest growing segment of the US population, these results have important public health implications.[46]

Unanswered Questions

Forthcoming papers will present data on the risk factors associated with diabetic retinopathy. In addition, longitudinal incidence and progression studies are needed in the Latino diabetic population.

Given that visual loss from diabetic retinopathy can be reduced with strict glycemic control and laser treatment, there will be an increased need for care and the implementation of culturally appropriate screening and prevention programs directed at Latinos.[46]

References

1. Daneman D, Drash A, Lobes LA, et al. Progressive retinopathy with improved control in diabetic dwarfism (Mauriac's syndrome). *Diabetes Care*. 1981;4:360–365.
2. Puklin JE, Tamborlane WV, Felig P, et al. Influence of long-term insulin infusion pump treatment of type I diabetes on diabetic retinopathy. *Ophthalmology*. 1982;89:735–747.
3. Lawson PM, Champion MC, Canny C, et al. Continuous Subcutaneous Insulin Infusion (CSII) does not prevent progression of proliferative and preproliferative retinopathy. *Br J Ophthalmol*. 1982;66:762–766.
4. Lauritzen T, Frost-Larsen K, Larsen HW, et al. Steno Study Group. Effect of 1 year of near-normal blood glucose levels on retinopathy. *Lancet*. 1983;1:200–204.
5. The Kroc Collaborative Study Group. Blood glucose control and the evolution of diabetic retinopathy and albuminuria: A multicenter trial. *N Engl J Med*. 1984;311:365–372.

6. van Ballegooie E, Hooymans JM, Timmerman Z, et al. Rapid deterioration of diabetic retinopathy during treatment with continuous subcutaneous insulin infusion. *Diabetes Care*. 1984;7:236–242.

7. Dahl-Jorgensen K, Brinchmann-Hansen O, Hanssen KF, et al. Aker Diabetes Group. Rapid tightening of blood glucose control leads to transient deterioration of retinopathy in insulin-dependent diabetes mellitus: The Oslo Study. *Br Med J*. 1985;290:811–815.

8. Diabetes Control and Complications Trial Research Group. The Diabetes Control and Complications Trial (DCCT): Design and methodologic considerations for the feasibility phase. *Diabetes*. 1986;35:530–545.

9. Diabetes Control and Complications Trial Research Group. The effect of intensive treatment of diabetes on the development and progression of long-term complications in insulin-dependent diabetes mellitus. *N Engl J Med*. 1993;329:977–986.

10. Diabetes Control and Complications Trial Research Group. Effect of intensive therapy on the development and progression of diabetic nephropathy in the Diabetes Control and Complications Trial. *Kidney Int*. 1995;47:1703–1720.

11. Diabetes Control and Complications Trial Research Group. Effect of intensive diabetes treatment on nerve conduction in the Diabetes Control and Complications Trial. *Ann Neurol*. 1995;38:869–880.

12. Diabetes Control and Complications Trial Research Group. The effect of intensive diabetes treatment on the progression of diabetic retinopathy in insulin-dependent diabetes mellitus. *Arch Ophthalmol*. 1995;113:36–51.

13. Diabetes Control and Complications Trial Research Group. The relationship of glycemic exposure (HbA$_{1c}$) to the risk of development and progression of retinopathy in the Diabetes Control and Complications Trial. *Diabetes*. 1995;44:968–983.

14. Diabetes Control and Complications Trial Research Group. Early worsening of diabetic retinopathy in the Diabetes Control and Complications Trial. *Arch Ophthalmol*. 1998;116:874–886.

15. Diabetes Control and Complications Trial Research Group. Progression of retinopathy with intensive versus conventional treatment in the Diabetes Control and Complications Trial. *Ophthalmology*. 1995;102:647–661.

16. Writing Team for the Diabetes Control and Complications Trial/Epidemiology of Diabetes Interventions and Complications Research Group. Effect of intensive therapy on the microvascular complications of type 1 diabetes mellitus. *JAMA*. 2002;287:2563–2569.

17. Diabetic Retinopathy Study Research Group. A modification of the Airlie House Classification of diabetic retinopathy. DRS Report No. 7. *Invest Ophthalmol Vis Sci*. 1981;21(1):210–226.

18. Klein R, Klein BEK, Moss SE. Visual impairment in diabetes. *Ophthalmology* 1984;91:1–9.

19. Klein R, Klein BEK, Moss SE, et al. The Wisconsin Epidemiologic Study of Diabetic Retinopathy II: Prevalence and risk of diabetic retinopathy when age at diagnosis is less than 30 years. *Arch Ophthalmol*. 1984;102:520–526.

20. Klein R, Klein BEK, Moss SE, et al. The Wisconsin Epidemiologic Study of Diabetic Retinopathy III: Prevalence and risk of diabetic retinopathy when age at diagnosis is 30 years or more. *Arch Ophthalmol*. 1984;102:527–532.

21. Klein R, Klein BEK, Moss SE, et al. The Wisconsin Epidemiologic Study of Diabetic Retinopathy IV: Diabetic macular edema. *Ophthalmology*. 1984;91:1464–1474.

22. Klein R, Klein BEK, Moss SE, et al. The Wisconsin Epidemiologic Study of Diabetic Retinopathy VI: Retinal photocoagulation. *Ophthalmology*. 1987;94:747–753.

23. Moss SE, Klein R, Klein BEK. The incidence of vision loss in a diabetic population. *Ophthalmology*. 1988;95:1340–1348.

24. Klein R, Klein BEK, Moss SE, et al. The Wisconsin Epidemiologic Study of Diabetic Retinopathy IX: Four-year incidence and progression of diabetic retinopathy when age at diagnosis is less than 30 years. *Arch Ophthalmol*. 1989;107:237–243.

25. Klein R, Klein BEK, Moss SE, et al. The Wisconsin Epidemiologic Study of Diabetic Retinopathy X: Four-year incidence and progression of diabetic retinopathy when age at diagnosis is 30 years or more. *Arch Ophthalmol*. 1989;107:244–249.

26. Moss SE, Klein R, Klein BEK. Ten-year incidence of visual loss in a diabetic population. *Ophthalmology*. 1994;101:1061–1070.

27. Klein R, Klein BEK, Moss SE, et al. The Wisconsin Epidemiologic Study of Diabetic

Retinopathy XIV: Ten-year incidence and progression of diabetic retinopathy. *Arch Ophthalmol.* 1994;112:1217–1228.

28. Moss SE, Klein R, Klein BEK. The 14-year incidence of visual loss in a diabetic population. *Ophthalmology* 1998;105:998–1003.

29. Klein R, Klein BEK, Moss SE, et al. The Wisconsin Epidemiologic Study of Diabetic Retinopathy XVII: The 14-year incidence and progression of diabetic retinopathy and associated risk factors in type 1 diabetes. *Ophthalmology* 1998;105:1801–1815.

30. Klein R, Klein BEK, Moss SE, et al. Glycosylated hemoglobin predicts the incidence and progression of diabetic retinopathy. *J Am Med Assoc.* 1988;260:2864–2871.

31. Klein R, Klein BEK, Moss SE, et al. Relationship of hyperglycemia to the long-term incidence and progression of diabetic retinopathy. *Arch Intern Med* 1994;154:2169–2178.

32. Klein BEK, Klein R, Moss SE, et al. A cohort study of the relationship of diabetic retinopathy to blood pressure. *Arch Ophthalmol.* 1995;113:601–606.

33. Klein BEK, Moss SE, Klein R, et al. The Wisconsin Epidemiologic Study of Diabetic Retinopathy XIII: Relationship of serum cholesterol to retinopathy and hard exudates. *Ophthalmology.* 1991;98:1261–1265.

34. Klein R, Moss SE, Klein BEK. Is gross proteinuria a risk factor for the incidence of proliferative diabetic retinopathy? *Ophthalmology.* 1993;100:1140–1146.

35. Klein R, Klein BEK, Moss SE, et al. Association of ocular disease and mortality in a diabetic population. *Arch Ophthalmol.* 1999;117:1487–1495.

36. Klein R, Klein BEK, Moss SE, et al. The Beaver Dam Eye Study. Retinopathy in adults with newly discovered and previously diagnosed diabetes mellitus. *Ophthalmology.* 1992;99:58–62.

37. Klein BEK, Klein R, Wang Q, et al. The Beaver Dam Eye Study. Older-onset diabetes and lens opacities. *Ophthalmic Epidemiol.* 1995;2:49–55.

38. Klein BEK, Klein R, Jensen SC. Open-angle glaucoma and older-onset diabetes. The Beaver Dam Eye Study. *Ophthalmology.* 1994;101:1173–1177.

39. Klein R, Klein BEK, Moss SE. Diabetes, hyperglycemia, and age-related maculopathy. The Beaver Dam Eye Study. *Ophthalmology.* 1992;99:1527–1534.

40. Klein R, Klein BE, Lee KE. Changes in visual acuity in a population. The Beaver Dam Eye Study. *Ophthalmology.* 1996;103:1169–1178.

41. Klein R, Klein BE, Lee KE, et al. Changes in visual acuity in a population over a 10-year period. The Beaver Dam Eye Study. *Ophthalmology* 2001;108:1757–1766.

42. Mitchell P, Smith W, Wang JJ, et al. Prevalence of diabetic retinopathy in an older community. The Blue Mountains Eye Study. *Ophthalmology.* 1998;105:406–411.

43. Rowe NG, Mitchell PG, Cumming RG, et al. Diabetes, fasting blood glucose and age-related cataract: The Blue Mountains Eye Study. *Ophthalmic Epidemiol.* 2000;7:103–114.

44. Mitchell P, Smith W, Chey T, et al. Open-angle glaucoma and diabetes. The Blue Mountains Eye Study, Australia. *Ophthalmology.* 1997;104:712–718.

45. Varma R, Paz SH, Azen SP, et al. Los Angeles Latino Study Group. The Los Angeles Latino Eye Study: Design, methods, and baseline data. *Ophthalmology.* 2004;111:1121–1131.

46. Varma R, Torres M, Pena F, et al. Los Angeles Latino Study Group. Prevalence of diabetic retinopathy in adult Latinos: The Los Angeles Latino Eye Study. *Ophthalmology.* 2004;111:1298–1306.

Diabetic Macular Edema: Clinical Trials

Dean Eliott, MD

Diabetic Macular Edema: Photocoagulation

Early Treatment Diabetic Retinopathy Study

Introduction

In the 1960s, diabetic retinopathy was a growing public health problem and an important cause of blindness, chiefly because of proliferative diabetic retinopathy (PDR) and diabetic macular edema (DME). The Diabetic Retinopathy Study (DRS) was successfully completed in the 1970s, and it served as the foundation for additional prospective, multicenter, randomized controlled trials (RCTs). The DRS (discussed in detail in the section on Proliferative Diabetic Retinopathy) conclusively demonstrated that scatter panretinal photocoagulation was effective in the treatment of PDR, and the remarkable benefit associated with treatment had important public health implications. Whereas the DRS results offered tremendous hope for patients with PDR, DME remained a significant clinical challenge, as macular edema was the leading cause of moderate visual loss in diabetic patients. It was in this historical context that the Early Treatment Diabetic Retinopathy Study (ETDRS) was organized.

Background

The ETDRS was established to address important questions related to diabetic retinopathy. Conducted in the 1980s, the ETDRS was even larger in scope and size than the recently completed DRS.

Before the ETDRS, there was no consensus regarding the optimum management of DME. Several small trials reported encouraging results using photocoagulation; however, it was suggested that treatment benefit might be limited to certain subgroups, such as eyes with focal rather than diffuse fluorescein leakage

or eyes with intact rather than damaged perifoveal capillaries.[1−4] One study involving macular photocoagulation sometimes used scatter treatment also, suggesting that scatter treatment itself might be beneficial for macular edema.[2] Questions regarding the roles of focal macular photocoagulation and scatter panretinal photocoagulation in the treatment of DME remained unanswered. The ETDRS was designed to address these questions, as well as questions involving the use of scatter panretinal photocoagulation in the treatment of earlier stages of retinopathy (mild to severe nonproliferative diabetic retinopathy [NPDR] and early PDR) and the use of aspirin.

The ETDRS sought to determine answers to three questions: Whether focal photocoagulation was effective in the treatment of DME, when scatter panretinal photocoagulation should be initiated to be most effective in the management of diabetic retinopathy, and whether aspirin was effective in altering the course of diabetic retinopathy. Each of these study questions is addressed separately. The management of DME is addressed in the subsequent text, and the other two arms of the ETDRS are reviewed in Chapter 6C.

Study Question

Is focal photocoagulation beneficial in the management of DME?

Patients Included in the Study

A total of 3,711 patients, with or without macular edema, and mild to severe NPDR or early PDR (less than high risk) were enrolled. Visual acuity criteria were 20/40 or better for eyes without macular edema and 20/200 or better for those with macular edema.

123

Eyes with macular edema were analyzed separately as one arm of the study.

Macular edema was defined as retinal thickening or hard exudates at or within one disc diameter of the center of the macula.[4,5] Clinically significant diabetic macular edema (CSDME) is defined in the following text. Definitions of mild, moderate, and severe NPDR and early PDR are included in the section discussing the early scatter treatment arm of the ETDRS (Chapter 6C).

Intervention and Outcome Measures

Eyes with macular edema were randomized to the immediate photocoagulation (focal and/or scatter) arm or the no treatment arm.

Specifically, eyes were divided among those without macular edema, those with macular edema and less severe retinopathy (mild or moderate NPDR), and those with macular edema and more severe retinopathy (severe NPDR or early PDR). One eye of each patient was randomized to deferral of treatment, and the other eye to early photocoagulation using different combinations of scatter panretinal and macular focal photocoagulation (see Figs. 6B.1A–C). If an eye assigned to treatment deferral developed high-risk proliferative retinopathy, then scatter panretinal laser was initiated as per the DRS recommendations.

In eyes with macular edema and less severe retinopathy, those assigned to early photocoagulation received one of four combinations: Immediate focal and delayed mild scatter photocoagulation, immediate focal and delayed full scatter photocoagulation, immediate mild scatter and delayed focal photocoagulation, or immediate full scatter and delayed focal photocoagulation (Fig. 6B.1B).[4] In eyes with macular edema and more severe retinopathy, those assigned to early photocoagulation received one of four combinations: Immediate mild scatter and immediate focal photocoagulation, immediate mild scatter and delayed focal photocoagulation, immediate full scatter and immediate focal photocoagulation, or immediate full scatter and delayed focal photocoagulation (Fig. 6B.1C).[4,6]

Focal photocoagulation (also called focal/grid) was performed using a combination of direct focal treatment to microaneurysms (see Fig. 6B.2) and/or grid photocoagulation to areas of diffuse fluorescein leakage or capillary nonperfusion (see Fig. 6B.3). Focal photocoagulation consisted of treatment to all focal points of leakage located between 500 μm and two disc diameters (3,000 μm) from the center of the

macula. Fifty- to 100-μm spots at 0.05 to 0.1-second duration were used. Focal lesions located between 300 and 500 μm from the center were treated only if the visual acuity was 20/40 or worse and if the treating ophthalmologist did not believe that treatment would destroy the remaining perifoveal capillary network (see Table 6B.1). Grid photocoagulation consisted of 50- to 200-μm spots at 0.05 to 0.1-second duration, placed at least 500 μm from the center of the macula and no closer than 500 μm from the edge of the optic disc. The argon blue–green wavelength was used initially, but the green wavelength was used later (Table 6B.1).[4–6]

Outcome measures included moderate visual loss, defined as a loss of 15 or more letters (3 lines on the ETDRS visual acuity chart) from baseline, which is equivalent to a doubling of the visual angle (for example, a decrease from 20/25 to 20/50 or from 20/50 to 20/100).

Major Findings

In patients with macular edema, the ETDRS identified features that were associated with a particularly high risk of visual loss, termed *clinically significant diabetic macular edema* (CSDME). CSDME was defined by the ETDRS as any one of the following: (a) Retinal thickening at or within 500 μm of the center of the macula; (b) hard exudates at or within 500 μm of the center of the macula, if associated with adjacent retinal thickening; (c) a zone or zones of retinal thickening of one disc area or larger in size, any part of which is within one disc diameter of the center of the macula (see Table 6B.2).[6] CSDME was assessed by stereo–contact lens biomicroscopy and stereo photography.

Eyes with macular edema demonstrated a considerable benefit from early focal photocoagulation, as treatment reduced the risk of moderate visual loss by approximately 50% (12% risk of moderate visual loss for treated eyes versus 24% untreated at 3 years). In eyes with CSDME, these differences were even greater. Of eyes with CSDME, a majority had central foveal involvement, and these eyes demonstrated the most benefit from treatment (13% risk of moderate visual loss for treated eyes versus 33% for untreated eyes at 3 years). In these eyes, early focal treatment was associated with a decrease in retinal thickening at the center of the macula. In eyes with CSDME but without central foveal involvement, treatment resulted in a lesser, but significant, benefit (6% for treated eyes

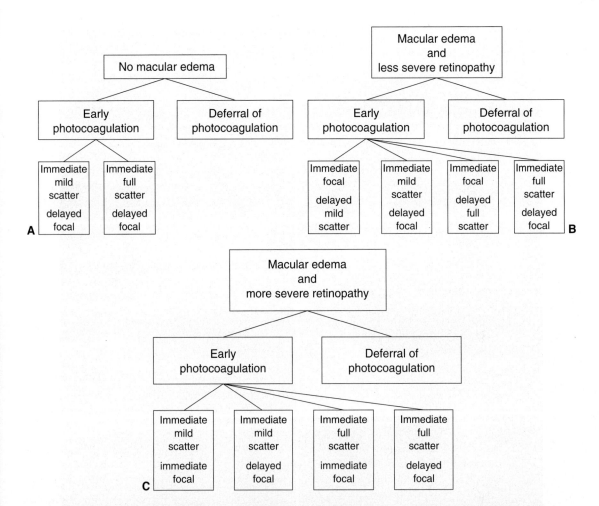

FIGURE 6B.1 ▪ **A:** Early Treatment Diabetic Retinopathy Study (ETDRS) photocoagulation treatment scheme for eyes without macular edema and moderate-to-severe nonproliferative or early proliferative retinopathy. Eyes were assigned randomly to early photocoagulation or deferral of photocoagulation. Eyes assigned to early photocoagulation were further assigned randomly to either mild or full scatter (panretinal) photocoagulation. (From Early Treatment Diabetic Retinopathy Study Research Group. Early Treatment Diabetic Retinopathy Study design and baseline characteristics. ETDRS Report No 7. *Ophthalmology*. 1991;98:741–756.) **B:** ETDRS photocoagulation treatment scheme for eyes with macular edema and less severe retinopathy (mild-to-moderate nonproliferative retinopathy). Eyes were assigned randomly to early photocoagulation or to deferral of photocoagulation. Eyes assigned to early photocoagulation were further assigned randomly to either mild or full scatter (panretinal) photocoagulation, and to either immediate focal or delayed focal treatment. For eyes assigned to immediate focal treatment, the assigned scatter treatment was not applied initially, but only if severe nonproliferative retinopathy or worse developed during follow-up. (From Early Treatment Diabetic Retinopathy Study Research Group. Early Treatment Diabetic Retinopathy Study design and baseline characteristics. ETDRS Report No 7. *Ophthalmology*. 1991;98:741–756.) **C:** ETDRS photocoagulation treatment scheme for eyes with macular edema and more severe retinopathy. Eyes were assigned randomly to early photocoagulation or to deferral of photocoagulation. Eyes assigned to early photocoagulation were further assigned randomly to either mild or full scatter (panretinal) photocoagulation, and to either immediate focal or delayed focal treatment for at least 4 months. (From Early Treatment Diabetic Retinopathy Study Research Group. Early Treatment Diabetic Retinopathy Study design and baseline characteristics. ETDRS Report No 7. *Ophthalmology*. 1991;98:741–756.)

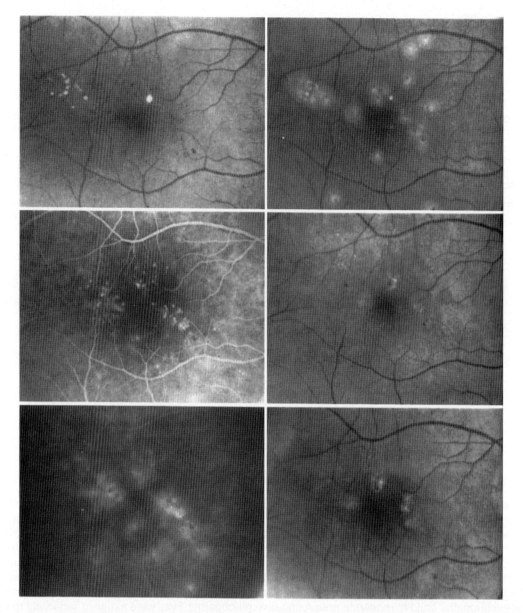

FIGURE 6B.2 ☐ Focal treatment of microaneurysms. The right eye of a 69-year-old woman with diabetes of 22 years' duration. *Top left*: At baseline visit, definite retinal thickening could be seen (with stereoscopic examination) nasal to the center of the macula and above it, probably involving the center. A few small microaneurysms and hard exudates are visible in the thickened area. Visual acuity was 20/30. *Center left*: Midphase angiogram shows microaneurysms surrounding the center of the macula, most of them within 1,000 μm of the center, and some within 500 μm. *Bottom left*: Late-phase angiogram shows leakage from the microaneurysms. *Top right*: Posttreatment photograph shows mild-to-moderate intensity focal treatment of most of the microaneurysms. The microaneurysms closest to the center have not been treated. *Center right*: One year after treatment, the center of the macula appears flat. Hard exudates and microaneurysms have decreased. Visual acuity was 20/50. *Bottom right*: Between the 1- and 2-year visits, additional focal photocoagulation was applied. At the 2-year visit, the center of the macula appears flat and no microaneurysms or hard exudates can be seen. Visual acuity was 20/25. (From Early Treatment Diabetic Retinopathy Study Research Group. Treatment techniques and clinical guidelines for photocoagulation of diabetic macular edema. Early Treatment Diabetic Retinopathy Study Report No 2. *Ophthalmology*. 1987;94:761–774.)

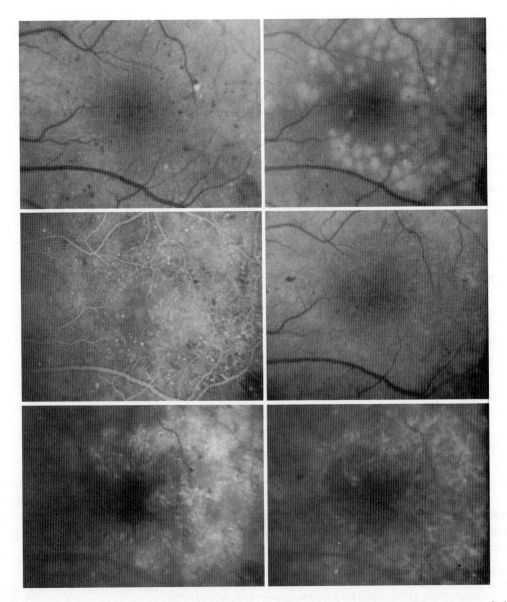

FIGURE 6B.3 ☐ Focal treatment of microaneurysms combined with a grid pattern to areas of diffuse fluorescein leakage and capillary dropout. The left eye of a 49-year-old man with diabetes of 22 years' duration. *Top left*: The pretreatment photograph shows extensive retinal thickening with a few scattered microaneurysms and small hard exudates temporal to the center of the macula. Retinal thickening at the center is mild. Visual acuity was 20/40. *Center left*: Midphase angiogram shows moderate capillary dilation above and temporal to the center of the macula, with mild perifoveal capillary dropout. Scattered microaneurysms are also present. *Bottom left*: Late-phase angiogram shows extensive small cystoid spaces above, below, and temporal to the center of the macula. Some of the large microaneurysms fill only partially with fluorescein. *Top right*: Posttreatment photograph shows focal burns to microaneurysms and a grid pattern of burns above, below, and temporal to the macula. *Center right*: Four months later, microaneurysms and hard exudates have decreased. Retinal thickening is less and no longer involves the center of the macula. Visual acuity was 20/25. *Bottom right*: Late-phase angiogram shows treatment scars but most of the microaneurysms and cystoid spaces have disappeared. (From Early Treatment Diabetic Retinopathy Study Research Group. Treatment techniques and clinical guidelines for photocoagulation of diabetic macular edema. Early Treatment Diabetic Retinopathy Study Report No 2. *Ophthalmology*. 1987;94:761–774.)

TABLE 6B.1 □ Specific Techniques for Scatter (Panretinal) and Focal Photocoagulation in the Early Treatment Diabetic Retinopathy Study

Scatter

Parameters	Full	Mild
Burn characteristics		
Size	500 μm (at retina)	500 μm (at retina)
Exposure	0.1 s	0.1 s
Intensity	Moderate	Moderate
Number	1200–1600	400–650
Placement	1/2 burn apart >2 disc diameters from fovea out to equator	≥1 burn apart >2 disc diameters from fovea out to equator
Number of episodes	≥2	1
Lesion treated directly	Patches of NVE <2 disc areas	Patches of NVE <2 disc areas
Indications for follow-up treatment	Recurrent or new NVE or high-risk proliferative retinopathy	Recurrent or new NVE or high-risk proliferative retinopathy

Focal

Parameters	Direct	Grid
Burn characteristics		
Size	50–100 μm	<200 μm (at retina)
Exposure	0.05–0.1 s	0.05–0.1 s
Intensity	Sufficient to whiten or darken large microaneurysms	Mild
Number	Sufficient to satisfactorily treat all focal leaks	Sufficient to cover areas of diffuse leakage and non-perfusion
Placement	500–3000 μm from center of fovea	Spaced greater than one burn width apart 500–3000 μm from center of fovea
Number of episodes	1	1
Indications for follow-up treatment	Presence of CSDME and treatable lesions at ≥4 mo	Presence of CSDME and treatable lesions at ≥4 mo

NVE, neovascularization elsewhere; CSDME, clinically significant diabetic macular edema.
From Early Treatment Diabetic Retinopathy Study Research Group. Early Treatment Diabetic Retinopathy Study design and Baseline Characteristics. ETDRS Report No 7. *Ophthalmology.* 1991;98:741–756.

vs. 16% for untreated eyes at 2 years). In contrast, in eyes with macular edema that did not meet the definition of CSDME, there was no benefit associated with treatment (see Fig. 6B.4).[5–7]

The beneficial response to early focal treatment was most apparent in eyes with CSDME and worse visual acuity at baseline (<20/40) as compared to those with better baseline acuity (20/25 to 20/40, 20/20 or better), but a treatment effect was demonstrated even in those with good initial visual acuity (see Fig. 6B.5).[7] Despite the reduced risk of visual loss with treatment, visual improvement was rare in the ETDRS (improvement of 15 letters occurred in <3%).

Therefore, the ETDRS recommendation was to consider prompt focal treatment for eyes with CSDME, regardless of visual acuity, to prevent visual loss.[6]

The ETDRS documented treatment-related side effects, which included a small, but not statistically significant, difference in visual field scores. Eyes assigned to focal photocoagulation demonstrated slightly more paracentral scotomata on Goldmann visual fields using the I-2 test object.[6]

Implications for Clinical Practice

Prompt focal photocoagulation was recommended for eyes with CSDME as defined by the ETDRS for

TABLE 6B.2 ☐ **Definition of Clinically Significant Diabetic Macular Edema**

Clinically Significant Diabetic Macular Edema—any one of the following:

1. Retinal thickening at or within 500 μm of the center of the macula
2. Hard exudates at or within 500 μm of the center of the macula, if associated with adjacent retinal thickening
3. A zone or zones of retinal thickening of one-disc area or larger, any part of which is within one-disc diameter of the center of the macula

patients who met the inclusion criteria. Treatment was recommended regardless of baseline visual acuity, since eyes in all categories of visual acuity (20/20 or better, 20/25 to 20/40, <20/40) were found to benefit from treatment. Treatment was recommended for eyes with or without thickening of the central macula, provided that they met the definition of CSDME. Treatment was most effective for those with worse visual acuity at baseline (<20/40) and for those with central macular thickening.

Focal photocoagulation, when applied using ETDRS treatment guidelines, resulted in a significant reduction in moderate visual loss. Since visual improvement was rare in this study, the ETDRS recommended that treatment be considered to prevent visual loss in patients with CSDME.

Macular edema often occurs in association with severe NPDR or PDR. The DRS and the ETDRS demonstrated that scatter panretinal photocoagulation may exacerbate macular edema and result in vision loss.[8,9] If panretinal photocoagulation can be safely delayed in a patient with CSDME and severe NPDR or early PDR, focal treatment should be applied followed by very close observation for proliferative changes. If panretinal laser cannot be safely delayed, or if a patient has CSDME and PDR with high-risk characteristics, both focal treatment and panretinal photocoagulation should be applied, but the scatter treatment should not be given before the focal treatment.

Beginning with the ETDRS, a new visual acuity chart was developed for use in prospective clinical research studies. This chart is still used today in clinical trials to evaluate visual acuity in a standardized manner (see Fig. 6B.6).[10–12]

Unanswered Questions

The ETDRS defined the standard of care (SOC) for the management of DME for over 20 years, and all current clinical trials continue to use ETDRS results for comparison. A direct comparison with new therapies, however, is often difficult because of the multitude of ocular and systemic variables that influence retinopathy.

Despite providing answers to critically important questions, the ETDRS results stimulated additional questions that remain unanswered. For example, the ETDRS did not evaluate eyes with visual acuity less than 20/200. The potential effect of focal treatment in eyes with macular edema and low vision is unknown. In addition, although the ETDRS was designed to determine whether laser was effective, it was not designed to determine the best time to apply laser, and the optimum timing of treatment remains unknown. Furthermore, the ETDRS used specific treatment guidelines for macular focal photocoagulation. Alternative laser treatment strategies have since been developed, including modified versions of the ETDRS protocol. The relative benefits of different treatment strategies are difficult to assess since a direct comparison with ETDRS results is not possible.

Retreatment with focal photocoagulation was allowed in the ETDRS if the edema persisted or recurred. There was no clear recommendation regarding the number of laser treatments that may be beneficial in eyes requiring retreatment, and the management of refractory DME remains one of the most challenging clinical problems today, 20 years after the initial ETDRS results were reported.

Diabetic Macular Edema: Emerging Pharmacologic Therapies

Steroids

Introduction

Intraocular corticosteroids are currently being evaluated for the treatment of DME. Triamcinolone, fluocinolone, and dexamethasone are promising pharmacologic agents that are in various phases of clinical trial development, and early results from these trials are available.

Triamcinolone acetonide is commonly being used off label for diabetic and other causes of macular edema, as it is not approved by the U.S. Food and Drug Administration (FDA) for this

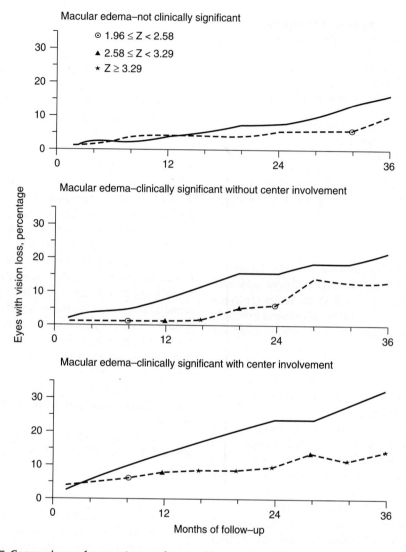

FIGURE 6B.4 ☐ Comparison of percentages of eyes with macular edema that experienced moderate visual loss classified by severity of macular edema and assigned to immediate focal treatment (broken line) or to deferral of treatment (solid line). (From Early Treatment Diabetic Retinopathy Study Research Group. Photocoagulation for diabetic macular edema. Early Treatment Diabetic Retinopathy Study Report No 4. *Int Ophthalmol Clin.* 1987;27:265–272.)

indication. Administered through an intravitreous injection, triamcinolone acetonide has been shown to be effective in improving visual acuity and reducing macular thickness measured by optical coherence tomography (OCT) in patients with DME.[13,14] Although this treatment is currently being evaluated in a multicenter, prospective, RCT (Intravitreous Steroid Injection Study [ISIS]), it has already become widely adopted by the medical community as the SOC.

In contrast, fluocinolone acetonide and dexamethasone are delivered through intravitreous sustained release devices, and these devices are not approved by the FDA for use in DME. These include the intravitreous fluocinolone acetonide implant (Retisert) and the intravitreous dexamethasone implant (Posurdex), both of which require surgical implantation and provide prolonged delivery of medication to the target tissue. These treatments are also currently being evaluated in

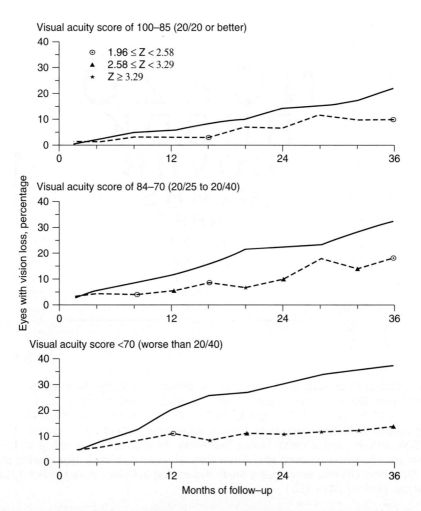

FIGURE 6B.5 ☐ Comparison of the percentages of eyes with clinically significant diabetic macular edema that experienced moderate visual loss classified by baseline visual acuity and assigned to immediate focal treatment (broken line) or to deferral of treatment (solid line). (From Early Treatment Diabetic Retinopathy Study Research Group. Photocoagulation for diabetic macular edema. Early Treatment Diabetic Retinopathy Study Report No 4. *Int Ophthalmol Clin.* 1987;27:265−272.)

multicenter, prospective, RCTs, and early results are available.

Corticosteroids act in a nonspecific manner. Although the exact mechanism of action in the treatment of DME is unknown, corticosteroids decrease the breakdown of the blood–retinal barrier, suppress inflammation, and downregulate the production of vascular endothelial growth factor (VEGF).

Intravitreous Steroid Injection Study

Background and Study Questions

This multicenter, prospective, randomized trial compared two doses of intravitreous triamcinolone acetonide (Kenalog-40, Bristol-Myers Squibb) (see Fig. 6B.7) in patients with macular edema from diabetes, vein occlusion, pseudophakia, and retinal telangiectasia. The 6-month results of this study were recently released. Only data for the DME arm of the study will be discussed.[15]

Patients Included in the Study

A total of 33 patients in the DME arm of the study were enrolled. Inclusion criteria were the presence of persistent clinically significant macular edema for at least 3 months after completion of what the treating physician considered maximal laser treatment and

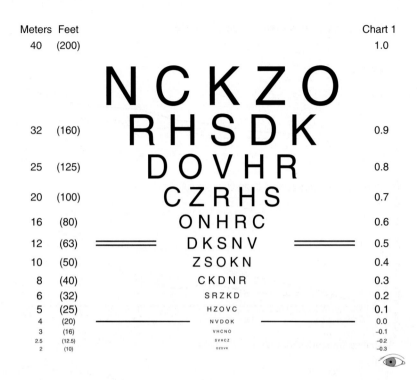

Meters Feet   Chart 1
40 (200)   1.0

FIGURE 6B.6 ☐ One of three Early Treatment Diabetic Retinopathy Study visual acuity charts. Four-meter testing distance with this chart yields the following Snellen equivalent lines: 20/10, 20/12.5, 20/16, 20/20, 20/25, 20/31.5, 20/40, 20/50, 20/63, 20/80, 20/100, 20/125, 20/160, and 20/200. At 1 m, the following additional Snellen equivalent lines of visual acuity could be measured: 20/250, 20/315, 20/400, 20/500, 20/630, and 20/800. Notice that every three lines is a doubling of the visual angle and that there are five letters on each line. (From Early Treatment Diabetic Retinopathy Study Research Group. Early Treatment Diabetic Retinopathy Study design and baseline characteristics. ETDRS Report No 7. *Ophthalmology*. 1991;98:741–756.)

ETDRS visual acuity ≤20/40. Patients with a history of intraocular pressure (IOP) elevation ≥30 mm Hg, steroid response, or ocular surgery within the previous 3 months were excluded.

Intervention and Outcome Measures

Patients were randomized to receive either 2 or 4 mg of intravitreous triamcinolone. Outcome measures included a three-line or greater improvement in visual acuity and total resolution of macular edema.

Major Findings

In the 2-mg group, a three-line or greater visual improvement in 23% at 3 months and 0% at 6 months was noted, compared with 33% at 3 months and 21% at 6 months for the 4-mg group. In the 2-mg group, there was total resolution of macular edema in 20% at 3 months and 10% at 6 months, compared with 54% at 3 months and 25% at 6 months for the 4-mg group. These data indicate a trend toward greater efficacy and longer duration with the 4-mg group when compared with the 2-mg group.

During analysis, eyes were grouped as cystoid and noncystoid foveal edema on the basis of a fluorescein angiogram graded in a masked manner. Interestingly, 62% of eyes with cystoid foveal edema showed a greater than or equal to 3-line improvement in vision compared with only 9% for those with noncystoid foveal edema, which is a statistically significant difference (see Figs. 6B.8 and 6B.9).

Adverse events included increased IOP. IOP elevation of ≥10 mm Hg was seen in 31% of patients, with a trend favoring the 4-mg group. A maximum IOP of ≥30 mm Hg (range 30–36) was recorded in 28% of patients. None of these patients

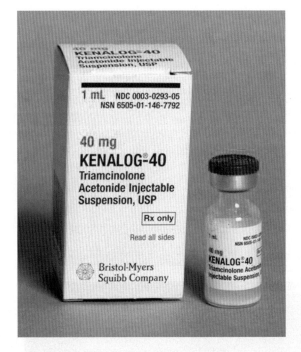

FIGURE 6B.7 ☐ Triamcinolone acetonide (Kenalog-40, Bristol-Myers Squibb). (Photograph courtesy of Ronald C. Gentile MD. New York.)

required glaucoma surgery. Follow-up of patients will continue.[15,16]

Implications for Clinical Practice

This study, which did not have a control group, demonstrates that there is potential for visual improvement after intravitreous triamcinolone injection in DME patients refractory to maximum laser treatment who met the inclusion criteria. There was a trend toward greater efficacy and longer duration with the 4-mg group when compared with the 2-mg group. This is a relatively cost-effective and technically easier procedure as compared with the steroid implants discussed below. However, as shown in this study, visual acuity tends to regress over time as the macular edema recurs and repeat injections are required.

In addition, the medication and the intraocular injection procedure have risks. Cataracts and glaucoma are well-known complications of steroid therapy. In this study with only 6 months of follow-up, progression of cataract was not observed and increases in IOP were controlled medically in all patients. The 4-mg dose was associated with a higher rate of IOP elevation. Infectious endophthalmitis is the most serious complication associated with the intravitreous injection procedure, although it did not occur in this small study. Additional follow-up is needed.

Unanswered Questions

The lack of a control group is a serious limitation. In addition, although the short follow-up results that are available for this study are encouraging, these data must be interpreted with caution. Additional follow-up is required to assess the potential need for retreatment as well as the potential for adverse events such as cataract and glaucoma.

The safety of intravitreous triamcinolone is yet to be established. The commercially available standard preparation (Kenalog-40) contains a preservative (benzyl alcohol) and an excipient (polysorbate-80), and is approved by the FDA only for intramuscular use. Benzyl alcohol and polysorbate-80 have been implicated in postinjection sterile endophthalmitis. In addition to the standard preparation, a preservative-free formulation is available from an independent compounding/pharmacy facility (New England Compounding Center).[14] Another preservative-free triamcinolone acetonide preparation (Allergan Inc) specifically formulated for intraocular use is currently being evaluated in clinical trials (SCORE: Standard Care vs. Corticosteroid for Retinal Vein Occlusion Study; and the Diabetic Retinopathy Clinical Research Network Study: A Randomized Trial Comparing Intravitreal Triamcinolone Acetonide and Laser Photocoagulation for Diabetic Macular Edema).

Fluocinolone Acetonide Implant (Retisert)

Background and Study Questions

Bausch & Lomb Inc. and Control Delivery Systems Inc have developed a sustained release device containing the steroid fluocinolone acetonide (Retisert) (see Fig. 6B.10). The fluocinolone drug pellet is enclosed in a polymer, and is similar to but smaller than the ganciclovir intravitreous implant (Vitrasert, Bausch & Lomb Inc./Control Delivery Systems Inc.) used for cytomegalovirus retinitis. The $3 \times 2 \times 5$ mm implant is inserted into the vitreous cavity through a pars plana incision and secured to the sclera with a suture. Fluocinolone is released at a constant rate for almost 3 years (initial rate 0.6 μg/day, decreasing over the

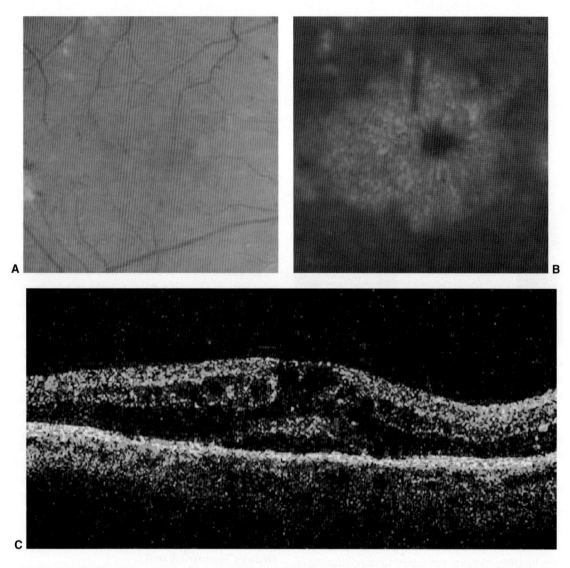

FIGURE 6B.8 □ The right eye of a 49-year-old man with diabetes of 18 years' duration. Clinically significant diabetic macular edema was present despite a history of prior focal photocoagulation. Visual acuity was 20/200. **A:** Fundus photograph of the macula shows cystoid retinal thickening, a few small retinal hemorrhages, and prior focal laser spots. **B:** Late-phase fluorescein angiogram shows leakage in a petalloid pattern. **C:** Optical coherence tomography shows cystic retinal thickening.

first month to a steady state 0.3–0.4 µg/day for 30 months). The fluocinolone implant has the advantage of maintaining therapeutic levels in the target tissue (the macula) with minimal systemic exposure and an associated reduction in systemic side effects. Retisert was recently approved by the FDA for the treatment of noninfectious posterior uveitis.

This multicenter, prospective, randomized, masked, controlled clinical trial (CDS FL-002)

compared the fluocinolone acetonide implant to SOC in patients with DME. The 24-month results of this phase III study were recently released.[16,17]

Patients Included in the Study

A total of 80 patients with DME were enrolled. Inclusion criteria were a history of at least one macular laser procedure at least 3 months before enrollment,

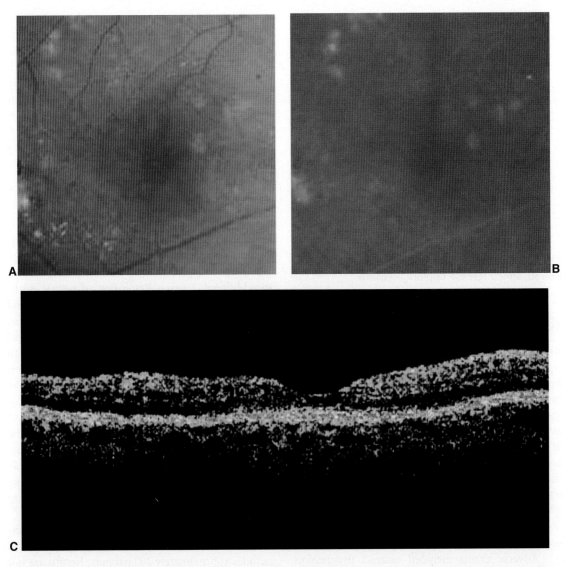

FIGURE 6B.9 □ The same patient as in Figure 6B.8, 3 months after intravitreous injection of triamcinolone acetonide, 4 mg. Visual acuity was 20/80. **A:** Fundus photograph shows the resolution of macular edema. **B:** Late-phase fluorescein angiogram shows the resolution of leakage. **C:** Optical coherence tomography shows the resolution of retinal thickening. (Three months later, the patient developed recurrent edema and underwent a repeat injection, with subsequent resolution of the edema.)

ETDRS visual acuity ≥20/400 and ≤20/50, and retinal thickening involving fixation and at least one disc area in size. Patients with a history of uncontrolled IOP or a history of ocular surgery within 3 months before enrollment were excluded.

Intervention and Outcome Measures

Patients were randomized into an implant group (0.59 mg, $n = 41$; or 2.1 mg, $n = 11$) and an SOC group (SOC, $n = 28$) that received either macular grid laser or was put on observation. The 2.1 mg implant was discontinued early in the study because it showed no advantage over the lower dose.

The primary end point evaluated from masked retinal photographs was the resolution of retinal thickening at the center of the macula. Secondary end points were changes in visual acuity from baseline, diabetic retinopathy score, and total area of hard exudates.

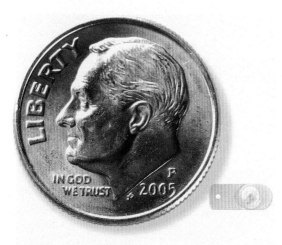

FIGURE 6B.10 ☐ Fluocinolone acetonide intravitreous sustained release implant (Retisert).

Major Findings

At 24 months, retinal edema at the center of the macula had resolved completely in 54% of the 0.59-mg group as compared to 29% of the SOC group, ($p = 0.039$). In addition, 46% (0.59-mg group) showed a >2-grade improvement in retinal thickness at the center of the macula as compared to 15% in the SOC group ($p = 0.006$). The mean change in visual acuity at 24 months was a gain of 9.3 ± 14.4 letters for the 0.59-mg implant group and a loss of 1.9 ± 15.2 letters for the SOC group ($p = 0.003$). The diabetic retinopathy severity scores either remained stable or improved in 88% of the 0.59-mg implant group as compared with 63% of the SOC group ($p = 0.61$).

Adverse events included cataract progression (78% in the 0.59-mg vs. 13% in the SOC group) and increased IOP (32% in the 0.59-mg vs. 0% in the SOC group). Rates of cataract extraction were 74% in the 0.59-mg implant group and 13% in SOC the group. Most of the patients with elevated IOP were managed with drops, although eight patients (19.5%) in the 0.59-mg implant group required trabeculectomy. Patient follow-up will continue for an additional 2 years.[16,17]

Implications for Clinical Practice

On the basis of the early results of this study, this device has the potential to reduce retinal thickening and improve visual acuity in patients with DME who met the specific inclusion criteria. The improvement in diabetic retinopathy severity may have favorable implications that are not readily apparent at the 2-year time point. This implant provides sustained levels of targeted fluocinolone and, as expected, is associated with a higher incidence of cataract and IOP elevation. All patients who were phakic at baseline required cataract surgery, and almost 20% of patients required trabeculectomy during the 2-year follow-up. The positive results seen so far may be limited by the adverse events associated with the progression of cataract and the development of glaucoma.

Unanswered Questions

The Retisert device releases fluocinolone acetonide for almost 3 years. Since this is a 4-year study, patient follow-up will continue at 3-month intervals for an additional 2 years. Resolution of retinal thickening and improvement in visual acuity are end points with tremendous clinical value. In contrast, the potential benefits associated with improvement in diabetic retinopathy severity as demonstrated in this study may not yet be clinically apparent. If this improvement is sustained, it is possible that this may decrease the risk of progression to PDR, and this would represent a significant development.

Although the 2-year data is encouraging, the potential adverse clinical effects associated with cessation of drug availability are unknown. It is possible to have multiple sequential implants in one eye; however, the necessity, optimum timing, and long-term effects of repeat implantation are also unknown.

A larger phase III study (CDS FL-005) with similar inclusion criteria is currently under way and includes approximately 200 patients. Results are not yet available.

Dexamethasone Sustained Release Implant (Posurdex)

Background and Study Questions

Allergan Inc. has developed a sustained release device containing the steroid dexamethasone (Posurdex) (see Fig. 6B.11). This is a biodegradable implant, delivering dexamethasone for approximately 6 to 8 weeks. The cylindrical pellet is inserted into the region of the vitreous base through a small sclerotomy. Similar to other sustained release devices, the dexamethasone implant has the advantage of maintaining therapeutic levels in the target tissue (the

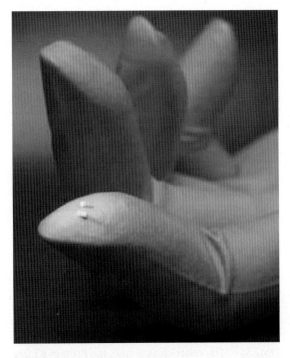

FIGURE 6B.11 ☐ Dexamethasone intravitreous sustained release implants (Posurdex), 350 and 700 μg doses.

macula) with minimal systemic exposure and an associated reduction in systemic side effects.

This multicenter, prospective, randomized, masked, controlled clinical trial compared the dexamethasone implant to observation alone in patients with persistent macular edema from a variety of causes. The 180-day results of this phase II study were recently released.[16,18]

Patients Included in the Study

A total of 306 patients with persistent macular edema from multiple causes were enrolled. Etiologies included DME ($n = 172$), retinal vein occlusion ($n = 103$), Irvine-Gass syndrome ($n = 27$), and uveitis ($n = 14$). Inclusion criteria were macular edema persisting at least 90 days following treatment (laser or medical management), visual acuity worse than 20/40 and attributable to macular edema, retinal thickening in the center of the fovea, and angiographic evidence of leakage involving the perifoveal capillary network. Patients with visual acuity worse than 20/200, retinal neovascularization, or a history of pars plana vitrectomy or glaucoma were excluded.

Intervention and Outcome Measures

Patients were randomized to receive either a single Posurdex implant containing 350 or 700 μg of dexamethasone or no treatment (observation). The primary efficacy end point was a two-line or greater improvement in visual acuity. Secondary end points were change in retinal thickness measured by OCT, change in contrast sensitivity, and improvement in fluorescein angiographic leakage as determined by masked grading.

Major Findings

The available results include all the etiological subgroups enrolled in this study (DME, vein occlusion, Irvine-Gass, and uveitis). Ninety days after receiving the implant, a statistically significant primary efficacy outcome of a 2-line improvement in visual acuity was achieved with the 700-μg dose, as compared to the observation group, and this effect persisted at the 180-day evaluation. Also, at 180 days, 19% of patients with the 700-μg implant showed an improvement of three or more lines as compared to 8% in the observation group ($p = 0.019$). Patients treated with the 350-μg implant showed a trend toward improvement in visual acuity, indicating a dose response. Measures of edema correlated with improvement in visual acuity with a statistically significant decrease in retinal thickness and fluorescein leakage in both the 700- and 350-μg groups. Ninety days after implantation, contrast sensitivity was significantly improved in the 700-μg group as compared with the observation group.

Ocular adverse events were more common in the implant groups and were mostly related to the implantation procedure. These included subconjunctival hemorrhage and vitreous hemorrhage, both of which were self-limited. Patients did not show the development or progression of cataract; however, 17% of treated patients (700-μg group) showed a ≥ 10 mm Hg IOP increase over baseline at some point during the study as compared with 3% in the observation group. All rises in IOP were treated with glaucoma drops alone.[16,18]

Implications for Clinical Practice

The results of this phase II study indicate that this device has the potential to reduce retinal edema and improve visual acuity in patients with macular edema from a variety of causes who met the specific inclusion criteria. The Posurdex implant provides sustained levels of dexamethasone and is associated with an increased incidence of IOP elevation. Pressure elevations were successfully treated with topical therapy, and trabeculectomy procedures were not required during the relatively short, 180-day trial. In addition, development or progression of cataract was not observed during the brief study period. The positive results seen so far must be weighed against the relatively short duration of drug availability and the potential for recurrent disease.

Unanswered Questions

The Posurdex device releases dexamethasone for 6 to 8 weeks. The 180-day data is encouraging; however, the clinical effects associated with cessation of drug availability are unknown. This device has a relatively short duration of action, and sustained treatment benefit may require multiple implants. Although it is possible to have multiple sequential implants in one eye, the necessity, timing, and sequelae of repeat implantation are unknown. Cataracts and glaucoma are of particular concern, since the risk of these complications increases with prolonged and repeated administration of intraocular steroids.

A single-use 22-gauge applicator preloaded with the implant has been developed for office-based insertion of the implant through the pars plana, and this may reduce the adverse events associated with conjunctival incision and sclerostomy. This applicator is currently being used in the ensuing larger phase III study. Results are not yet available.

Anti-VEGF Agents

Introduction

New pharmacologic interventions at the molecular level show great promise in treating visually disabling conditions such as DME and PDR. Two of the molecules being targeted in current clinical trials are VEGF and protein kinase C (PKC). VEGF, a vascular endothelial cell mitogen and potent permeability factor, is produced by glial cells, retinal pigment epithelial cells, and vascular endothelial cells, and is normally present in the retina and vitreous in low levels. Retinal hypoxia upregulates VEGF production, resulting in abnormal angiogenesis and a marked increase in vascular permeability. The PKC family is a group of enzymes involved in signal transduction. The β isoform has been shown to have an important

role in regulating vascular permeability and is an important signaling component for VEGF. The chronic hyperglycemia due to uncontrolled diabetes leads to increased cellular levels of diacylglycerol, which in turn activates PKC, especially the β isoform. PKC β increases the synthesis of VEGF, and also contributes to the microvascular abnormalities in diabetic retinopathy. Inhibition of either VEGF or PKC β moderates the microvascular complications seen in experimental animal models. In addition, PKC β inhibitors given orally have the potential to influence other diabetic complications such as renal insufficiency and peripheral neuropathy.[16]

Ruboxistaurin Mesylate (Arxxant, Eli Lilly and Co.)

Background and Study Questions

One of the clinical trials that have evaluated the role of ruboxistaurin mesylate is the Protein Kinase C β Inhibitor Diabetic Macular Edema Study (PKC-DMES).[19] The other clinical trial, the Protein Kinase C β Diabetic Retinopathy Study (PKC-DRS), is discussed in Chapter 6C. The PKC-DMES is a multicenter, double-masked, placebo-controlled study that evaluated the progression of DME in patients who were treated with ruboxistaurin or placebo.

Patients Included in the Study

A total of 686 patients with DME that was not imminently sight threatening were enrolled. Eligibility criteria included visual acuity of 20/32 or better and no prior photocoagulation.

Intervention and Outcome Measures

Patients were randomized to placebo or to ruboxistaurin 4, 16, or 32 mg orally per day for ≥ 30 months. The primary outcome was progression of DME to involve or imminently threaten the center of the macula or application of focal/grid photocoagulation. Eligibility and outcomes were assessed using stereoscopic fundus photographs taken at 3- to 6-month intervals. Analysis was based on time to occurrence of the primary outcome using the intent-to-treat population.

Major Findings

At 36 months, there was no statistically significant difference between the placebo and the ruboxistaurin groups with regard to DME progression. When subgroup analysis of these patients was conducted on the basis of baseline HbA1c (HbA1c at baseline ≤10%, ≤75th percentile), placebo and ruboxistaurin (32 mg) event rates were 45% and 31%, respectively, indicating a risk reduction in the progression of DME of 31% ($p = 0.019$). Ruboxistaurin was well tolerated with no significant adverse events noted.[19]

Implications for Clinical Practice

Treatment with ruboxistaurin did not prevent the primary end point of progression of DME to involve or imminently threaten the center of the macula or application of focal/grid photocoagulation in patients with nonimminently sight-threatening DME who met the inclusion criteria. However, when patients with very poor glycemic control at enrollment (HbA1c >10%) were excluded from the analysis, ruboxistaurin 32 mg was associated with a reduction in DME progression.

When considering systemic therapy, the safety profile of the medication is critical. A prior study using a nonspecific inhibitor of multiple kinases and PKC isoforms was limited by hepatotoxicity and gastrointestinal side effects. In contrast, ruboxistaurin is selective for the β isoform of PKC, and it was well tolerated and not associated with significant adverse events.

Unanswered Questions

The apparent lack of efficacy of ruboxistaurin in preventing the progression of DME to involve or imminently threaten the center of the macula or the application of focal/grid photocoagulation could have occurred for a variety of reasons. PKC β activation occurs very early in diabetes, and it is possible that in patients with very poor glycemic control (HbA1c >10%), the pathologic retinal changes are no longer amenable to PKC β inhibition. Alternatively, the drug may not be potent enough to overcome these changes. When patients with very poor glycemic control were excluded, ruboxistaurin 32 mg was associated with a reduction in DME progression. Although a statistically significant benefit was achieved in these patients who were treated with ruboxistaurin according to the study protocol, the optimum time to initiate therapy and the optimum duration of therapy remain unknown.

The PKC-DME clinical trial has demonstrated the potential for the use of ruboxistaurin in the treatment of diabetic microvascular retinal complications, especially with regard to clinically important outcomes such as the reduction of DME in patients with better glycemic control. The results support further evaluation of this approach.

Pegaptanib Sodium (Macugen)

Background and Study Questions

Pegaptanib sodium is an aptamer (a synthetic oligonucleotide that binds to a target molecule) that selectively binds to the pathologic isoform of VEGF, VEGF165. The aptamer is pegylated (bound to polyethylene glycol) to delay its metabolism *in vivo*. This increases the half-life of the drug and allows administration every 6 weeks. The medication is delivered through intravitreous injection. Macugen is currently approved by the FDA for neovascular age-related macular degeneration.[20]

Results of a phase II prospective, randomized, placebo-controlled, double-masked, dose-ranging, multicenter trial using pegaptanib in eyes with DME are now available.[21] The study compared three different doses of pegaptanib with sham injection to evaluate its safety and efficacy in patients with DME over a 36-week period.

Patients Included in the Study

A total of 172 patients who were otherwise eligible for thermal laser therapy for DME were enrolled. Subjects included were individuals with visual acuity between 20/50 and 20/320 and retinal thickening involving the center of the macula for whom the investigators judged that photocoagulation could be safely withheld for 16 weeks.

Intervention and Outcome Measures

Patients received varying doses (0.3, 1, and 3 mg) of pegaptanib through an intravitreous injection or sham injection every 6 weeks for at least 12 weeks with additional injections and/or focal laser at the discretion of the investigators for another 18 weeks. Final assessments were conducted at 36 weeks.

Main outcomes were visual acuity, central retinal thickness as assessed by OCT, and additional treatment with laser between weeks 12 and 36.

Major Findings

The data were statistically significant for the 0.3-mg dose of pegaptanib as compared to sham with respect to the following outcomes at 36 weeks. Median visual acuity was 20/50 with pegaptanib as compared with 20/63 in the sham group ($p = 0.04$). A gain of >10 letters was experienced in 34% of pegaptanib patients as compared to 10% of sham patients ($p = 0.003$). Mean central retinal thickness decreased by 68 μm with pegaptanib as compared to an increase of 4 μm with sham ($p = 0.02$). Larger proportions of those receiving pegaptanib had an absolute decrease of both >75 μm (49% vs. 19%, $p = 0.008$) and >100 μm (42% vs. 16%, $p = 0.02$). Photocoagulation was deemed necessary in fewer patients who received pegaptanib as compared with sham (25% vs. 48%, $p = 0.04$).

All pegaptanib doses were well tolerated. Endophthalmitis occurred in 1 of 652 injections (0.15% per injection) out of 130 patients who received an injection (0.8% per patient), and it was not associated with severe visual loss.[21]

Implications for Clinical Practice

In this phase II study, patients who received pegaptanib experienced better visual outcomes, were more likely to show reduction in central retinal thickness on OCT, and were deemed less likely to need additional laser treatment during the 36-week period. The specific inhibition of VEGF-165 in this study was accomplished with an aptamer, a new therapeutic class of nonbiologic agents that possess an exceedingly high degree of target selectivity and binding affinity. Aptamers show promise as therapeutic agents, and the data suggest that inhibiting VEGF-165 with an aptamer was beneficial for patients with DME who met the specific inclusion criteria. VEGF-165 is the isoform most associated with pathologic ocular neovascularization and retinal vascular permeability, and its inhibition may result in a clinically meaningful benefit. The lowest efficacious dose of pegaptanib that was evaluated in this trial was 0.3 mg per injection. This form of therapy requires repeated injections, and although the drug appears to be well tolerated, there are potential risks associated with the injection procedure.

In a prior study comprising approximately 1,200 patients with age-related macular degeneration, there was a favorable safety profile for pegaptanib at all three doses.[20] Most adverse events in the study were mild, transient, and attributed by investigators to the injection procedure rather than to the study drug. Risks of the injection procedure include endophthalmitis, retinal detachment, and vitreous hemorrhage. Endophthalmitis is a rare complication when simple precautions are implemented, such as the use of topical 5% betadine and a sterile lid speculum. Nevertheless, the decision to undertake long-term administration by repeated injections should be made carefully.

Unanswered Questions

The control group in this trial consisted of sham injection, with deferral of photocoagulation for at least 16 weeks. The current SOC for most cases of CSDME is prompt initiation of focal/grid laser after the diagnosis is established. A more appropriate comparison would involve pegaptanib injections as compared to prompt initiation of laser therapy, thereby avoiding deferral of laser for 16 weeks. In some patients with DME, retinal thickening is confined to the foveal avascular zone, and laser is contraindicated in these patients. Intravitreous triamcinolone injections are typically performed in these patients, and a comparison between pegaptanib and steroid injections would be appropriate. In this manner, pegaptanib therapy could be compared with control groups that represent the current standards of care, as opposed to the natural history of DME, and a more accurate assessment of its safety and efficacy could be attained.

Currently there is no long-term safety or efficacy data available for pegaptanib use in patients with DME. It is unknown whether the beneficial outcomes demonstrated in this study would persist through at least 3 years, as has been shown for focal laser. Final assessments in this study were conducted at 36 weeks; however, diabetes is a chronic disease and DME may be refractory to treatment or may recur. The necessity, duration, and sequelae of repeated pegaptanib injections in this condition are unknown.

A larger, phase III trial investigating the use of pegaptanib sodium in the treatment of DME is currently under way.

Conclusion

Tremendous advances have been made in the treatment of DME. The ETDRS conclusively demonstrated that focal photocoagulation was effective in the treatment of DME, and it proved that for eyes with CSDME, the risk of moderate visual loss was substantially reduced. The ETDRS defined the SOC for over 20 years, and all DME clinical trials continue to use ETDRS results for comparison.

Emerging pharmacologic therapies in various phases of clinical trial development hold great promise in the treatment of DME. Steroids such as triamcinolone, fluocinolone, and dexamethasone, and anti-VEGF agents such as ruboxistaurin (Arxxant) and pegaptanib (Macugen) represent new approaches to the management of DME, and the early clinical trial results are encouraging. Additional medications such as ranibizumab (Lucentis) and bevacizumab (Avastin) have not undergone controlled clinical trial testing for DME, but they also offer tremendous potential.

Sustained release drug delivery devices such as Retisert and Posurdex represent first-generation devices in a field that is rapidly expanding. The future will likely involve oral and intravitreous (probably via sustained release devices) administration of new pharmacologic agents, and emphasis will likely be on prevention and early treatment. The visual morbidity associated with DME will hopefully, one day, be eliminated.

References

1. Patz A, Schatz H, Berkow JW, et al. Macular edema – an overlooked complication of diabetic retinopathy. *Trans Am Acad Ophthalmol Otolaryngol*. 1973;77:OP34–OP42.
2. Cheng H, Kohner EM, Keen H, et al. Photocoagulation in treatment of diabetic maculopathy. Interim report of a multicentre controlled study. *Lancet*. 1975;2:1110–1113.
3. Blankenship GW. Diabetic macular edema and argon laser photocoagulation: A prospective randomized study. *Ophthalmology*. 1979;86:69–78.
4. Early Treatment Diabetic Retinopathy Study Research Group. Early Treatment Diabetic Retinopathy Study design and baseline characteristics. ETDRS Report No 7. *Ophthalmology*. 1991;98:741–756.
5. Early Treatment Diabetic Retinopathy Study Research Group. Treatment techniques and clinical guidelines for photocoagulation of diabetic macular edema. Early Treatment Diabetic Retinopathy Study Report No 2. *Ophthalmology*. 1987;94:761–774.
6. Early Treatment Diabetic Retinopathy Study Research Group. Photocoagulation for diabetic macular edema. Early Treatment Diabetic

Retinopathy Study Report No 1. *Arch Ophthalmol*. 1985;103:1796–1806.
7. Early Treatment Diabetic Retinopathy Study Research Group. Photocoagulation for diabetic macular edema. Early Treatment Diabetic Retinopathy Study Report No 4. *Int Ophthalmol Clin*. 1987;27:265–272.
8. Ferris FL, Podgor MJ, Davis MD, et al. Macular edema in Diabetic Retinopathy Study patients. Diabetic Retinopathy Study Report No 12. *Ophthalmology*. 1987;94:754–760.
9. Early Treatment Diabetic Retinopathy Study Research Group. Early photocoagulation for diabetic retinopathy. ETDRS Report No 9. *Ophthalmology*. 1991;98:766–785.
10. Ferris FL, Kassoff A, Bresnick GH, et al. New visual acuity charts for clinical research. *Am J Ophthalmol*. 1982;94:91–96.
11. Ferris FL, Sperduto RD. Standardized illumination for visual acuity testing in clinical research. *Am J Ophthalmol*. 1982;94:97–98.
12. Ferris FL, Freidlin V, Kassoff A, et al. Relative letter and position difficulty on visual acuity charts from the Early Treatment Diabetic Retinopathy Study. *Am J Ophthalmol*. 1993;116:735–740.
13. Martidis A, Duker JS, Greenberg PB. Intravitreal triamcinolone for refractory diabetic macular edema. *Ophthalmology*. 2002;109:920–927.
14. Bakri SJ, Shah A, Falk NS, et al. Intravitreal preservative-free triamcinolone acetonide for the treatment of macular oedema. *Eye*. 2004; http://www.ncbi.nlm.nih.gov/entrez/query.fcgi?db=pubmed&cmd=Retrieve&dopt=Abstract&list_uids=15332099&query_hl=1&itool=pubmed_docsum.
15. Pollack JS. Intravitreous steroid injection study: Diabetic macular edema. Presented at the *22nd Retina Society meeting*. Baltimore. August 16-20, 2004.
16. Buddi R, Eliott D. Emerging treatments for diabetic eye disease: Update on clinical trials. *Ret Phys*. 2004;18–23.
17. Pearson P, Baker C, Eliott D, et al. Fluocinolone acetonide intravitreous implant for diabetic macular edema: 2 year results. Presented at *The Annual Association for Research in Vision and Ophthalmology meeting*. Ft. Lauderdale. April 25-29, 2004.
18. Haller JA. The Steroid Device: The Oculex Study. Presented at the Retina Subspecialty Day.

American Academy of Ophthalmology meeting. Anaheim. November 15-18, 2003.

19. Aiello LP, Davis MD, Milton RC, et al. Initial results of the protein kinase C beta inhibitor diabetic macular edema study (PKC-DMES). *Diabetologia.* 2003;46(suppl 2):A42.

20. Gragoudas ES, Adamis AP, Cunningham ET Jr, et al. VEGF Inhibition Study in Ocular Neovascularization Clinical Trial Group. Pegaptanib for neovascular age-related macular degeneration. *N Engl J Med.* 2004;351:2863–2865.

21. Macugen Diabetic Retinopathy Study Group. A phase II randomized double-masked trial of pegaptanib, an anti-vascular endothelial growth factor aptamer, for diabetic macular edema. *Ophthalmology.* 2005;112:1747–1757.

CHAPTER **6C**

Proliferative Diabetic Retinopathy: Clinical Trials

Dean Eliott, MD

Diabetic Retinopathy Study

Introduction

Eyes that develop proliferative diabetic retinopathy (PDR) have at least a 50% probability of becoming blind within 5 years without treatment.[1-3] Retinal photocoagulation, introduced by Meyer-Schwickerath in 1960 with the xenon arc, appeared to have a beneficial effect on neovascularization; however, there was uncertainty as to its exact role.[4] The xenon arc was used to treat patches of surface neovascularization directly, while the ruby laser and, subsequently, the argon laser, were used in the same manner as well as in an indirect scatter pattern. Results of several small clinical trials in the late 1960s suggested that photocoagulation might be a promising new treatment for retinal neovascularization.[5] The Diabetic Retinopathy Study (DRS) was organized in the 1970s to determine the effect of photocoagulation on diabetic retinopathy. This was the first prospective, multicenter, randomized controlled trial (RCT) sponsored by the newly formed National Eye Institute of the National Institutes of Health. In addition to its historical importance, the DRS has contributed tremendously to our understanding of the role of photocoagulation in the management of PDR.[6,7]

Background and Study Questions

When the DRS was organized, visual loss from diabetic retinopathy was a growing public health problem. There was no consensus regarding the treatment of PDR and diabetic macular edema (DME), the two major causes of blindness in patients with diabetes. The DRS, which attempted to seek answers to an important public health issue, was unprecedented in its scope and size.

To describe fundus findings in a consistent manner, the DRS used a modified version of the Airlie House Classification of diabetic retinopathy.[8] The original Airlie House Classification was developed in 1968 at a symposium where the most up-to-date knowledge of diabetic retinopathy was discussed. Despite a symposium among more than 50 international experts in retinal disease, the best approach in the management of diabetic retinopathy was unknown.[9,10]

It was in this historical context that the DRS was established. The DRS sought to determine whether photocoagulation (xenon or argon) was effective in the treatment of diabetic retinopathy. Specifically, it attempted to determine whether photocoagulation could prevent severe visual loss in eyes with PDR, whether there was a difference in safety and efficacy between xenon arc and argon laser, and whether certain stages of retinopathy demonstrated different responses to treatment.[6,7]

Patients Included in the Study

Approximately 1,750 patients with PDR in at least one eye or severe nonproliferative diabetic retinopathy (NPDR) in both eyes, and visual acuity of at least 20/100 in both eyes were enrolled.[11]

Severe NPDR was defined by the DRS as cotton-wool spots (see Fig. 6C.1), venous beading (see Fig. 6C.2), and intraretinal microvascular abnormalities (see Fig. 6C.3) in at least two of four contiguous photographic fields or two of these findings and moderately severe hemorrhages and/or microaneurysms (see Fig. 6C.4) in at least one photographic field. There are seven standard 30-degree photographic fields (see Fig. 6C.5).[8,11]

143

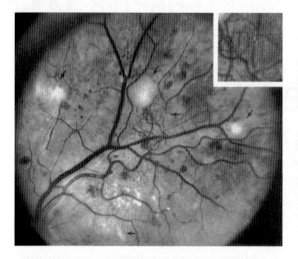

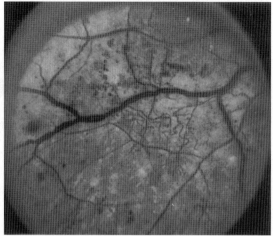

FIGURE 6C.1 □ Diabetic Retinopathy Study standard photograph 5, the more severe of two standards for soft exudates. There are four soft exudates (cotton-wool spots) in the upper half of this photograph: Two (almost confluent) at the 9:30 position, one just above the center, and one at the 3 o'clock position. This photograph also shows hard exudates (lipid) below the center of the picture and a small segment of arteriolar sheathing (*inset*). Some of the abnormal vessels at the center of the photograph are intraretinal microvascular abnormalities and some are new vessels. (From Diabetic Retinopathy Study Research Group. A modification of the Airlie House Classification of diabetic retinopathy. DRS Report No. 7. *Invest Ophthalmol Vis Sci.* 1981;21(1):210–226 and from Early Treatment Diabetic Retinopathy Study Research Group. Grading diabetic retinopathy from stereoscopic color fundus photographs—an extension of the modified Airlie House Classification. ETDRS Report No. 10. *Ophthalmology.* 1991;98:786–806.)[11a]

FIGURE 6C.2 □ Diabetic Retinopathy Study standard photograph 6B, more severe standard for venous beading. Most venous branches, both large and small, are involved by severe beading. (From Diabetic Retinopathy Study Research Group. A modification of the Airlie House Classification of diabetic retinopathy. DRS Report No. 7. *Invest Ophthalmol Vis Sci.* 1981;21(1):210–226 and from Early Treatment Diabetic Retinopathy Study Research Group. Grading diabetic retinopathy from stereoscopic color fundus photographs—an extension of the modified Airlie House Classification. ETDRS Report No. 10. *Ophthalmology.* 1991;98:786–806.)[11a]

Neovascularization of the disc (NVD) was defined by the DRS as the presence of abnormal vessels on or within one-disc diameter of the optic disc (see Fig. 6C.6), and neovascularization elsewhere (NVE) as the presence of abnormal vessels located more than one-disc diameter from the disc (see Fig. 6C.7).

Intervention and Outcome Measures

One eye of each patient was randomized to receive treatment, either with the xenon arc or the argon blue–green laser, and the other eye served as a control and was observed without treatment. All treated eyes received both direct photocoagulation to surface neovascularization (NVE only) and scatter panretinal photocoagulation from the vascular arcades to beyond the equator (laser burns separated by one burn width). In addition, eyes randomized to argon laser treatment also had NVD treated directly only in the initial part of the study (this was not possible with xenon). Argon laser burns were generally smaller and less intense than xenon arc burns (see Fig. 6C.8).

Outcome measures included severe visual loss, defined as visual acuity less than 5/200 at each of two consecutive visits 4 months apart.

Major Findings

The DRS demonstrated a 50% reduction in severe visual loss in eyes that received photocoagulation (see Fig. 6C.9).[12,13] This finding was so impressive that the protocol was amended to allow the control group to receive photocoagulation.[13]

The study also identified features that were associated with a particularly high risk of severe visual loss.[13–16] These risk factors were based on the presence, location, and severity of neovascularization, as

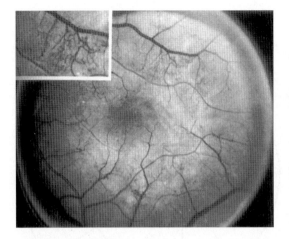

FIGURE 6C.3 ☐ Diabetic Retinopathy Study standard photograph 8B, more severe standard for intraretinal microvascular abnormalities (IRMA). This photograph shows IRMA in all quadrants. Inset shows IRMA superotemporal to the center of the macula. (From Diabetic Retinopathy Study Research Group. A modification of the Airlie House Classification of diabetic retinopathy. DRS Report No. 7. *Invest Ophthalmol Vis Sci.* 1981;21(1):210–226 and from Early Treatment Diabetic Retinopathy Study Research Group. Grading diabetic retinopathy from stereoscopic color fundus photographs—an extension of the modified Airlie House Classification. ETDRS Report No. 10. *Ophthalmology.* 1991; 98:786–806.)[11a]

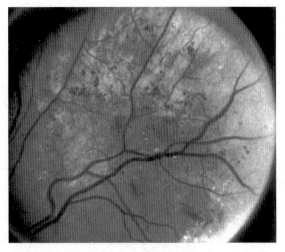

FIGURE 6C.4 ☐ Diabetic Retinopathy Study standard photograph 2B, severe standard for hemorrhages and microaneurysms. (From Diabetic Retinopathy Study Research Group. A modification of the Airlie house classification of diabetic retinopathy. DRS Report No. 7. *Invest Ophthalmol Vis Sci.* 1981;21(1):210–226 and from Early Treatment Diabetic Retinopathy Study Research Group. Grading diabetic retinopathy from stereoscopic color fundus photographs—an extension of the modified Airlie House Classification. ETDRS Report No. 10. *Ophthalmology.* 1991;98:786–806.)[11a]

well as the presence of vitreous or preretinal hemorrhage. Specifically, these risk factors were defined as (a) the presence of new vessels; (b) the location of new vessels on or within one-disc diameter of the optic disc (NVD); (c) the severity of new vessels, defined for NVD as equal to or greater than one-fourth to one-third disc area in extent (equal to or greater than standard photograph 10A) (Fig. 6C.6),[8] or for NVE, equal to or greater than one-half disc area; and (d) preretinal or vitreous hemorrhage. Eyes with at least 3 of these risk factors were considered to be at high risk for severe visual loss, and these eyes demonstrated the most benefit from photocoagulation (see Table 6C.1, Fig. 6C.10).

After 2 years of follow-up in the DRS, severe visual loss occurred in 26% of eyes in the control group as compared with 11% in the treated group for eyes with high-risk characteristics (HRC). After 4 years, 44% of control eyes and 20% of treated eyes developed severe visual loss, and the unequivocal benefit of photocoagulation was substantiated in all

additional reports with longer follow-up.[17,18] Prompt photocoagulation was recommended for eyes with HRC.

For eyes with PDR and less than high-risk retinopathy, the risk of developing severe visual loss at 2 years was 7% for the control group and 3% for the treated group. For eyes with severe NPDR, these rates were even lower. The DRS did not recommend prompt treatment for these categories of eyes.

Regarding the safety and efficacy of argon versus xenon photocoagulation, the DRS demonstrated that decreased visual acuity and constricted visual fields were more common in the xenon group. Persistent visual acuity loss of one line occurred in 19% of xenon-treated eyes as compared with 11% in the argon group; a loss of two or more lines occurred in 11% for xenon and 3% for argon. A modest loss of visual field (measured on Goldmann perimetry using the largest test object, IVe4) occurred in 25% of xenon-treated eyes as compared with 5% of argon-treated eyes; more severe field loss occurred in an additional 25% in the xenon group.[13,17]

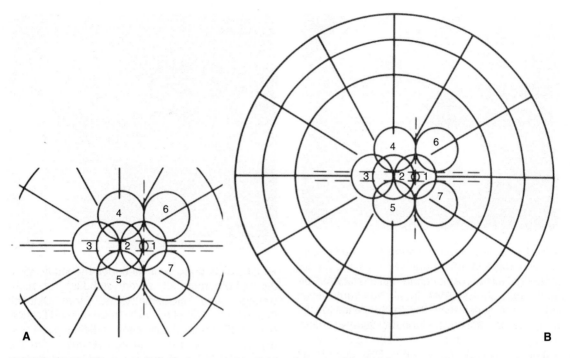

FIGURE 6C.5 ☐ Seven standard photographic fields of the modified Airlie House Classification shown for the right eye. Field 1 is centered on the optic disc; field 2 on the macula; field 3 temporal to the macula. Fields 4 through 7 are tangential to horizontal lines passing through the superior and inferior edges of the optic disc and to a vertical line passing through its center. (From Diabetic Retinopathy Study Research Group. A modification of the Airlie House Classification of diabetic retinopathy. DRS Report No. 7. *Invest Ophthalmol Vis Sci.* 1981;21(1):210–226 and from Olk RJ, Lee CM. Review of national collaborative studies. In: *Diabetic retinopathy: Practical management.* Philadelphia, PA: JB Lippincott Co; 1993:22.)

Implications for Clinical Practice

The DRS conclusively demonstrated that photocoagulation was effective in the treatment of PDR, and the overwhelming benefit associated with treatment had important public health implications.

The DRS identified four retinopathy risk factors for severe visual loss in eyes with PDR that met the inclusion criteria. Eyes with at least three of these risk factors were considered to be at high risk. Since these eyes demonstrated a 50% reduction of severe visual loss with photocoagulation, prompt treatment was recommended for eyes with PDR and HRC as defined by the DRS.

Three clinical situations were thus characteristic of eyes with high-risk retinopathy: (a) NVD equal to or greater than one-fourth to one-third disc area (greater than photograph 10A); (b) less extensive NVD with preretinal or vitreous hemorrhage; (c) NVE equal to or greater than one-half disc area with preretinal or vitreous hemorrhage (Table 6C.1).

For high-risk eyes, the risk of severe visual loss was substantially reduced at 2 years and 4 years using either xenon or argon photocoagulation, and the beneficial effects far outweighed the side effects of either modality. Nevertheless, argon was recommended rather than xenon arc because of similar benefits and less harmful effects.

Before a protocol amendment, the initial DRS protocol included direct treatment of NVD in eyes randomized to argon laser. Since this was associated with an increased risk of hemorrhage at the time of treatment without an increase in NVD regression, this treatment technique was discontinued.

Unanswered Questions

Although prompt photocoagulation was recommended for eyes with PDR and HRC as defined by the DRS, the DRS did not provide a clear recommendation for eyes with early PDR or those with severe NPDR. The question remained as to whether

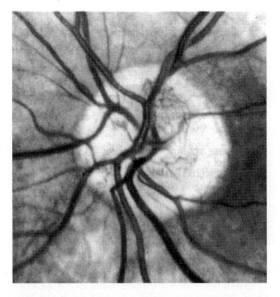

FIGURE 6C.6 ▢ Diabetic Retinopathy Study standard photograph 10A demonstrating neovascularization of the disc, one-fourth to one-third disc area in extent. (From Diabetic Retinopathy Study Research Group. Photocoagulation treatment of proliferative diabetic retinopathy: the second report of Diabetic Retinopathy Study findings. *Am J Ophthalmol.* 1978;85:82−106 and from Early Treatment Diabetic Retinopathy Study Research Group. ETDRS Report No. 10. Grading diabetic retinopathy from stereoscopic color fundus photographs−an extension of the modified Airlie house classification. *Ophthalmology.* 1991;98:786−806.)[11a]

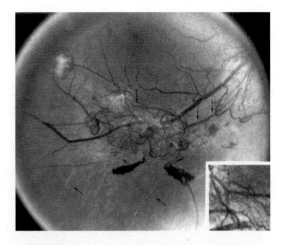

FIGURE 6C.7 ▢ Diabetic Retinopathy Study standard photograph 7 demonstrating the lower boundary of severe new vessels elsewhere. This photograph also shows new vessels within 1 disc diameter from the disc (Neovascularization of the disc) in the upper right part of the picture, focal arteriolar narrowing, arteriolar sheathing, "white threads" (completely opaque arteriolar branches), and small preretinal hemorrhages. (From Diabetic Retinopathy Study Research Group. A modification of the Airlie House Classification of diabetic retinopathy. DRS Report No. 7. *Invest Ophthalmol Vis Sci.* 1981;21(1):210−226 and from Early Treatment Diabetic Retinopathy Study Research Group. Grading diabetic retinopathy from stereoscopic color fundus photographs−an extension of the modified Airlie house classification. ETDRS Report No. 10. *Ophthalmology.* 1991;98:786−806.)[11a]

photocoagulation performed at an earlier stage of retinopathy would be more beneficial. At the other end of the spectrum, the DRS did not address the surgical management of late complications of diabetic retinopathy, such as severe fibrovascular proliferation and vitreous hemorrhage.

In addition to PDR, DME remained a significant cause of visual loss in diabetic patients. In the DRS, panretinal scatter photocoagulation was associated with progression of macular edema in some patients.[19] The DRS did not adequately assess this effect, nor did it evaluate the potential benefit of focal photocoagulation.

Diabetic Retinopathy Vitrectomy Study

Introduction

The Diabetic Retinopathy Vitrectomy Study (DRVS) has provided tremendous value in our understanding of the sight-threatening complications related to PDR. While the DRS addressed laser treatment for eyes with PDR and severe NPDR, the DRVS sought to evaluate the surgical management of eyes with more severe complications, and it attempted to define the role and timing of vitrectomy. Specifically, the DRVS was established by the National Eye Institute to evaluate the risks and benefits of performing early pars plana vitrectomy in eyes with advanced PDR.

Conducted in the late 1970s and early 1980s, this multicenter, prospective, RCT comprised three studies.[20−24] One was a natural history study that included eyes with severe PDR but without severe vitreous hemorrhage, and these eyes were followed up with conventional management.[20] The other two studies were RCTs involving vitrectomy. The first of these randomized trials compared early vitrectomy (before 6 months)

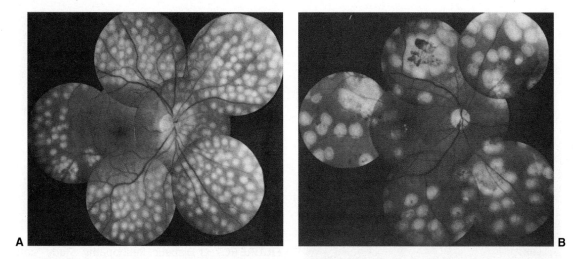

FIGURE 6C.8 ☐ **A:** Twenty-four-hour posttreatment photographs after Diabetic Retinopathy Study argon technique. Note extensive 500-μ scatter burns, focal treatment of neovascularization of the disc adjacent to the disc, and confluent focal treatment of two small patches of neovascularization elsewhere (NVE) along the inferotemporal artery inferotemporal to the macula. **B:** Twenty-four-hour posttreatment photographs after DRS xenon technique. Scatter burns are less evenly spaced than the argon burns in Figure 6C.8A. Confluent focal treatment has been applied to four patches of NVE. A small preretinal hemorrhage within the NVE superotemporal to the disc has occurred since treatment. Focal treatment has been applied to microaneurysms (thought to be the cause of mild macular edema) temporal to the macula. (From Diabetic Retinopathy Study Research Group. Photocoagulation of proliferative diabetic retinopathy: clinical applications of DRS findings. DRS Report 8. *Ophthalmology*. 1988;88:583–600.)

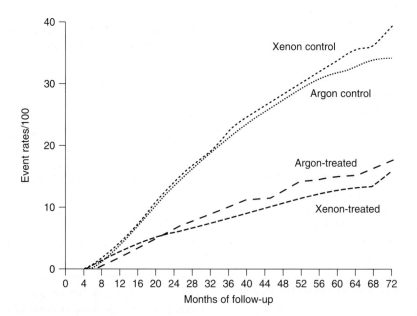

FIGURE 6C.9 ☐ Cumulative rates of severe visual loss for argon-treated and xenon-treated groups and controls. (From Diabetic Retinopathy Study Research Group. Photocoagulation of proliferative diabetic retinopathy: clinical applications of DRS findings. DRS Report 8. *Ophthalmology*. 1988;88:583–600.)

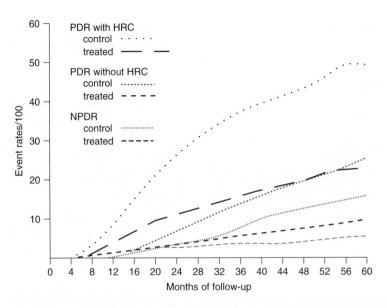

FIGURE 6C.10 ☐ Cumulative rates of severe visual loss for eyes classified to have proliferative diabetic retinopathy (PDR), high-risk characteristics (HRC), and nonproliferative diabetic retinopathy (NPDR) at baseline. Argon and xenon groups combined. (From Diabetic Retinopathy Study Research Group. Photocoagulation of proliferative diabetic retinopathy: clinical applications of DRS findings. DRS Report 8. *Ophthalmology*. 1988;88:583–600.)

versus deferral of surgery (1 year) in eyes with severe nonclearing vitreous hemorrhage,[21,24] and the second compared early vitrectomy versus conventional management in eyes with advanced, active PDR (severe fibrovascular proliferation) and useful vision.[22,23] Each of these studies will be addressed separately.

TABLE 6C.1 ☐ **Eyes with at least three of these risk factors (high risk characteristics) were considered to be at high risk for severe visual loss, and these eyes demonstrated the most benefit from photocoagulation**

Features associated with a particularly high risk of severe visual loss

1. The presence of new vessels
2. The location of new vessels on or within one-disc diameter of the optic disc (NVD)
3. The severity of new vessels (one of the following):
   a. NVD equal to or greater than one-fourth to one-third disc area in extent (equal to or greater than standard photograph 10A)
   b. Equal to or greater than one-half disc area
4. Preretinal or vitreous hemorrhage

High-risk characteristics of severe visual loss.
NVD, neovascularization of the disc.

Natural History Study

Background and Study Questions

Despite the early success obtained with vitrectomy, the procedure had a high rate of complications and some patients lost all perception of light. As technical advances were made, vitrectomy was offered to an increasing number of patients with the sequelae of PDR. It was difficult for clinicians to determine the proper role of vitrectomy because of a lack of sufficient information regarding the natural course of the disease.

It was in this historical context that a natural history study was undertaken. Eyes with severe PDR but without severe vitreous hemorrhage were followed up with conventional management for two years.

Patients Included in the Study

A total of 744 eyes (622 patients) with very severe PDR were enrolled. There were three subgroups, defined by the dominant retinopathy at baseline: Eyes with severe new vessels at least four disc areas in size and visual acuity 10/50 or better, eyes with extramacular traction retinal detachment at least four disc areas in extent and visual acuity 10/50 or better, and eyes with vitreous hemorrhage obscuring at least one-half of at least three standard photographic fields with visual acuity 10/200 or better or between 5/200 and hand motion.

Intervention and Outcome Measures

Patients were followed up with conventional management, including photocoagulation, over a 2-year period. Patients were offered vitrectomy only if they developed retinal detachment involving the center of the macula or if they developed severe vitreous hemorrhage that did not clear after one year of follow-up. The primary outcome measure was visual acuity, assessed at 1 and 2 years. Good vision was defined as 10/20 or better, and poor vision was less than 5/200.

Major Findings

Decreases in visual acuity were more frequent during the first year of follow-up than during the second year, and were related to retinopathy severity and baseline visual acuity. In eyes with more than four disc areas of new vessels and visual acuity of 10/30 to 10/50 at baseline, visual acuity decreased to <5/200 in 45% at 2 years. In contrast, in eyes with traction retinal detachment not involving the center of the macula and without active new vessels or fresh vitreous hemorrhage at baseline, visual acuity decreased to <5/200 in only 14%. Vitrectomy, which was required only if a macula-involving retinal detachment occurred or if severe vitreous hemorrhage did not clear after 1 year, was performed in 25% of eyes during the 2-year follow-up period.[20]

Implications for Clinical Practice

When the DRVS was planned, most surgeons followed up patients with severe vitreous hemorrhage for at least 1 year before recommending vitrectomy. Because of the high rate of visual loss and the high likelihood of the need for vitrectomy in the natural history study, investigators suggested evaluating the benefit of early vitrectomy (before 6 months) in patients with severe vitreous hemorrhage. The relatively good prognosis of eyes with traction retinal detachment not involving the center of the macula did not justify surgical intervention for this indication.

Unanswered Question

Does early vitrectomy (before 6 months) offer any benefit compared with vitrectomy performed after 1 year for severe vitreous hemorrhage?

Severe Nonclearing Vitreous Hemorrhage

Background and Study Questions

Of historical interest, the first pars plana vitrectomy ever performed was by Robert Machemer in 1970 for a nonclearing diabetic vitreous hemorrhage of 5 years' duration, resulting in improvement in visual acuity from 2/200 to 20/50.[25] Vitreous hemorrhage from retinal neovascularization is a frequent complication of PDR, and a report from 1977 indicated that this was the most common indication for diabetic vitrectomy.[26]

Since the optimal timing of vitrectomy was unknown, this study compared early vitrectomy (<6 months) to deferral of surgery (1 year) in patients with severe nonclearing vitreous hemorrhage.

Patients Included in the Study

A total of 616 eyes were enrolled. Severe vitreous hemorrhage was defined as central vitreous hemorrhage reducing visual acuity to 5/200 or less for at least 1 month. Patients were classified as having type I diabetes if diabetes was diagnosed at or before age 20 and if they were receiving insulin at the time of entry into the study. Type II diabetes included patients aged 40 or older at diagnosis (regardless of insulin use) and patients with diabetes diagnosed at a younger age if they were not receiving insulin. An intermediate group comprised patients diagnosed between 21 and 39 years of age, inclusive, who were receiving insulin.

Intervention and Outcome Measures

Patients were randomized into one of two groups. The early vitrectomy group underwent vitrectomy within a few days of randomization (from 1 to 6 months after the onset of severe vitreous hemorrhage), and the deferral group was offered surgery 1 year after randomization (if severe vitreous hemorrhage persisted at 1 year, or sooner if macular detachment occurred). The primary outcome measure was visual acuity, with particular regard to recovery of good vision (10/20 or better) and no light perception.

Major Findings

After two years of follow-up, the DRVS demonstrated that in eyes with severe vitreous hemorrhage, early vitrectomy resulted in final visual acuity of 20/40 or better in 25% of cases, compared with 15%

of cases in the group with deferred surgery. Early vitrectomy helps in the recovery of good vision, as was most apparent in type I diabetics, as 36% of eyes in this group achieved visual acuity of 20/40 or better, whereas only 12% of eyes in the deferral group achieved this level. In the type II and intermediate groups, however, there was little difference between early vitrectomy and deferral of surgery regarding the recovery of good vision (16% vs. 18%).[21] After 4 years of follow-up, the advantage for the early-vitrectomy group persisted.[24]

This study also demonstrated that progression to no light perception was similar for the early-vitrectomy and deferral groups at 2-year follow-up (25% vs. 19%). For patients with type I diabetes, the risk of losing light perception was the same with either treatment strategy, but for the type II and intermediate groups, there was a (nonsignificant) trend toward less frequent visual acuity of no light perception in the deferral group.

Implications for Clinical Practice

For patients with type I diabetes, the more favorable visual results after early vitrectomy were attributed to their more advanced retinopathy, as these patients had greater severity of new vessels, fibrous proliferations, and vitreoretinal adhesions. Progression of new vessels, contraction of fibrous proliferations, and worsening of traction retinal detachment during the waiting period would be expected to be more severe in the type I group, thereby reducing their potential for recovery of good vision without vitrectomy.

The prevalence of severe, nonclearing vitreous hemorrhage has been reduced by the more widespread use of panretinal photocoagulation; however, it still remains a major indication for vitrectomy. When adequate fundus visualization is present despite vitreous hemorrhage, panretinal photocoagulation is always performed in an attempt to stabilize or achieve regression of neovascularization. The use of krypton or diode lasers may facilitate treatment through hemorrhage, because red and infrared wavelengths are transmitted through hemoglobin pigments better than the blue and green wavelengths of argon. Alternatively, the laser indirect delivery system may allow treatment when slit lamp delivery is not possible. Restricting patient activity and elevating the head of the patient's bed are additional conservative measures that are usually initially recommended.

When vitreous hemorrhage is of sufficient density to preclude visualization of fundus details, echography is essential to detect the need for earlier intervention. If retinal detachment involving the center of the macula, combined traction/rhegmatogenous retinal detachment, or severe fibrovascular proliferation is identified at any time, vitrectomy is indicated. If spontaneous clearing of a dense vitreous hemorrhage does not occur, vitrectomy is considered, especially for patients with type I diabetes. Surgical goals include removal of vitreous hemorrhage to provide a clear media, excision of the posterior hyaloid and epiretinal fibrovascular membranes to relieve vitreoretinal traction, and application of endolaser photocoagulation to achieve regression of proliferative tissue.[27]

An important point is that the DRVS results were obtained before the development of endolaser photocoagulation. Furthermore, surgery was performed in this study without the benefit of using glucose-fortified infusion solutions to reduce the intraoperative development of cataract. These advances, as well as countless others, have contributed to the more favorable results noted recently. In the DRVS, one-fifth to one-quarter of all patients progressed to no light perception vision; however, using current vitreoretinal instrumentation and techniques, this rate is much lower.

Unanswered Questions

While this study provided information of tremendous clinical value, progressive advances in surgical instrumentation and technique have favorably altered the risk-benefit ratio, and the optimal timing of vitrectomy is constantly evolving. Although a variety of ocular and systemic factors influence the decision to perform vitrectomy, in general, the recommended timing of vitrectomy for severe diabetic vitreous hemorrhage is approximately 3 months. More recently, vitrectomy was advocated by some surgeons even earlier. It is certain that modern advances will continue to alter practice patterns.

Severe Proliferative Diabetic Retinopathy (Severe Fibrovascular Proliferation)

Background and Study Questions

When laser treatment was growing in popularity, it was noted that in some patients, active neovascular and fibrovascular proliferations progressed rapidly

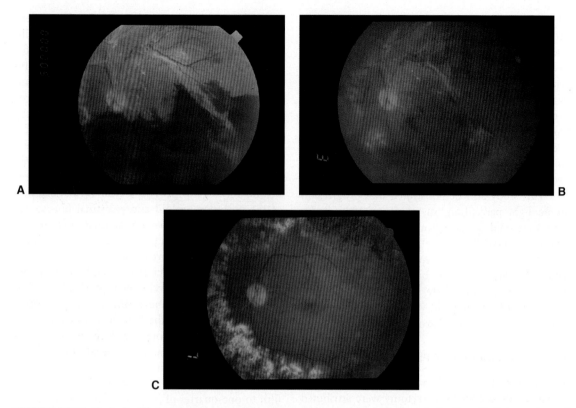

FIGURE 6C.11 ☐ **A:** Proliferative diabetic retinopathy with extensive neovascularization. **B:** Progression of fibrovascular proliferation and vitreous hemorrhage despite panretinal photocoagulation. **C:** Postoperative appearance after vitrectomy for severe fibrovascular proliferation. Visual acuity is 20/20. (From Eliott D, Lee MS, Abrams GW. Proliferative Diabetic Retinopathy: Principles and techniques of surgical treatment. In: Ryan SJ, ed. *Retina,* 3rd ed. St Louis, MO: Mosby, 2000:2444. Fig. 146−8.)

despite extensive panretinal photocoagulation (see Fig. 6C.11A, B). This typically occurred in young patients with poorly controlled type I diabetes and in patients with an attached hyaloid, as the role of formed vitreous contact with the retina in the development of neovascular proliferation was well known.[28] The fibrovascular tissue usually underwent contraction resulting in vitreous hemorrhage, macular distortion, and/or retinal detachment.

Once a macula-involving traction retinal detachment developed, surgical attempts at retinal reattachment often failed to restore good vision. Surgeons noted that in patients with progressive fibrovascular proliferation, neovascularization rarely occurred after surgical excision of the posterior cortical vitreous (Fig. 6C.11C). Thus, when proliferation was severe and vision was not yet significantly impaired, early vitrectomy had the potential to stop the proliferative process and preserve vision. These potential

benefits were offset by the potential for severe surgical complications, including progression to no light perception vision.

Since the optimal timing of surgical intervention was unknown, this study evaluated the outcome of early vitrectomy versus conventional management in eyes with advanced, active PDR (extensive, active neovascular or fibrovascular proliferations) and useful vision.

Patients Included in the Study

A total of 370 eyes with visual acuity of 10/200 or better and extensive, active, neovascular or fibrovascular proliferations were enrolled. This was defined as severe new vessels (four or more disc areas) and severe fibrous proliferations (two or more disc areas at the disc, or 4 or more disc areas total); severe new vessels and red vitreous hemorrhage (any preretinal or vitreous hemorrhage); or moderate new vessels (two or more disc areas), severe fibrous proliferations, and red vitreous hemorrhage.

Intervention and Outcome Measures

Patients were randomized to early vitrectomy or conventional management. Conventional management included observation, photocoagulation, and vitrectomy only after traction macular detachment or 6 months of nonclearing vitreous hemorrhage. The primary outcome was visual acuity at each year for a total of 4 years, with particular regard to good vision (10/20 or better), poor vision (less than 5/200), and no light perception.

Major Findings

In eyes with severe fibrovascular proliferation (extensive, active neovascular or fibrovascular proliferations) and useful vision (10/200 or better), early vitrectomy resulted in final visual acuity of 20/40 or better in 44% of cases (at 4-year follow-up), compared with 28% of cases managed conventionally (observation, photocoagulation, or vitrectomy only after traction macular detachment or 6 months of nonclearing vitreous hemorrhage). The advantage of early vitrectomy in the recovery of good vision was most apparent in eyes with the most severe proliferation at baseline. With increasing severity of neovascularization, the outcome with conventional management worsened for each end point. In contrast, the outcome did not worsen by increasing severity for eyes treated with early vitrectomy, accounting for the more favorable results. There was no significant difference between the two treatment groups in the development of poor vision or no light perception vision, although more eyes progressed to no light perception in the early vitrectomy group. Prior photocoagulation increased the chances of good vision.[22,23,27]

Implications for Clinical Practice

The more favorable visual results after early vitrectomy for advanced, active PDR were attributed to the removal of severe fibrovascular proliferations before their contracture led to distortion or detachment of the macula. Eyes most suitable for early vitrectomy are those in which both fibrous proliferations and at least moderately severe new vessels are present, and in which extensive panretinal photocoagulation has already been carried out or is precluded by vitreous hemorrhage.

Unanswered Questions

As noted previously, the DRVS was performed before the development of endolaser photocoagulation. The instrumentation and techniques of vitrectomy surgery have been constantly evolving, and results today are much more favorable than in the past. Although the optimal timing of vitrectomy is constantly changing, the findings from the DRVS serve as the foundation for the decision to perform vitrectomy in the modern era.

Early Treatment Diabetic Retinopathy Study

Background

Because of the overwhelming success of the DRS in finding answers to an important public health problem, the Early Treatment Diabetic Retinopathy Study (ETDRS) was established to address additional questions related to diabetic retinopathy. Conducted in the 1980s, the ETDRS was even larger in scope and size than the recently completed DRS.

The DRS demonstrated that photocoagulation was beneficial for eyes with PDR and HRC, as previously noted. The DRS, however, did not provide a clear recommendation for eyes with early PDR or those with severe NPDR. The question remained as to whether photocoagulation performed at an earlier stage of retinopathy would be even more beneficial. The ETDRS was designed to address this question, as well as questions involving the treatment of DME and the use of aspirin.

The ETDRS sought to determine when panretinal photocoagulation should be initiated to be most effective in the management of diabetic retinopathy, whether focal photocoagulation was effective in the treatment of DME, and whether aspirin was effective in altering the course of diabetic retinopathy. Each of these study questions is addressed separately. The management of DME is addressed in Chapter 6B, and the other two arms of the ETDRS are discussed in the subsequent text.

Study Question

When should scatter panretinal photocoagulation be initiated to be most effective in the management of diabetic retinopathy?

Patients Included in Study

A total of 3,711 patients with mild-to-severe NPDR or early PDR (less than high risk), with or without DME, were enrolled. Visual acuity criteria were 20/40 or better for eyes without macular edema and 20/200 or better for those with macular edema.

Mild NPDR was defined by the ETDRS as the presence of at least one microaneurysm.[29]

Moderate NPDR was defined as hemorrhages and/or microaneurysms greater than standard photograph 2A (see Fig. 6C.12); and/or the presence of soft exudates, venous beading, or intraretinal microvascular abnormalities (IRMA).[29]

Severe NPDR was defined as soft exudates, venous beading, and IRMA in at least two of fields four through seven; or two of these findings in at least two of these fields and hemorrhages and microaneurysms in all four of these fields (greater than standard photograph 2A in 1 field); or IRMA in all four of these fields (greater than standard photograph 8A in 2 fields) (see Fig. 6C.13).[29]

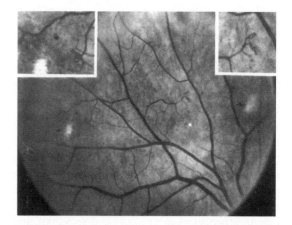

FIGURE 6C.13 □ Diabetic Retinopathy Study standard photograph 8A, less severe of two standards for intraretinal microvascular abnormalities (IRMA) and soft exudates. This photograph shows four areas of IRMA: two near the soft exudate at the 9 o'clock position (*inset*), one below these at the 7:30 position, and one near the center of the photograph along the 2 o'clock meridian (*inset*). (From Diabetic Retinopathy Study Research Group. A modification of the Airlie House Classification of diabetic retinopathy. DRS Report No. 7. *Invest Ophthalmol Vis Sci.* 1981;21(1):210–226 and from Early Treatment Diabetic Retinopathy Study Research Group. Grading diabetic retinopathy from stereoscopic color fundus photographs—an extension of the modified Airlie house classification. ETDRS Report No. 10. *Ophthalmology.* 1991;98:786–806.)[11a]

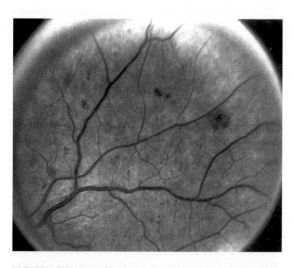

FIGURE 6C.12 □ Diabetic Retinopathy Study standard photograph 2A, intermediate standard for hemorrhages and microaneurysms. (From Diabetic Retinopathy Study Research Group. A modification of the Airlie House Classification of diabetic retinopathy. DRS Report No. 7. *Invest Ophthalmol Vis Sci.* 1981;21(1):210–226 and from Early Treatment Diabetic Retinopathy Study Research Group. Grading diabetic retinopathy from stereoscopic color fundus photographs—an extension of the modified Airlie House Classification. ETDRS Report No. 10. *Ophthalmology.* 1991;98:786–806.)[11a]

Early PDR was defined as proliferative retinopathy but without DRS HRC.[29] The definition of high-risk proliferative retinopathy is included in Table 6C.1.

Intervention and Outcome Measures

Eyes were randomized to immediate scatter panretinal photocoagulation (either mild or full scatter) or to no treatment. Specifically, eyes were divided among those without macular edema, those with macular edema and less severe retinopathy (mild or moderate NPDR), and those with macular edema and more severe retinopathy (severe NPDR or early PDR). One eye of each patient was randomized to deferral of treatment and the other eye to early photocoagulation using different combinations of scatter panretinal and macular focal photocoagulation. If an eye assigned to treatment deferral developed high-risk proliferative retinopathy, then scatter panretinal laser was initiated as per the DRS recommendations.[6]

In eyes without macular edema, those assigned to early photocoagulation received one of two combinations: Immediate mild scatter and delayed focal photocoagulation or immediate full scatter and delayed focal photocoagulation (see Fig. 6C.14A).[29]

In eyes with macular edema and less severe retinopathy, those assigned to early photocoagulation received one of four combinations: Immediate focal and delayed mild scatter photocoagulation, immediate focal and delayed full scatter photocoagulation, immediate mild scatter and delayed focal photocoagulation, or immediate full scatter and delayed focal photocoagulation (Fig. 6C.14B).[29]

In eyes with macular edema and more severe retinopathy, those assigned to early photocoagulation received one of four combinations: Immediate mild scatter and immediate focal photocoagulation, immediate mild scatter and delayed focal photocoagulation, immediate full scatter and immediate focal photocoagulation, or immediate full scatter and delayed focal photocoagulation (Fig. 6C.14C).[29]

Treatment was performed using the argon blue–green or green laser, although the krypton red laser was allowed if cataract or vitreous hemorrhage was present. Full scatter panretinal photocoagulation involved 1,200 to 1,600 burns applied in two or more sessions, and mild scatter involved 400 to 650 burns delivered in a single session. A 500-μ spot size was achieved using the Goldmann contact lens (500-μ setting) or the Rodenstock lens (300-μ setting).[30]

Outcome measures included moderate visual loss, defined as a loss of 15 or more letters from baseline, equivalent to a doubling of the visual angle, and severe visual loss, defined as visual acuity <5/200 at each of two consecutive follow-up visits 4 months apart.

Major Findings

Although the combination of early photocoagulation involving immediate full scatter reduced the rate of progression to high-risk retinopathy by 50%, and those involving immediate mild scatter reduced the rate by 25%, the overall risk for severe visual loss was low for all eyes.[31] Early photocoagulation also reduced the need for vitrectomy.[32]

In eyes without macular edema, there was no significant difference in the rates of moderate or severe visual loss between deferral of treatment or early photocoagulation using either treatment strategy.[31]

In eyes with macular edema and less severe retinopathy, early photocoagulation was associated with a reduced rate of severe visual loss at 5 years compared with deferral of treatment, but the rate was very low in all groups and the difference was not significant. Since the rate of progression to severe visual loss was so low in eyes with mild-to-moderate NPDR, treatment benefits were not considered sufficient to compensate for the side effects associated with photocoagulation, and treatment was not recommended.[31]

In eyes with macular edema and more severe retinopathy, early photocoagulation was associated with a reduced rate of severe visual loss at 5 years (3.8% to 4.7%) compared with deferral of treatment (6.5%), but the rate was low in all groups and the difference was not significant. Nevertheless, treatment benefits were encouraging, and it was suggested that scatter treatment should be considered in eyes with severe NPDR and early PDR.[31] This recommendation was supported by a subsequent report that demonstrated an even greater treatment effect in patients with type II diabetes.[33]

Similar to the DRS, the ETDRS demonstrated treatment-related side effects. Early scatter photocoagulation, especially full scatter treatment, was associated with visual field constriction and an increased rate of moderate visual loss. Moderate visual loss was increased only during the first year of follow-up (except in eyes with macular edema that received early focal treatment); subsequently, there was a lower rate of moderate visual loss for all combinations of early photocoagulation.

The ETDRS also provided information on the rates of progression from earlier stages of retinopathy to PDR with HRC.[31,34] Eyes with mild NPDR had a 1% risk of developing high-risk retinopathy at 1 year and a 15% risk at 5 years.[35,36] Eyes with moderate NPDR had a 3% risk at 1 year and a 27% risk at 5 years. These rates of progression for mild and moderate NPDR were considered relatively low, and although panretinal photocoagulation was not suggested by the ETDRS, close follow-up was recommended.

In contrast, severe NPDR was associated with a much higher risk of progression to high-risk PDR, and specific characteristics were identified that were especially predictive. The 4-2-1 rule was developed, and an eye with one of the following features was considered to have severe NPDR: Microaneurysms or hemorrhages in 4 quadrants; venous beading in 2

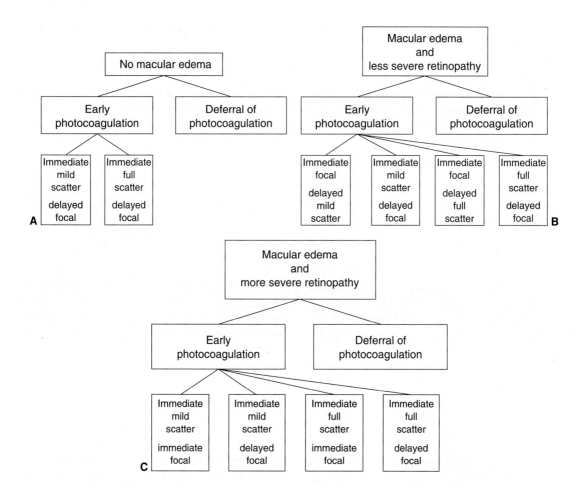

FIGURE 6C.14 □ **A:** Early Treatment Diabetic Retinopathy Study photocoagulation treatment scheme for eyes without macular edema and moderate-to-severe nonproliferative or early proliferative retinopathy. Eyes were assigned randomly to early photocoagulation or deferral of photocoagulation. Eyes assigned to early photocoagulation were further assigned randomly to either mild or full scatter (panretinal) photocoagulation. (From Early Treatment Diabetic Retinopathy Study Research Group. Early Treatment Diabetic Retinopathy Study design and baseline characteristics. ETDRS Report No 7. *Ophthalmology.* 1991;98:741−756.) **B:** Early Treatment Diabetic Retinopathy Study photocoagulation treatment scheme for eyes with macular edema and less severe retinopathy (mild-to-moderate nonproliferative retinopathy). Eyes were assigned randomly to early photocoagulation or to deferral of photocoagulation. Eyes assigned to early photocoagulation were further assigned randomly to either mild or full scatter (panretinal) photocoagulation, and to either immediate focal or delayed focal treatment. For eyes assigned to immediate focal treatment, the assigned scatter treatment was not applied initially, but only if severe nonproliferative retinopathy or worse developed during follow-up. (From Early Treatment Diabetic Retinopathy Study Research Group. Early Treatment Diabetic Retinopathy Study design and baseline characteristics. ETDRS Report No 7. *Ophthalmology.* 1991;98:741−756.) **C:** Early Treatment Diabetic Retinopathy Study photocoagulation treatment scheme for eyes with macular edema and more severe retinopathy. Eyes were assigned randomly to early photocoagulation or to deferral of photocoagulation. Eyes assigned to early photocoagulation were further assigned randomly to either mild or full scatter (panretinal) photocoagulation, and to either immediate focal or delayed focal treatment for at least 4 months. (From Early Treatment Diabetic Retinopathy Study Research Group. Early Treatment Diabetic Retinopathy Study design and baseline characteristics. ETDRS Report No 7. *Ophthalmology*. 1991;98:741−756.)

TABLE 6C.2 ☐ **The features in the 4-2-1 rule are associated with a high rate of progression to high-risk proliferative diabetic retinopathy. Any one of these features constitutes severe nonproliferative diabetic retinopathy, while any two features constitutes very severe nonproliferative diabetic retinopathy. See figures 12, 15, and 13 for Diabetic Retinopathy Study standard photographs 2A, 6A, and 8A, respectively**

4-2-1 Rule
4 quadrants of hemorrhages or microaneurysms equal to or greater than DRS standard photograph 2A
2 quadrants of venous beading equal to or greater than DRS standard photograph 6A
1 quadrant of intraretinal microvascular abnormalities equal to or greater than DRS standard photograph 8A

Features of the 4-2-1 rule.
DRS, diabetic retinopathy study.

quadrants; and IRMA in 1 quadrant (see Table 6C.2).[6,37] Eyes with severe NPDR as defined here had a 15% risk of developing HRC at 1 year and a 56% risk at 5 years. An additional category was identified, very severe NPDR, and included eyes having two findings of the 4-2-1 rule. These eyes had a 45% risk at 1 year and a 71% risk at 5 years. The ETDRS recommended that the benefits of early photocoagulation should be considered in eyes with severe or very severe NPDR and in those with early PDR.

Implications for Clinical Practice

Since there was a low rate of severe visual loss and a relatively low rate of progression to high-risk retinopathy in eyes with mild-to-moderate NPDR assigned to deferral of treatment, the ETDRS concluded that the adverse effects of panretinal photocoagulation (visual field constriction, early transient moderate visual loss) probably outweighed the small benefits of early treatment, and close follow-up was recommended.

In contrast, in eyes with more severe retinopathy (severe or very severe NPDR and early PDR), the recommendation was that early photocoagulation should be considered since these eyes had a high likelihood of progressing to PDR with HRC. Early treatment or deferral of treatment until progression

of retinopathy occurred was considered a reasonable option. This recommendation was based on the assumption of adequate and reliable patient follow-up. If there was any question about a patient's likelihood of returning for follow-up, early photocoagulation was strongly suggested.

Unanswered Questions

The ETDRS recommendation was to consider early treatment in eyes with severe or very severe NPDR and in eyes with early PDR (less than HRC), and reasonable options included early photocoagulation or deferral of treatment until progression of retinopathy occurred. The ETDRS did not provide a clear recommendation, except in circumstances where there was doubt about a patient's ability to return for adequate and timely follow-up. The decision regarding when to treat a patient with these more advanced stages of retinopathy was left to the discretion of the treating physician.

Early Treatment Diabetic Retinopathy Study

Introduction

In the 1970s, a variety of medical therapies for diabetic retinopathy had been proposed, including aspirin, dipyridamole, vitamins, and calcium dobesilate. The most promising agents seemed to be the ones that reduced platelet aggregation, because patients with diabetes demonstrated alterations in platelet function. The increased platelet adhesiveness was possibly related to the increased arachidonic acid metabolites prostaglandin E_2 and thromboxane E_2, and these alterations were thought to be potentially responsible for the capillary closure observed in diabetic retinopathy.[29]

Background

Aspirin therapy was a potential treatment, since it blocked cyclo-oxygenase and thus inhibited prostaglandin production and platelet aggregation. In addition, there was some clinical evidence that patients with diabetes who were treated with aspirin, usually for arthritis, had reduced prevalence of retinopathy.[29] Questions related to the potential benefit of aspirin regarding retinopathy progression were offset by those relating to the potential adverse consequences, such as increased hemorrhage. The ETDRS was designed to address these questions, as well

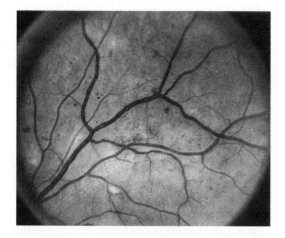

FIGURE 6C.15 ☐ Diabetic Retinopathy Study standard photograph 6A, less severe of two standards for venous beading. Two main branches of the superotemporal vein show definite, but not severe, beading. (From Diabetic Retinopathy Study Research Group. A modification of the Airlie House Classification of diabetic retinopathy. DRS Report No. 7. *Invest Ophthalmol Vis Sci.* 1981;21(1):210–226 and from Early Treatment Diabetic Retinopathy Study Research Group. Grading diabetic retinopathy from stereoscopic color fundus photographs—an extension of the modified Airlie House Classification. ETDRS Report No. 10. *Ophthalmology.* 1991;98:786–806.)[11a]

as questions involving the treatment of DME and questions involving the use of scatter treatment for earlier stages of retinopathy (mild-to-severe NPDR and early PDR).

The ETDRS sought to determine answers to three questions: Whether focal photocoagulation was effective in the treatment of DME, when panretinal photocoagulation should be initiated to be most effective in the management of diabetic retinopathy, and whether aspirin was effective in altering the course of diabetic retinopathy. Each of these study questions is addressed separately. This section will review the aspirin arm of the ETDRS.

Study Question

Is aspirin effective in altering the course of diabetic retinopathy?

Patients Included in Study

A total of 3,711 patients with mild-to-severe NPDR or early PDR (less than high risk), with or without DME,

were enrolled. Visual acuity criteria were 20/40 or better for eyes without macular edema and 20/200 or better for those with macular edema.

Intervention and Outcome Measures

Patients were randomized to receive 650 mg of aspirin per day or placebo (see Fig. 6C.16). The ETDRS used a factorial study design for aspirin use (patients randomized) and photocoagulation (eyes randomized). As indicated above for the other two arms of the ETDRS (DME, early scatter treatment) eyes were grouped into those without macular edema, those with macular edema and less severe retinopathy (mild or moderate NPDR), and those with macular edema and more severe retinopathy (severe NPDR or early PDR). One eye of each patient was randomized to early photocoagulation using different combinations of scatter panretinal and macular focal photocoagulation, and the other eye had deferral of treatment. If an eye assigned to treatment deferral developed high-risk proliferative retinopathy, then scatter panretinal laser was initiated as per the DRS recommendations.

Outcome measures included the progression to high-risk retinopathy (PDR with HRC), the development of vitreous hemorrhage, and visual loss. Moderate visual loss was defined as a loss of 15 or more letters from the baseline, equivalent to a doubling of the visual angle, and severe visual loss was defined as visual acuity <5/200 at each of two consecutive follow-up visits 4 months apart. Additional end points were the development of cardiovascular disease and mortality.

Major Findings

No difference was found in the progression to high-risk retinopathy, the development of vitreous hemorrhage, and the risk of visual loss between eyes of patients who received aspirin or placebo, despite randomization to immediate photocoagulation or to deferral of treatment.[38,39] Therefore, there was no contraindication to the use of aspirin in patients with mild-to-severe NPDR or early PDR who met the inclusion criteria of the ETDRS.

Interestingly, aspirin use was associated with a 17% decrease in morbidity and mortality from cardiovascular disease, and the benefits of aspirin use in patients with diabetes were evident.[40]

Since aspirin use was not associated with a treatment effect for ocular outcomes, and since its use had no interaction with photocoagulation, the ETDRS results for the other two arms of the study

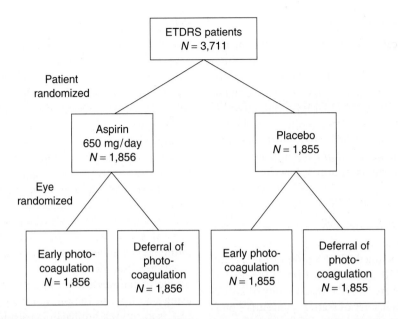

FIGURE 6C.16 ☐ Randomization scheme of Early Treatment Diabetic Retinopathy Study patients to aspirin or placebo treatment, and of eyes to photocoagulation strategies. (From Early Treatment Diabetic Retinopathy Study Research Group. Early Treatment Diabetic Retinopathy Study design and baseline characteristics. ETDRS Report No 7. *Ophthalmology*. 1991;98:741–756.)

(DME, early scatter treatment) were reported using the combined aspirin and placebo groups.

Implications for Clinical Practice

The ETDRS recommended that aspirin use, when prescribed for nonophthalmic medical conditions, was not contraindicated in patients with mild-to-severe NPDR or those with early PDR who met the inclusion criteria.

Unanswered Questions

The ETDRS did not evaluate the use of aspirin in patients with more advanced retinopathy (PDR with HRC), and there was no clear recommendation regarding the use of aspirin in these patients.

Proliferative Diabetic Retinopathy: Emerging Pharmacologic Therapies

Ruboxistaurin Mesylate (Arxxant, Eli Lilly and Co.)

Introduction

New pharmacologic interventions at the molecular level show great promise in treating the major causes of visual loss in diabetics: PDR and DME. As previously noted in Chapter 6B, two of the molecules being targeted are vascular endothelial growth factor (VEGF) and protein kinase C (PKC). VEGF is a vascular endothelial cell mitogen and potent permeability factor, and it is produced by glial cells, retinal pigment epithelial cells, and vascular endothelial cells. VEGF is normally present in the retina and vitreous in low levels; however, retinal hypoxia upregulates VEGF production, resulting in abnormal angiogenesis and a marked increase in vascular permeability. The PKC family is a group of enzymes involved in signal transduction. The β- isoform has been shown to have an important role in regulating vascular permeability and is an important signaling component for VEGF. The chronic hyperglycemia of uncontrolled diabetes leads to increased cellular levels of diacylglycerol that, in turn, activates PKC, especially the β-isoform. PKC-β increases the synthesis of VEGF, and also contributes to the microvascular abnormalities in diabetic retinopathy. Inhibition of either VEGF or PKC-β moderates the microvascular complications seen in experimental animal models. In addition, PKC-β inhibitors given orally have the potential to influence other diabetic complications such as renal insufficiency and peripheral neuropathy.[41]

Background and Study Questions

One of the clinical trials that have evaluated the role of ruboxistaurin mesylate is the PKC-β Inhibitor Diabetic Retinopathy Study (PKC-DRS).[42] The other clinical trial, the Protein Kinase C beta Diabetic Macular Edema Study (PKC-DMES), is discussed in Chapter 6B. The PKC-DRS is a multicenter, double-masked, placebo-controlled study that evaluated progression of diabetic retinopathy in patients who were treated with ruboxistaurin or placebo.

Patients Included in the Study

A total of 252 patients with moderately severe to very severe NPDR in at least one eye were enrolled. Eligibility criteria included ETDRS retinopathy severity level between 47B and 53E inclusive (moderately severe to very severe NPDR), visual acuity of 20/125 or better, and no history of scatter (panretinal) photocoagulation.

Intervention and Outcome Measures

Patients were randomized to placebo or ruboxistaurin 8, 16, or 32 mg orally per day for 36 to 46 months. The primary outcome was progression of retinopathy ($\geq$2-step worsening in the ETDRS retinopathy eye severity scale for patients with one study eye, >3-step worsening in the ETDRS retinopathy person severity scale for patients with two study eyes, or application of scatter photocoagulation). Secondary study outcomes were moderate visual loss (visual acuity loss > 15 letters, doubling or more of the visual angle), and sustained moderate visual loss (loss of > 15 letters observed at each of two consecutive visits 6 or more months apart).

Eligibility and outcomes were assessed using stereoscopic fundus photographs taken at 6-month intervals. Analysis was based on time to occurrence of the outcome measures using the intent-to-treat population.

Major Findings

Ruboxistaurin did not prevent the progression of diabetic retinopathy, but it reduced the risk of visual loss. Moderate visual loss was lower in the 32-mg group compared with placebo. Sustained moderate visual loss was lower in the 32-mg group only in eyes with definite DME at baseline. Ruboxistaurin was well tolerated with no significant adverse events noted.[42]

Implications for Clinical Practice

Selective systemic inhibition of PKC-β represents a new approach to the treatment of diabetic microvascular retinal complications. Although this study did not demonstrate a treatment effect on the primary end point of progression of diabetic retinopathy in patients who met the inclusion criteria and were treated with ruboxistaurin, it showed that clinically relevant outcomes such as moderate visual loss might be affected by this treatment approach. Ruboxistaurin showed a beneficial effect in reducing moderate visual loss on an oral administration of 32 mg per day, and sustained moderate visual loss was also reduced using this dose, especially in eyes with more severe retinopathy and definite DME at baseline.

When considering systemic therapy, the safety profile of the medication is critical. A prior study using a nonspecific inhibitor of multiple kinases and PKC isoforms was limited by hepato-toxicity and gastrointestinal side effects.[43] In contrast, ruboxistaurin is selective for the β-isoform of PKC, and it was well tolerated and not associated with significant adverse events.

Unanswered Questions

The apparent lack of efficacy of ruboxistaurin in preventing progression of retinopathy could have occurred for several reasons. PKC-β activation occurs very early in diabetes, and it is possible that in this study of moderately severe to very severe NPDR patients, the pathologic retinal changes are no longer amenable to PKC-β inhibition. Alternatively, the drug may not be potent enough to overcome these changes. Although PKC-β is involved in mediating the effects of VEGF, it is not primarily a VEGF inhibitor, and its antiproliferative activity is weaker than its antipermeability effect.[42] It is possible that ruboxistaurin use in patients with less severe retinopathy may have a different effect on retinopathy progression. Similarly, earlier use of ruboxistaurin may have a different effect on moderate visual loss and sustained moderate visual loss. The optimal time to initiate therapy and the optimal duration of therapy remain unknown.

The PKC-DRS clinical trial has demonstrated the potential for ruboxistaurin use in the treatment of diabetic microvascular retinal complications, especially with regard to clinically important outcomes such as the reduction of moderate visual loss. The results supported further evaluation of this approach, and the Protein Kinase C-β Inhibitor Diabetic Retinopathy Study 2 (PKC-DRS2) was initiated.

Preliminary results from the PKC-DRS2 trial have just become available.[44] Inclusion criteria were similar to those of the PKC-DRS, and patients were randomized to receive placebo or 32 mg of ruboxistaurin per day ($n = 684$). There was a reduction in the occurrence of sustained moderate visual loss from 9.1% in the placebo group to 5.5% in the ruboxistaurin group at 36 months ($p < 0.05$). Mean baseline to end point change in visual acuity (ETDRS letters) was −2.6 for placebo and −0.9 for ruboxistaurin ($p < 0.05$).[44]

Ovine Hyaluronidase (Vitrase)

Introduction

Current management options for vitreous hemorrhage include observation and vitrectomy. A pharmacologic approach such as enzymatic vitreolysis has the potential benefit of earlier clearance of vitreous hemorrhage compared with conventional treatment. This would result in earlier visualization of the retina and more timely treatment of the underlying pathology.

Hyaluronidase cleaves glycosidic bonds of hyaluronic acid, a major component of vitreous. Dissolution of the hyaluronic acid and collagen complex increases the diffusion of red blood cells and phagocytes because of vitreous liquefaction, thereby facilitating erythrocyte lysis and phagocytosis. Vitrase (ISTA Pharmaceuticals, Inc, Irvine, CA) is a highly purified preservative-free ovine hyaluronidase, and it has recently been evaluated as an intravitreous pharmacotherapy for the treatment of vitreous hemorrhage.

Background and Study Questions

Ovine hyaluronidase has been approved by the U.S. Food and Drug Administration (FDA) for use as a spreading or diffusing agent to increase the absorption and dispersion of other injected drugs. Although this medication is not approved for intravitreous use at this time, pooled data is available from two phase-III clinical trials that evaluated ovine hyaluronidase administered through intravitreous injection in patients with vitreous hemorrhage. These randomized, double-masked, placebo-controlled, multinational studies were designed to assess the safety and efficacy of intravitreous ovine hyaluronidase for the treatment of diabetes and other causes of vitreous

hemorrhage.[45,46] The trials were conducted in North America (Vit-02 Study) and outside of North America (Vit-03 Study).

Patients Included in the Study

Over 1,300 patients with severe vitreous hemorrhage for at least 1 month and visual acuity worse than 20/200 were enrolled. Severe vitreous hemorrhage was defined as the density sufficient to obscure fundus visualization on indirect ophthalmoscopy such that no retinal details were visible posterior to the equator. Patients whose hemorrhages were possibly due to trauma or sickle cell disease were excluded.

Intervention and Outcome Measures

Patients were randomized to 55 IU or 75 IU of ovine hyaluronidase or saline (50 microliters injection volume for all groups). The primary outcome was a reduction in hemorrhage density sufficient to enable a diagnosis and, when indicated, to perform laser treatment in at least 6 clock hours (for PDR or central retinal vein occlusion) or at least 3 clock hours (for branch retinal vein occlusion) by month 3. Secondary outcomes were visual acuity improvement >3 lines, hemorrhage density reduction assessment using a grading scale, and therapeutic utility assessment (clearance sufficient to diagnose, but without the requirement to treat the underlying pathology). Outcomes were measured at 1, 2, and 3 months.

Major Findings

Efficacy data was evaluated in 1,125 patients from the above indicated dose groups (in one of the two trials, 181 patients received a 7.5 IU dose, and these patients were excluded from the pooled efficacy data).[45] At enrollment, 90% of patients had counting finger vision or worse and 76% were patients with diabetes (60% type I, 40% type II). Mean hemorrhage duration was 120 days.

For the primary end point, efficacy was achieved for the 55 IU dose group at months 1 and 2, but not at month 3 (month 1: 13.2% vs. 5.5%; month 2: 25.5% vs. 16.2%; month 3: 32.9% vs. 25.6% for 55 IU vs. saline). The secondary end points confirmed the treatment effect at both doses and all time points.[45]

Safety data was evaluated in 1,362 patients.[46] Hyaluronidase was used in 966 patients, saline in 378, and 18 received no treatment (the initial version of one of the two trials contained an observational control group). Pooled safety data was collected until at least month 3, with some patients followed up to 32 months. Iritis was the most common adverse event in both the saline (33% of patients) and hyaluronidase groups (60% of patients), occurring in patients who received hyaluronidase in a dose–response manner. Most cases were mild-to-moderate and were easily managed; however, some patients (1.6% in the 55 IU group) developed sterile, self-limited hypopyon. No eyes developed infectious endophthalmitis. The incidence of rhegmatogenous retinal detachment was not statistically different between groups. No serious safety issues were reported.[46]

Implications for Clinical Practice

While the primary outcome was to be achieved by month 3, it was seen with statistical significance as early as month 1 and through month 2 (but not at month 3) in patients who met the inclusion criteria and were treated with a single intravitreous injection of 55 IU of ovine hyaluronidase. The secondary end points were reached by month 1 and persisted through month 3. The fact that the greatest treatment effect was seen by month 1 may be consistent with the relatively short half-life of ovine hyaluronidase (60 to 112 hours in ocular tissues), and this may allow earlier diagnosis and treatment of the underlying pathology while minimizing risk. These results suggest a potential clinically useful new pharmacologic approach to the management of vitreous hemorrhage due to diabetes and other causes.

Unanswered Questions

These studies included patients with vitreous hemorrhage from a variety of causes. In addition to PDR, etiologies included central retinal vein occlusion, branch retinal vein occlusion, exudative macular degeneration, hemorrhagic posterior vitreous detachment, and macroaneurysm. The published results are inclusive of all causes, and outcomes in the subset of diabetic patients have not been reported.

It is possible that the saline injection control (required by the FDA) may have had a treatment effect, for example, by mechanical induction of a posterior vitreous detachment. Comparison with a sham injection would be of interest. In addition, only a single injection of ovine hyaluronidase was allowed in these studies. The potential benefits and complications of additional injections of ovine hyaluronidase are unknown.

Conclusion

Over the past several decades, significant advances have been made in the management of PDR. The DRS conclusively demonstrated that photocoagulation was effective in the treatment of PDR, and it proved that for eyes with HRC, the risk of severe visual loss was substantially reduced. The DRVS showed that early vitrectomy was beneficial for eyes with non-clearing vitreous hemorrhage and for eyes with severe PDR (severe fibrovascular proliferation). The ETDRS established that photocoagulation should be considered for eyes with severe or very severe NPDR and for eyes with early PDR, and that aspirin did not alter the course of diabetic retinopathy. As a result of these overwhelmingly successful multicenter, randomized, controlled clinical trials, laser photocoagulation and vitrectomy surgery have remained the standards of care for years, and countless patients have avoided the blinding sequelae of PDR.

Emerging pharmacologic therapies such as ruboxistaurin mesylate (Arxxant) and ovine hyaluronidase (Vitrase) represent new approaches to the prevention and management of PDR, and the results of clinical trials are encouraging. Additional new medications such as pegaptanib (Macugen), ranibizumab (Lucentis), and bevacizumab (Avastin) have not been subjected to controlled clinical trials for PDR, but they offer tremendous potential in the treatment of retinal disease since they target specific molecules. A greater understanding of the molecular pathways underlying diabetic retinopathy will enable new pharmacologic interventions. The future will likely involve oral and intravitreous (probably via sustained release devices) administration of new drugs, and emphasis will likely be on prevention.

References

1. Beetham WP. Visual prognosis of proliferative diabetic retinopathy. *Br J Ophthalmol.* 1963; 47:611–619.
2. Caird FI, Burditt AF, Draper GJ. Diabetic retinopathy: A further study of prognosis for vision. *Diabetes.* 1968;17:121–123.
3. Deckert T, Simonsen SE, Poulson JE. Prognosis of proliferative retinopathy in juvenile diabetics. *Diabetes.* 1967;16:728–733.
4. Meyer-Schwickerath G. *Light coagulation.* (translated by Drance SM), St Louis, MO: Mosby; 1960.
5. Ederer F, Hiller R. Clinical trials, diabetic retinopathy and photocoagulation: A reanalysis of five studies. *Surv Ophthalmol.* 1975;19:267–286.

6. Olk RJ, Lee CM. Review of National Collaborative Studies. In: *Diabetic retinopathy: Practical management.* Philadelphia, PA: JB Lippincott Co; 1993.

7. Ferris FL, Davis MD, Aiello LM, et al. Clinical studies on treatment of diabetic retinopathy. In: Flynn HW, Smiddy WE, eds. *Diabetes and ocular disease: Past, present, and future therapies.* San Francisco, CA: The Foundation of the American Academy of Ophthalmology; 2000.

8. Diabetic Retinopathy Study Research Group. A modification of the Airlie house classification of diabetic retinopathy. DRS Report No. 7. *Invest Ophthalmol Vis Sci.* 1981;21(1):210–226.

9. Goldberg MF, Fine SL, eds. *Symposium on the treatment of diabetic retinopathy.* (Airlie House, 1968) Washington, DC: Public Health Service Publ. No. 1890, US Govt Printing Office; 1969.

10. Goldberg MF, Jampol LM. Knowledge of diabetic retinopathy before and 18 years after the Airlie house symposium on treatment of diabetic retinopathy. *Ophthalmology.* 1987;94:741–746.

11. Diabetic Retinopathy Study Research Group. Design, methods, and baseline results. DRS Report No. 6. *Invest Ophthalmol Vis Sci.* 1981;21:149–209.

11a. Grading diabetic retinopathy from stereoscopic color fundus photographs—an extension of the modified Airlie House Classification. ETDRS Report No. 10. *Ophthalmology.* 1991;98:786–806.

12. Diabetic Retinopathy Study Research Group. Preliminary report on effects of photocoagulation therapy. *Am J Ophthalmol.* 1976;81:383–396.

13. Diabetic Retinopathy Study Research Group. Photocoagulation of proliferative diabetic retinopathy: Clinical applications of DRS findings. DRS Report No. 8. *Ophthalmology.* 1988;88:583–600.

14. Diabetic Retinopathic Study Research Group. Photocoagulation treatment of proliferative diabetic retinopathy: The second report of diabetic retinopathy/vitrectomy study findings. *Am J Ophthalmol.* 1978;85:82–106.

15. Diabetic Retinopathy Study Research Group. Four risk factors for severe visual loss in diabetic retinopathy. DRS Report No. 3. *Arch Ophthalmol.* 1979;97:654–655.

16. Diabetic Retinopathy Study Research Group. Photocoagulation treatment of proliferative diabetic retinopathy: Relationship of adverse treatment effects to retinopathy severity. DRS Report No. 5. *Dev Ophthalmol.* 1981;2:248–261.

17. Diabetic Retinopathy Study Research Group. Diabetes 1979. International Congress Series No. 500. DRS Report No. 4. *Proceedings of the 10th congress of the internal diabetes federation.* Vienna, Austria, September 1979;789–794.

18. Diabetic Retinopathy Study Research Group. Indications for photocoagulation treatment of diabetic retinopathy. DRS Report No. 14. *Int Ophthalmol Clin.* 1987;274:239–252.

19. Ferris FL, Podgor MJ, Davis MD. Diabetic Retinopathy Study Research Group. Macular edema in diabetic retinopathy study patients. DRS Report No. 12. *Ophthalmology.* 1987;94:754–760.

20. Diabetic Retinopathy Vitrectomy Study Research Group. Two-year course of visual acuity in severe proliferative diabetic retinopathy with conventional management. Diabetic Retinopathy Vitrectomy Study (DRVS) Report No. 1. *Ophthalmology.* 1985;92:492–502.

21. Diabetic Retinopathy Vitrectomy Study Research Group. Early vitrectomy for severe vitreous hemorrhage in diabetic retinopathy. Two-year results of a randomized trial. Diabetic Retinopathy Vitrectomy Study Report 2. *Arch Ophthalmol.* 1985;103:1644–1652.

22. Diabetic Retinopathy Vitrectomy Study Research Group. Early vitrectomy for severe proliferative diabetic retinopathy in eyes with useful vision. Results of a randomized trial - Diabetic Retinopathy Vitrectomy Study Report 3. *Ophthalmology.* 1988;95:1307–1320.

23. Diabetic Retinopathy Vitrectomy Study Research Group. Early vitrectomy for severe proliferative diabetic retinopathy in eyes with useful vision. Clinical application of results of a randomized trial - Diabetic Retinopathy Vitrectomy Study Report 4. *Ophthalmology.*1988;95:1321–1334.

24. Diabetic Retinopathy Vitrectomy Study Research Group. Early vitrectomy for severe vitreous hemorrhage in diabetic retinopathy. Four-year results of a randomized trial. Diabetic Retinopathy Vitrectomy Study Report 5. *Arch Ophthalmol.* 1990;108:958–964.

25. Machemer R, Buettner H, Norton EWD, et al. Vitrectomy for proliferative diabetic retinopathy: A pars plana approach. *Trans Am Acad Ophthalmol Otolaryngol.* 1971;75:813.

26. Aaberg TM. Vitrectomy for diabetic retinopathy. In: Freeman HM, Hirose T, Schepens CL, eds. *Vitreous surgery and advances in fundus diagnosis and treatment*. New York: Appleton-Century-Crofts, 1977.

27. Eliott D, Lee MS, Abrams GW. Proliferative diabetic retinopathy: Principles and techniques of surgical treatment. In: Ryan SJ, ed. *Retina*, 3rd ed. St Louis, MO: Mosby; 2000:2436–2476.

28. Davis MD. Vitreous contraction in proliferative diabetic retinopathy. *Arch Ophthalmol*. 1965; 74:741.

29. Early Treatment Diabetic Retinopathy Study Research Group. Early Treatment Diabetic Retinopathy Study design and baseline patient characteristics. ETDRS Report No. 7. *Ophthalmology*. 1991;98:741–756.

30. Early Treatment Diabetic Retinopathy Study Research Group. Techniques for scatter and focal photocoagulation treatment of diabetic retinopathy. ETDRS Report No. 3. *Int Ophthalmol Clin*. 1987;27:254–264.

31. Early Treatment Diabetic Retinopathy Study Research Group. Early photocoagulation for diabetic retinopathy. ETDRS Report No. 9. *Ophthalmology*. 1991;98:766–785.

32. Flynn HW, Chew EY, Simons BD, et al. Pars plana vitrectomy in the Early Treatment Diabetic Retinopathy Study. ETDRS Report No. 17. *Ophthalmology*. 1992;99:151–1357.

33. Ferris F. Early photocoagulation in patients with either type I or type II diabetes. *Trans Am Ophthalmol Soc*. 1996;94:505–537.

34. Early Treatment Diabetic Retinopathy Study Research Group. Fundus photographic risk factors for progression of diabetic retinopathy. ETDRS Report No. 12. *Ophthalmology*. 1991; 98:823–833.

35. Early Treatment Diabetic Retinopathy Study Research Group. Photocoagulation for diabetic macular edema. ETDRS Report No. 4. *Int Ophthalmol Clin*. 1987;27:265–272.

36. Kinyoun J, Barton F, Fisher M, et al. Detection of diabetic macular edema: Ophthalmoscopy vs. photography. ETDRS Report No. 5. *Ophthalmology*. 1989;96:746–751.

37. Diabetes 2000 symposium. *At the Annual meeting of the American Academy of ophthalmology*. Anaheim, CA: 1991.

38. Early Treatment Diabetic Retinopathy Study Research Group. Effects of aspirin treatment on diabetic retinopathy. ETDRS Report No 8. *Ophthalmology*. 1991;98:757–765.

39. Chew EY, Klein ML, Murphy RP, et al. Effects of aspirin on vitreous/preretinal hemorrhage in patients with diabetes mellitus. ETDRS Report No 20. *Arch Ophthalmol*. 1995;113:52–55.

40. Early Treatment Diabetic Retinopathy Study Investigators. Aspirin effects on mortality and morbidity in patients with diabetes mellitus. ETDRS Report No 14. *JAMA*. 1992; 268:1292–1300.

41. Buddi R, Eliott D. Emerging treatments for diabetic eye disease: Update on clinical trials. *Ret Phys*. 2004:18–23.

42. The PKC-DRS Study Group. The effect of ruboxistaurin on visual loss in patients with moderately severe to very severe nonproliferative diabetic retinopathy: Initial results of the protein kinase C beta inhibitor diabetic retinopathy study (PKC-DRS) multicenter randomized clinical trial. *Diabetes*. 2005;54:2188–2197.

43. Campochiaro PA. Reduction of diabetic macular edema by oral administration of the kinase inhibitor PKC412. *Invest Ophthalmol Vis Sci*. 2004;45:922–931.

44. Aiello LP, Vignati L, Sheetz MJ, et al. PKC-DRS2 Study Group. The effect of the PKC-beta inhibitor ruboxistaurin on moderate visual loss: The PKC-DRS2 trial baseline characteristics and preliminary results. *Presented at the American Academy of Ophthalmology annual meeting*. Chicago, IL, November 2005.

45. Kuppermann BD, Thomas EL, de Smet MD, et al. The Vitrase for Vitreous Hemorrhage Study Groups. Pooled efficacy results from two multinational randomized controlled clinical trials of a single intravitreous injection of highly purified ovine hyaluronidase (Vitrase®) for the management of vitreous hemorrhage. *Am J Ophthalmol*. 2005;140:573–584.

46. Kuppermann BD, Thomas EL, de Smet MD, et al. The Vitrase for Vitreous Hemorrhage Study Groups. Safety results of two phase III trials of an intravitreous injection of highly purified ovine hyaluronidase (Vitrase®) for the management of vitreous hemorrhage. *Am J Ophthalmol*. 2005; 140:585–597.

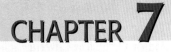

CHAPTER **7**

Clinical Trials in Age-Related Macular Degeneration

Sophie J. Bakri, MD and Peter K. Kaiser, MD

Age-related macular degeneration (AMD) is the leading cause of blindness in patients over the age of 65, with the neovascular (exudative) form accounting for >80% of the cases with severe visual loss.[1,2] Over the last 10 years, there has been a dramatic increase in the armamentarium of available treatments for AMD. Accepted treatments for exudative macular degeneration include observation, thermal laser photocoagulation, verteporfin photodynamic therapy (PDT), and anti-VEGF agents. In addition, surgical management of AMD has been explored, including macular translocation and submacular surgery. Many other therapies for exudative AMD, in particular pharmacologic therapy, are under clinical investigation. This chapter will summarize the main clinical trials for AMD.

The Macular Photocoagulation Study

The Macular Photocoagulation Study (MPS) was a group of randomized, controlled, multicenter clinical trials performed in the 1980s to address whether direct thermal laser photocoagulation of a choroidal neovascular membrane (CNV) prevented loss of visual acuity (VA) as compared to observation alone. Later, MPS reports were published that examined the incidence, risk factors, and value of repeating photocoagulation for persistent and recurrent CNV. The effect of laser wavelength was also evaluated. Only one eye of each eligible participant was randomized to either laser treatment or no treatment, even if both eyes were eligible for the study. Results of the MPS were classified according to whether the CNV was extrafoveal (≥200 and <2,500 μm from the center of the foveal avascular zone [FAZ]), juxtafoveal (1 to 199 μm from the center of the FAZ) or subfoveal (under the center of the FAZ) at baseline.

Major Inclusion Criteria

All three studies (extrafoveal, juxtafoveal, and subfoveal studies) required that participants be aged at least 50 years, have evidence of AMD in the form of drusen, and have visual symptoms related to the presence of CNV. Additional inclusion criteria were:

Extrafoveal study

1. Fluorescein angiography obtained <96 hours before randomization showing a well-demarcated CNV between 200 and 2,500 μm from the center of the FAZ
2. Early Treatment Diabetic Retinopathy Study (ETDRS) best corrected visual acuity (BCVA) of 20/100 or better

Juxtafoveal study

1. Fluorescein angiography obtained <96 hours before randomization showing:
   - A well-demarcated CNV between 1 and 199 μm from the center of the FAZ, or
   - CNV >200 μm from the FAZ with adjacent blood or pigment extending within 200 μm of the FAZ
2. ETDRS BCVA of 20/100 or better

Subfoveal study

1. Fluorescein angiography obtained <96 hours before randomization, showing CNV with well-demarcated boundaries under the center of the FAZ
2. CNV area <3.5 MPS disc areas with most of the lesion composed of either classic or occult CNV
3. VA of 20/40 to 20/320

165

Major Exclusion Criteria

- Prior laser photocoagulation
- Coexisting ocular disease that may potentially affect VA

Subfoveal Recurrent Choroidal Neovascular Membrane (CNV) Study

Fluorescein angiography obtained <96 hours before randomization, showing one of the following:

- CNV under the center of the FAZ, contiguous with a prior laser treatment scar
- CNV within 150 μm from the center of the FAZ, contiguous with a scar that had crept under the fovea
- The area of CNV greater than the area of the scar
- VA at study entry of 20/40 to 20/320

Following proposed laser treatment, some part of the retina within 1.5 mm from the center of the FAZ

would remain untreated, and the total area treated by previous and new lasers would be <6 MPS disc areas.

Major Exclusion Criteria

- Prior laser photocoagulation involving the center of the FAZ

Primary Outcome

The primary outcome was "severe visual loss" defined as a loss of six or more lines of VA (quadrupling of the visual angle) on the Bailey-Lovie chart. Other outcomes included reading speed and contrast threshold.

Laser Photocoagulation Methods
Extrafoveal Treatment

After retrobulbar anesthesia, argon laser burns were used to produce a retinal whitening over the CNV and extending 100 to 125 μm beyond its borders (see Figs. 7.1 and 7.2). The extension beyond the

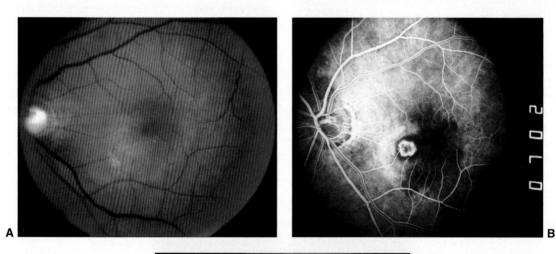

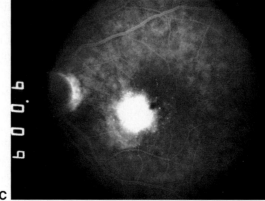

FIGURE 7.1 ☐ Color photograph **(A)** and fluorescein angiogram **(B, C)** of an extrafoveal choroidal neovascular membrane before laser treatment.

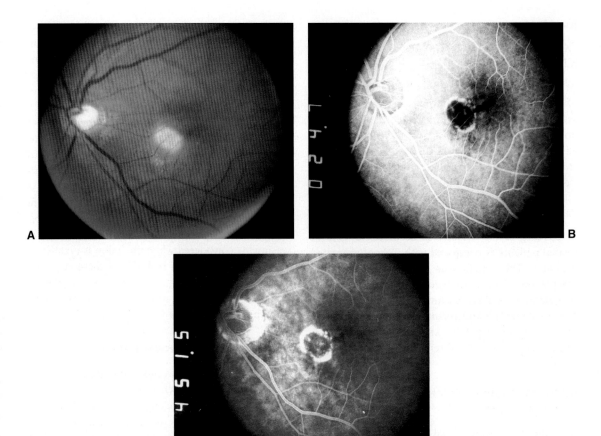

FIGURE 7.2 ◻ Color photograph **(A)** and fluorescein angiogram **(B, C)** of an extrafoveal choroidal neovascular membrane after laser treatment.

lesion was not required if the lesion extended within 200 to 300 μm from the center of the FAZ. Spot size was 200 to 500 μm with a duration of 0.5 seconds. Within 350 μm of the FAZ, burns were 100 μm in size, with a duration of 0.1 to 0.2 seconds. Peripapillary CNV was eligible for treatment only if laser photocoagulation would spare a minimum of one and a half clock hours of the peripapillary nerve fiber layer. Figures 7.1 and 7.2 illustrate an extrafoveal CNV before and after argon laser treatment.

Juxtafoveal Treatment

This was done with retrobulbar anesthesia and a krypton red laser. Treatment was extended for 100 μm beyond the lesion, except on the foveal side, where treatment beyond the borders of the lesion was required only if the leakage

extended further than 100 μm from the center of the FAZ.

Subfoveal Treatment

Retrobulbar anesthesia was optional, and patients ($n = 373$) were randomized to be treated with either krypton red ($n = 92$ eyes) or argon green ($n = 97$ eyes). Treatment was extended for 100 μm beyond the lesion, and for thick blood the burns were extended up to but not beyond the lesion borders.

Subfoveal Recurrent Neovascularization Treatment

This was similar to the initial subfoveal treatment. Treatment was extended for 300 μm into the prior laser scar to cover any visible feeder vessel, for 100 μm on either side of the vessel, and to extend 300 μm beyond the vessel base.

Results

Extrafoveal Choroidal Neovascular Membrane (CNV) Study

At 6 months, severe visual loss, defined as ≥6 lines of vision loss, occurred in 25% of treated patients as compared with 60% of untreated patients.[3] This positive VA benefit persisted at 3 years (52% vs. 68%)[4] and at 5 years (46% vs. 64%).[5] Unfortunately, choroidal neovascularization recurred in 54% of treated patients by the end of 5 years.[5]

Juxtafoveal Krypton Laser Study

At 3 years, severe visual loss occurred in 49% of treated patients as compared with 58% of untreated patients.[6] The benefit was greatest in normotensive patients. Persistent choroidal neovascularization (angiographic leakage within 6 weeks) occurred in 32% of patients,[7] and recurrent choroidal neovascularization occurred in 41.7% by 5 years. At 5 years, recurrence or persistence occurred in 78% of patients.[8]

Subfoveal Argon or Krypton Laser Photocoagulation

At 3 months, severe visual loss occurred in 20% of laser-treated eyes as compared with 11% of untreated eyes.[9] Despite the eventual visual benefit of subfoveal laser treatment over observation, subfoveal laser treatment always resulted in an immediate, permanent VA loss (three lines on average). Long-term results from the MPS showed that untreated patients continued to lose vision, whereas VA in treated eyes remained relatively stable after the immediate decline. At 24 months, severe visual loss occurred in 20% of treated eyes as compared with 37% of untreated eyes, and at 4 years severe visual loss occurred in 22% of treated eyes as compared with 47% of untreated eyes.[10] Among eligible patients who were treated, the recurrence rate was 51% and the most recurrent neovascular lesions were subfoveal.[9] The MPS concluded that photocoagulation should be considered for subfoveal lesions when the lesion is well-demarcated, has evidence of classic CNV, and is small (<3.5 MPS disc areas).[11,12]

Recurrent Subfoveal Choroidal Neovascular Membrane (CNV) Study

The MPS study also evaluated the outcome of treatment of recurrent subfoveal CNV.[13] At 24 months, severe visual loss had occurred in 9% of laser-treated eyes as compared with 28% of untreated eyes, and at 36 months, in 12% of laser-treated eyes as compared with 36% of untreated eyes.[10] The persistent choroidal neovascularization occurred in 13% of eyes, and the recurrence rate at 3 years[14] was 35%.

The MPS showed that laser treatment of CNV in AMD has significant pitfalls and limitations. Only a very small proportion of patients with neovascular AMD are eligible for laser treatment, as the CNV has to be classified angiographically as well defined. Moreover, because of the immediate and significant—albeit stable—visual loss that accompanies subfoveal treatment, laser treatment can only be reasonably considered when the lesion is juxtafoveal or extrafoveal; and the majority of these cases will have subfoveal recurrences after photocoagulation. Thus, other treatment modalities for CNV due to AMD have been explored.

Photodynamic Therapy Trials

PDT involves the intravenous injection of a photosensitizing drug, which is activated by light from a laser source at a wavelength corresponding to an absorption peak of the drug. The laser light activates the photosensitizer molecules, exciting them to a higher-energy triplet state, without producing any thermal damage (photocoagulation). The triplet-state molecules then transfer their energy to surrounding molecules through two pathways. The first is transferring energy through a free radical mechanism to form cytotoxic intermediates (type I reaction). The other mechanism is transferring energy to nearby oxygen molecules, exciting them to a higher and more reactive state called singlet oxygen while returning the photosensitizer to the ground state (type II reaction). The type II reaction usually predominates and is the reason that oxygen is required for PDT action. The free radicals and singlet oxygen rapidly oxidize nearby chemicals including lipid membranes (lipid peroxidation), organelles, mitochondrial enzymes, lysozymes, proteins, and nucleic acids, leading to the disruption of cellular structures. Tissue damage is mediated through the release of thromboxane, histamines, and tumor necrosis factors. In addition, there is platelet aggregation, vasoconstriction, immunologic effects, and direct endothelial damage. The culmination of these events is eventually vessel thrombosis and vascular occlusion.[15,16] Currently, verteporfin (Visudyne,

Predominantly classic CNV

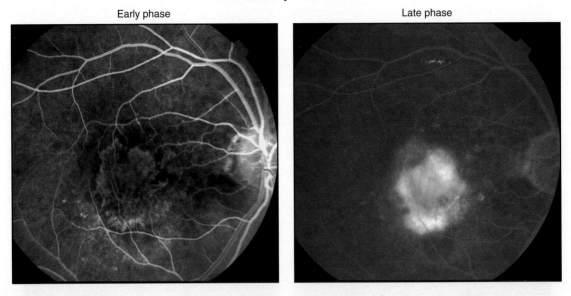

Early phase

Late phase

FIGURE 7.3 ◻ Early and late views of a fluorescein angiogram of a predominantly classic choroidal neovascularization lesion demonstrating early well-defined hyperfluorescence with leakage beyond the edges of the original leakage in the late views.

Novartis AG) is the only U.S. Food and Drug Administration (FDA)-approved photosensitizer used in ocular PDT.

Visudyne Photodynamic Therapy Protocol (PDT)

The standard published PDT protocol consists of an infusion of 6 mg per m^2 verteporfin over a 10-minute period followed by laser irradiation using a 689-nm diode laser (light dose: 50 J per cm^2; power density: 600 mW per cm^2; duration: 83 seconds) 15 minutes after the start of the infusion.

Treatment of Age-Related Macular Degeneration with Photodynamic Therapy (TAP) Study

The Treatment of Age-Related Macular Degeneration with PDT (TAP) Study was initiated in December 1996 at 22 clinical centers in North America and Europe.[17] It consisted of two simultaneous, double-masked, placebo-controlled, multicenter, randomized studies in patients with classic-containing subfoveal CNV secondary to AMD.

Important definitions in the PDT trials include describing the CNV lesions as classic, occult, or a

mixture. These descriptions are based on angiographic leakage patterns. Classic CNV is an area of well-demarcated hyperfluorescence that appears very early in the angiogram, increases in intensity, and extends beyond its boundaries in the later phases of the angiogram (see Fig. 7.3). There are two patterns of occult CNV hyperfluorescence: A fibrovascular pigment epithelial detachment (FVPED) and a "late leakage of an undetermined source." An FVPED shows stippled hyperfluorescence in an irregularly elevated pigment epithelial detachment (PED). In the late phases of the angiogram, the fluorescein collects in the FVPED or pools in the subretinal space overlying the FVPED (see Fig. 7.4). Late leakage of an undetermined source refers to late choroidal leakage usually in a stippled pattern where no corresponding early leakage is seen (see Fig. 7.5).

Major Inclusion Criteria

- Age ≥50 years
- ETDRS BCVA between 20/40 and 20/200
- New or recurrent subfoveal CNV due to AMD
- Fluorescein angiography showing the lesion to have some evidence of classic CNV
- Lesion components such as blood, blocked fluorescence, or a serous detachment of the

Occult with no classic CNV
Type 1

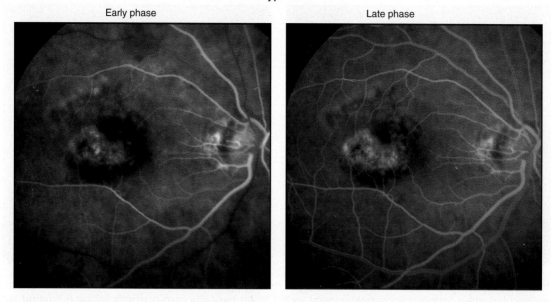

FIGURE 7.4 ☐ Early and late views of a fluorescein angiogram of a type-1 occult with no classic choroidal neovascularization (CNV) lesion demonstrating early, stippled hyperfluorescence with leakage evident in late views that does not extend beyond its boundaries—like a classic CNV. This is a fibrovascular pigment epithelial detachment.

Occult with no classic CNV
Type 2

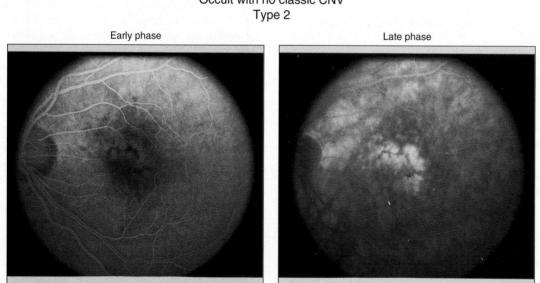

FIGURE 7.5 ☐ Early and late views of a fluorescein angiogram of a type-2 occult with no classic choroidal neovascularization lesion demonstrating late, stippled hyperfluorescence with minimal leakage evident in early views consistent with late leakage of a type-2 occult lesion (late leakage of undetermined origin).

retinal pigment epithelium not more than 50% of the entire lesion

- The greatest linear dimension of the entire lesion 5,400 μm or less

Major Exclusion Criteria

- Previous subfoveal laser photocoagulation

Study Design

A total of 609 patients (402 assigned to verteporfin, 207 to placebo) were enrolled in the two studies. During these studies, PDT was allowed every 3 months if fluorescein angiograms showed any recurrence or persistence of leakage. The placebo control (sham treatment) consisted of intravenous administration of dextrose 5% in water (D5W), followed by light application identical to that used for verteporfin therapy.

Primary Outcome

Percentage of patients with a <15-letter decrease in VA (approximately <3 lines)

Results

Enrollment included 609 patients (311 in Study A and 298 in Study B) in the TAP study (December 1996 to October 1997). Of the eyes treated with verteporfin, 61.2% lost <15 letters (p <0.001) at 12 months, as compared with 46.4% of the eyes administered placebo. Figure 7.6 shows the Kaplan-Meier estimates of the cumulative proportion of eyes treated with verteporfin or given placebo with moderate VA loss (15 letters or approximately 3 lines) at each 3-month study visit over time.

- The average change in VA differed by 1.3 lines, in favor of the eyes treated with verteporfin at 12 months
- Verteporfin-treated eyes were more likely to have improvements of one or more lines in vision (16% eyes) than placebo-treated eyes (7%)

Subgroup Analyses

Predominantly classic CNV:

- There was a larger treatment benefit when the classic component of the CNV occupied 50% or more of the area of the entire lesion

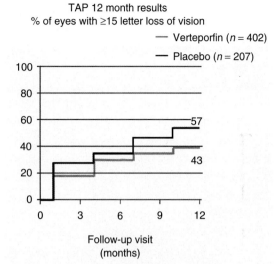

TAP 12 month results
% of eyes with ≥15 letter loss of vision
— Verteporfin ($n = 402$)
— Placebo ($n = 207$)

FIGURE 7.6 □ Kaplan-Meier estimates of the cumulative proportion of eyes treated with verteporfin or given placebo with moderate VA loss (≥15 letters or approximately 3 lines) at each 3-month study visit over time. (Reproduced from: Treatment of Age-Related Macular Degeneration with Photodynamic Therapy (TAP) Study Group. Photodynamic therapy of subfoveal choroidal neovascularization in age-related macular degeneration with verteporfin one-year results of two randomized controlled trials (RCTs)—TAP report 1. *Arch Ophthalmol.* 1999;117:1329–1345.)

(Fig. 7.3), with 33% of the 159 verteporfin-treated eyes losing three or more lines at 12 months as compared with 61% of the placebo-treated eyes.

- In eyes with 100% classic CNV, 23% of those treated with verteporfin and 73% of those given placebo lost 3 or more lines (p <0.001).

Minimally classic CNV:

- There was no appreciable VA benefit seen in eyes where classic CNV occupied <50% of the lesion (see Fig. 7.7).

Occult CNV:

- Eyes with 100% occult CNV appeared to have a treatment benefit, but the number of patients was too small to reach a statistically viable conclusion. More importantly, these patients should not have been enrolled in the clinical study since the inclusion criteria

Minimally classic CNV
(Retinal angiomatous proliferation)

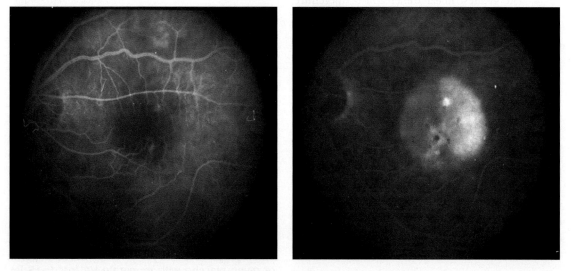

FIGURE 7.7 ☐ Early and late views of a fluorescein angiogram of a minimally classic choroidal neovascularization (CNV) lesion demonstrating a small area of early well-defined hyperfluorescence with leakage beyond the edges of the original leakage in late views, surrounded by a larger area of pooling into a pigment epithelial detachment. Since the area of classic CNV is smaller than the occult component this is a minimally classic lesion.

required some classic component of the CNV lesion.

Safety

Few ocular or other systemic adverse events were seen with Visudyne therapy. Less than 2% of patients withdrew from the TAP study because of adverse events. The most common adverse events were injection-site reaction (13.4%), mild to moderate decreased vision (2%), infusion-related back pain (2%), and self-resolving photosensitivity reactions within 24 hours (3%).

Two-Year Results of the Treatment of Age-Related Macular Degeneration with Photodynamic Therapy (TAP) Study

The 2-year results of the TAP Study[18] included 351 (87%) of the 402 patients in the verteporfin-treated group as compared with 178 (86%) of the 207 patients in the placebo-treated group, who completed the 24-month examination. In the verteporfin-treated group, 213 (53%) of the eyes as compared with 78 (38%) of the placebo-treated eyes lost <3 lines of VA. Figure 7.8 shows a Kaplan-Meier estimate of the cumulative probability of eyes treated with verteporfin or given placebo with moderate VA loss of 15 letters or approximately three lines) at each 3-month study visit over time. Figure 7.9 shows the mean change in vision over time during the first 24 months of the study. In subgroup analyses for predominantly classic lesions at baseline, 94 (59%) of the 159 verteporfin-treated eyes as compared with 26 (31%) of 83 placebo-treated eyes lost <3 lines at 24 months. For minimally classic lesions there was no statistically significant difference: 47.5% of 202 verteporfin-treated eyes as compared to 44.2% of 104 placebo-treated patients lost <3 lines at 24 months. The mean number of PDT treatments in the TAP Study was 3.5 in year 1 and 2.3 in year 2.

Treatment of Age-Related Macular Degeneration with Photodynamic Therapy (TAP) Extension Study

The TAP study was extended into an open-label extension study for another 3 years[19] to evaluate safety and visual outcomes between months 24 and 60. Of the 609 patients enrolled in the TAP Investigation, 156 of 207 (75.4%) patients assigned to placebo therapy

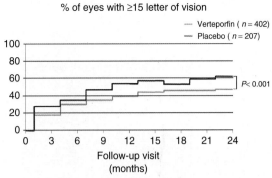

TAP 24 month results

% of eyes with ≥15 letter of vision

— Verteporfin (n = 402)
— Placebo (n = 207)

P < 0.001

Follow-up visit
(months)

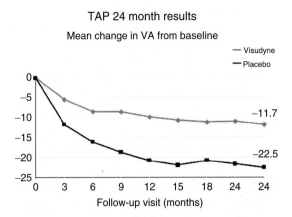

TAP 24 month results

Mean change in VA from baseline

— Visudyne
— Placebo

−11.7

−22.5

Follow-up visit (months)

FIGURE 7.8 ☐ Kaplan-Meier estimate of the cumulative probability of eyes treated with verteporfin or given placebo with moderate VA loss (≥15 letters or approximately 3 lines) at each 3-month study visit over time. (Reproduced from: Bressler NM. Treatment of Age-Related Macular Degeneration with Photodynamic Therapy (TAP) Study Group. Photodynamic therapy of subfoveal choroidal neovascularization in age-related macular degeneration with verteporfin: Two-year results of two randomized controlled trials-TAP report 2. *Arch Ophthalmol.* 2001;119(2):198–207.)

FIGURE 7.9 ☐ Mean change in vision from the TAP Study over time for the first 24 months of the clinical study.

at baseline, and 320 of 402 (79.6%) patients assigned to verteporfin therapy at baseline participated in the open-label extension study.

The 105 patients with a predominantly classic lesion at baseline who completed the 36-month examination received an average of 1.3 treatments between months 24 and 36. An average of 0.5 of a maximum possible four treatments was given to the patients with predominantly classic CNV at baseline from the month 36 examination (inclusive) up to, but not including, the month 48 follow-up examination. A visual loss of three lines or more occurred in 41.9% of patients at month 36 as compared with 37.5% at month 24. An average loss of 0.1 line of VA occurred between months 24 and 36. The TAP Study group identified no safety concerns to preclude repeating verteporfin PDT. The 48-month results show that there is very little change in VA from the month 24 and month 36 examinations. No additional safety concerns were identified during the open-label extension up to the 48-month follow-up.[20] The TAP Study group identified no safety concerns to preclude repeating verteporfin PDT.

Verteporfin in Photodynamic Therapy Study

The Verteporfin in Photodynamic Therapy (VIP) Study was a placebo-controlled, randomized, multicenter trial that evaluated patients who were not originally eligible for the TAP Study. It consisted of one group of patients with pathologic myopia that was enrolled and analyzed separately from the two groups of patients with AMD: Occult, with no classic CNV and classic-containing CNV with good VA.

Major Inclusion Criteria

- Age ≥50 years
- Subfoveal CNV secondary to AMD (<9 MPS disc areas in size, including lesion components)
- ETDRS BCVA of 20/40 to 20/100 in patients with occult and no classic CNV.
- An ETDRS VA score of at least 70 (Snellen equivalent 20/40 or better) for patients with classic CNV
- Evidence of recent disease progression defined as either subretinal hemorrhage (but comprising no more than 50% of the lesion), documented evidence of 5 or more letters of vision loss (ETDRS) during the previous 12 weeks, or documented increase in size of 10% or more of greatest linear dimension within the previous 12 weeks for patients with occult and no classic CNV

- Lesion components such as blood, blocked fluorescence, or a serous detachment of the retinal pigment epithelium that could occupy no more than 50% of the entire lesion
- The greatest linear dimension of the entire lesion of 5,400 μm or less

Major Exclusion Criteria

- Previous subfoveal laser photocoagulation

Primary Outcome

- Percentage of patients with a <15-letter decrease in VA (approximately <3 lines)

Secondary Outcomes

- Percentage of patients with <30-letter decrease in VA (approximately <6 lines)
- Percentage of patients with a VA score of 35 letters or worse or 20/200 or worse
- Mean change in VA
- Mean change in contrast threshold

Results

Of the 225 verteporfin-treated patients, 49% versus 46% of the 114 placebo-treated patients lost <15 letters of vision at the month-12 examination ($p = 0.517$). However, by the month-24 examination, 46% of verteporfin-treated patients as compared with 33% of the placebo-treated patients lost <15 letters ($p = 0.023$). When the patients with occult and no classic CNV lesions (75% of the patients) were analyzed separately a similar treatment benefit was seen at month 24. In these patients, moderate vision loss occurred in 29% of verteporfin-treated patients and 47% of placebo-treated patients ($p = 0.004$). The mean lesion size decreased from 4,122 to 3,025 μm by month 24 in the verteporfin-treated patients, while it increased from 4,337 to 4,472 μm in the placebo-treated patients ($p < 0.001$). The mean number of PDT required was 3.1 treatments in year 1 and 1.9 in year 2.

Subgroup Analysis

Logistic regression analysis of moderate vision loss confirmed that both baseline lesion size and baseline VA had statistically significant interactions with the treatment benefits (see Figure 7.10). The greatest benefit was seen in patients with *either* smaller lesions

VIP 24 month results
Difference between verteporfin and placebo

FIGURE 7.10 ☐ In the VIP Study, both smaller baseline lesions (≤4 Macular Photocoagulation Study [MPS] disc areas) and lower levels of visual acuity (20/50 or worse) had a statistically significant influence on the treatment benefit.

(≤4 MPS disc areas) *or* lower levels of VA (20/50 or worse).

Safety

One important adverse effect seen in the trial was the occurrence of acute severe vision decrease (ASVD) (defined as a documented loss of at least 20 letters on an ETDRS chart within 7 days of treatment as compared with the VA pretreatment) in 10 out of 225 patients (4.4%) of the verteporfin-treated group and none of the placebo group in the first year of the study. The acute loss of vision was due to subretinal fluid, subretinal pigment epithelial blood, or no obvious cause. Half of these patients did not have persistent loss of vision because by the next 3-month examination, 4/10 recovered to a <20-letter loss, 5/10 still had a ≥20-letter loss, and 1/10 had a 3-letter gain. In the second year of the study no further episodes of ASVD were noted.

Photodynamic Therapy Trials Exploratory Analyses

Exploratory analyses were done in patients with predominantly classic or minimally classic lesions at enrollment in the TAP Study and in AMD patients with occult but no classic CNV in the VIP Study.[21] Baseline characteristics of patients among these three lesion compositions were compared. In addition, multiple linear regression modeling was used to explore the effect of baseline lesion size, VA, and lesion composition on the mean change in VA from baseline to 24 months.

At baseline, the mean size of predominantly classic lesions (3.4 disc areas) was smaller than that of minimally classic (4.7 disc areas) and occult with no classic lesions (4.3 disc areas). In the multiple linear regression model of individual lesion compositions, there was a significant treatment-by-lesion-size interaction for minimally classic and occult with no classic lesions, but not for predominantly classic lesions. Small verteporfin-treated lesions lost less vision than large verteporfin-treated lesions in each lesion composition. In the multiple linear regression model that included all lesion compositions, lesion size was a more significant predictive factor for the magnitude of treatment benefit than either lesion composition or VA. Smaller (4.0 disc areas or less) minimally classic and occult with no classic lesions had VA outcomes similar to those observed in predominantly classic lesions.

Verteporfin In Minimally Classic (VIM) Choroidal Neovascularization Study

Multiple linear regression analysis suggested a treatment benefit for smaller minimally classic lesions and the TAP Study showed a treatment benefit for smaller lesions, especially with lower levels of VA ($\geq 20/50$). Thus, the goal of the Verteporfin In Minimally Classic (VIM) Choroidal Neovascularization study was to compare the treatment effect and safety of PDT using a standard (SF; 600 mW per cm^2) or reduced (RF; 300 mW per cm^2) light fluence rate with that of placebo therapy in patients with smaller, subfoveal minimally classic CNV with AMD. This was a phase II, multicenter, double-masked, placebo-controlled, RCT that took place in 19 clinical centers in Europe and North America.

Major Inclusion Criteria

- Age ≥ 50 years
- Subfoveal CNV (new: No prior treatment) from AMD
- Lesion composition: Minimally classic
- Lesion size: ≤ 6 MPS disc areas
- Baseline protocol ETDRS BCVA (approximate Snellen equivalent):
  - 20/250 or better for lesions ≤ 4 MPS disc areas
  - 20/50 to 20/250 for lesions >4 and ≤ 6 MPS disc areas

Major Exclusion Criteria

- Prior treatment for subfoveal CNV

Study Design

This was a phase II RCT in which 117 patients were randomly assigned (1:1:1) to verteporfin infusion (6 mg per m^2 and light application with an RF rate (300 mW per cm^2) for 83 seconds (light dose of 25 J per cm^2) or an SF rate (600 mW per cm^2) for 83 seconds (light dose of 50 J per cm^2) or to placebo infusion with RF or SF. Treatment was repeated every 3 months if the treating physician noted fluorescein leakage from CNV on angiography. Patients in whom a predominantly classic lesion developed could receive open-label standard verteporfin treatment with SF. The best-corrected VA was measured every 3 months, and angiographic changes were assessed through the 3-month examination unless an ocular adverse event or conversion to a predominantly classic lesion was identified by an investigator.

Results

One-hundred and three (88%) of 117 patients completed the 24-month examination. Twelve (30%) of the 40 patients assigned to placebo received open-label standard verteporfin treatment after confirmation of the presence of predominantly classic CNV.

At month 12, a loss of at least 3 lines of VA occurred in 5 (14%) of 36 eyes assigned to RF and 10 (28%) of 36 eyes assigned to SF, as compared with 18 (47%) of 38 eyes assigned to placebo (RF, $p = 0.002$; SF, $p = 0.08$; RF + SF, $p = 0.004$). Severe vision loss (≥ 6 lines) was seen in 0% of patients assigned to RF, 8% of patients assigned to SF, and 16% of patients receiving placebo. The mean change in vision from the baseline was -3 letters in patients assigned to RF, -8.3 letters in patients assigned to SF, and -14.4 letters in patients receiving placebo.

At month 24, moderate visual loss occurred in 9 (26%) of 34 eyes assigned to RF and 17 (53%) of 32 assigned to SF, as compared with 23 (62%) of 37 eyes assigned to placebo (RF, $p = 0.003$; SF, $p = 0.45$; RF + SF, $p = 0.03$). Progression to predominantly classic CNV by 24 months was more common in the placebo group (11 [28%] of 39 patients compared with 2 [5%] of 38 in the RF group and 1 [3%] of 37 in the SF group). No unexpected ocular or systemic adverse events were identified. Treatment-related, usually transient visual disturbances were 13% with SF, 10% with placebo, and 5% with RF. The difference in the mean VA score change between the fluence groups was approximately 1 line or less at the 12- and 24-month examinations. On the basis of these results, there is no accepted standard of care of reduced fluence as compared with the standard fluence for minimally classic lesions.

This trial concluded that PDT safely reduced the risks of losing at least 15 letters ($\geq$3 lines) of VA and progression to predominantly classic CNV for at least 2 years in individuals with subfoveal minimally classic lesions due to AMD measuring six MPS disc areas or less. The sample size of the VIM Trial was not powered to detect a difference between reduced and standard fluence. Further studies are required to explore this difference. Until that time, verteporfin PDT should be performed with standard fluence.

Verteporfin In Occult (VIO) Choroidal Neovascularization Study

The Verteporfin In Occult (VIO) Choroidal Neovascularization Study was performed to assess whether PDT in eyes with occult but no classic subfoveal CNV due to AMD can safely and effectively reduce the risk of vision loss as compared with the placebo.

Study Design

This was a phase III randomized, placebo-controlled, double-masked clinical trial. Patients were randomized 2:1 to Visudyne and placebo, and follow-up examinations, including VA, color fundus photography, and fluorescein angiography, were performed every 3 months.

Major Inclusion Criteria

- Age $\geq$50 years
- Presence of subfoveal occult with no classic CNV due to AMD
- Area of occult CNV occupies $\geq$50% of total lesion
- Evidence of recent disease progression within preceding 3 months:
  - Presence of subretinal blood *or*
  - Recent documented vision loss within the past 12 weeks of either
  - $\geq$6-letter loss (ETDRS) or $\geq$3-line (Snellen) VA loss, *or*

- Growth of lesions $\geq$10% within the last 12 weeks
- Lesion size $\leq$6 MPS disc area
- VA Snellen equivalent 20/40 to 20/200

Primary Outcome

Percentage of patients with a <15-letter decrease in VA (approximately <3 lines)

Results

A total of 364 patients were enrolled in the study with 244 assigned to verteporfin and 120 to placebo. The study did not meet its primary end point. There was no statistically significant difference between the two groups with 62.7% ($n = 153$) of PDT-treated as compared with 55% ($n = 66$) of placebo-treated patients losing 15 or fewer letters from baseline at 12 months, and 53% ($n = 130$) as compared with 48% ($n = 57$), respectively at 24 months. During the first year, an average of 2.84 treatments were delivered. The VIO study did not meet its primary end point, although VA and angiographic characteristics were better in the PDT-treated group.

Photodynamic Therapy and Intravitreal Triamcinolone

Steroids have antipermeability, antiangiogenic and antifibrotic properties. There are several case reports indicating that combining PDT and intravitreal triamcinolone may have added benefits, including lower retreatment rates and greater visual gain. There are several multicenter clinical trials underway (VERITAS, VERTACL, RETINA) to assess this combination treatment approach.

Antivascular Endothelial Growth Factor Studies

Vascular endothelial growth factor (VEGF) is a potent cause of vascular leakage in the retina. It has also been shown to be a critical rate-limiting step in the development of ocular neovascularization. In addition, it functions as a survival factor for newly formed blood vessels. VEGF is mainly upregulated by hypoxia and other factors. There are five major isoforms of VEGF that arise from alternate splicing of a single gene; however, $VEGF_{165}$ is the predominant and most abundant isoform. VEGF is present in surgically excised CNV[22,23] and in the aqueous and vitreous humor in eyes with proliferative retinal vascular disorders.[24] VEGF therefore represents an ideal target of antiangiogenic therapy.

Macugen (Pegaptanib Sodium, OSI-Eyetech Pharmaceuticals)

The Anti-VEGF pegylated aptamer Macugen (pegaptanib sodium, formerly NX1838; OSI-Eyetech Pharmaceuticals) is a polyethylene-glycol (PEG) conjugated oligonucleotide with high specificity and affinity for the major soluble human VEGF isoform, $VEGF_{165}$. Pegylation decreases the clearance of the drug from the vitreous following intravitreal injection. Aptamers are chemically synthesized short strands of RNA or deoxyribonucleic acid (oligonucleotides) designed to bind to specific molecular targets on the basis of their three-dimensional structure, and are made using Systematic Evolution of Ligands by EXponential enrichment (SELEX) technology. Pegaptanib sodium is an aptamer composed of 28 nucleotide bases that avidly binds and inactivates $VEGF_{165}$. An aptamer binds target proteins with high specificity and affinity. Pegaptanib sodium is approximately 50 kD in size and is thus small enough to diffuse across the internal limiting membrane and retina into the subretinal space.

Vascular Endothelial Growth Factor Inhibition Study In Ocular Neovascularization (VISION) Study

Study Design

The Vascular Endothelial Growth Factor Inhibition Study In Ocular Neovascularization (VISION) study was a phase III clinical trial,[25] in which patients were randomized to intravitreal injection or sham injection given every 6 weeks for 54 weeks. Two separate trials were conducted, one in North America and the other in Europe. Patients received either 0.3, 1.0, or 3.0 mg of pegaptanib sodium or sham injection in 1:1:1:1 randomization.

Patients with predominantly classic CNV could receive combination treatment with verteporfin ocular PDT based on the discretion of the investigator.

Major Inclusion Criteria

- Age ≥50 years
- Subfoveal CNV secondary to AMD
- Lesion size <12 MPS disc areas including lesion components

- CNV >50% of entire lesion
- Any lesion composition
- ETDRS BCVA between 20/40 and 20/320 in the study eye and better or equal to 20/800 in the fellow eye
- For patients with minimally classic or purely occult CNV, there had to be evidence of recent disease progression defined as:
  - subretinal hemorrhage (but comprising no more than 50% of the lesion) and/or lipid and/or
  - documented evidence of three or more lines of Snellen vision loss during the previous 12 weeks

Primary Outcome

Proportion of subjects who lose <15 letters at month 12 compared with the baseline in the best-corrected VA score.

Results

A total of 1,186 patients were included in the efficacy analysis; 7,545 intravitreal injections of pegaptanib and 2,557 sham injections were administered. Approximately 90% of the patients in each treatment group completed the study. An average of 8.5 injections were administered per patient out of a possible total of nine injections.

Efficacy was demonstrated, without a dose–response relationship, for all three doses of pegaptanib. The 0.3-mg group was the lowest effective dose and is, therefore, the dose used in clinical practice. In this group, 70% of patients lost <15 letters of VA, as compared with 55% of controls (p <0.001) at month 12. The risk of severe loss of VA (loss of 30 letters or more) was reduced from 22% in the sham group to 10% in the group receiving 0.3 mg of pegaptanib (p <0.001). More patients receiving pegaptanib 0.3 mg, compared with sham injection, maintained or gained VA (33% vs. 23%; p = 0.003). At all subsequent points from 6 weeks after beginning therapy, the mean VA among those receiving 0.3 mg of pegaptanib was better than in those receiving sham injections (p <0.002) (see Table 7.1 and Figure 7.11). There was no evidence that any angiographic subtype of the lesion, the size of the lesion, or the level of VA at baseline precluded a treatment benefit. In the study, 78% of patients never received PDT. A

TABLE 7.1 ☐ **Rate of Visual-Acuity Loss, Measured as the Loss of Fewer Than 15 Letters, in 1,186 Patients**

Time	0.3 mg Pegaptanib (n = 294)		1.0 mg Pegaptanib (n = 300)		3.0 mg Pegaptanib (n = 296)		Sham Injection (n = 296)
	No. (%)	p Value vs. Sham Injection	No. (%)	p Value vs. Sham Injection	No. (%)	p Value vs. Sham Injection	No. (%)
Week 12	256 (87)	0.01	259 (86)	0.04	251 (85)	0.13	237 (80)
Week 24	242 (82)	<0.001	239 (80)	<0.001	224 (76)	0.003	190 (64)
Week 36	220 (75)	<0.001	229 (76)	<0.001	222 (75)	<0.001	175 (59)
Week 54	206 (70)	<0.001	213 (71)	<0.001	193 (65)	0.03	164 (55)

Reproduced from VISION trial: Gragoudas ES, Adamis AP, Cunningham ET Jr, et al. VEGF inhibition study in ocular neovascularization clinical trial group. Pegaptanib for neovascular age-related macular degeneration. *N Engl J Med.* 2004;351(27):2805–2816.

slightly higher proportion of patients receiving sham injections than those receiving pegaptanib received PDT after baseline, suggesting a possible bias against pegaptanib.

Safety

The most common and serious adverse events were endophthalmitis (in 1.3% of patients—0.16% per injection), traumatic injury to the lens (in 0.7% of patients), and retinal detachment (in 0.6% of patients).

Results from the Second Year of the Vascular Endothelial Growth Factor Inhibition Study In Ocular Neovascularization (VISION) Study

Of the 1,186 patients in the study, 1,053 participated in the second year of the trial. Patients were re-randomized to continue receiving pegaptanib or stop treatment in the second year of the study. The mean number of injections in the 2-year period was 15.6 out of a possible 17. Patients treated with pegaptanib sodium in the second year lost a mean of 9.4 ETDRS letters, as compared with patients in

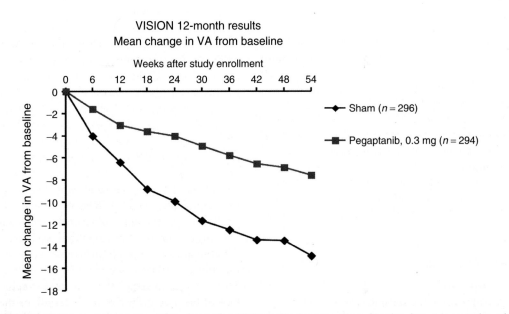

FIGURE 7.11 ☐ Mean change in vision from the VISION Study over time for the first 12 months of the clinical study.

the usual care group, who lost 17 ETDRS letters. The treatment benefit between years 1 and 2 was small, but statistically significant. In the patients receiving 1 year of treatment, there were 35 instances of visual loss of 15 ETDRS letters or more, as compared with 21 instances in the patients treated for 2 years with pegaptanib sodium.

Lucentis (Ranibizumab, Genentech)

Lucentis (ranibizumab; Genentech) is a humanized, antigen-binding fragment (Fab) of a second-generation, recombinant mouse monoclonal antibody directed toward VEGF. It consists of two parts: A nonbinding human sequence (humanized), making it less antigenic in humans, and a high-affinity binding epitope (Fab fragment) derived from the mouse, which serves to bind the antigen.[26] Ranibizumab with a molecular weight of 48 kD, is a much smaller molecule than the full-length RhuMab VEGF (Avastin, bevacizumab, Genentech) with a molecular weight of 148 kD that is currently approved for the treatment of colorectal cancer. Ranibizumab has been shown to completely penetrate the retina and enter the subretinal space after intravitreal injection.[26,27] Ranibizumab has high specificity and affinity for all the soluble human isoforms of VEGF.

Ranibizumab has been studied in three phase I/II trials in humans and two pivotal phase III clinical trials in patients with neovascular AMD and subfoveal CNV.

Phase III Trials

There are two pivotal phase III clinical trials in patients with neovascular AMD and subfoveal CNV.

Minimally Classic/Occult Trial of Antivascular Endothelial Growth Factor Antibody RhuFab V2 in the Treatment of Neovascular Age-Related Macular Degeneration (MARINA) Study

Study Design

In the Minimally Classic/Occult Trial of Anti-VEGF Antibody RhuFab V2 in the Treatment of Neovascular Age-Related Macular Degeneration Trial (Study FVF2598g), patients were randomized (1:1:1) to receive 24 monthly ranibizumab 300 or 500 μg or a sham intravitreal injections in minimally classic or occult with no classic, subfoveal CNV.

Primary Outcome

Proportion of subjects who lose <15 letters at month 12 compared with the baseline in the best-corrected VA score.

Major Inclusion Criteria

- Age ≥50 years
- ETDRS BCVA (Snellen equivalent) between 20/40 and 20/320 in the study eye
- Subfoveal CNV secondary to AMD
- No prior PDT
- Lesion composition by fluorescein angiography:
  - Area of CNV must be ≥50% of total lesion
  - Minimally classic or occult with no classic CNV
  - Evidence of presumed recent disease progression as evidenced by new subretinal hemorrhage, recent growth by fluorescein angiography or recent VA loss
  - Lesion size ≤12 disc areas

Results

Twelve-month data showed that in the study group, 452 of 478 (95%) patients lost 15 or less ETDRS letters as compared with 62% of patients in the sham group (Miller JW, American Society of Retina Specialists, Montreal, Canada, July 2005). Of the patients treated with ranibizumab, 25% of those receiving 0.3 mg and 34% of those treated with 0.5 mg gained at least 15 letters of vision as compared with 5% in the control group. Almost 40% of patients treated with ranibizumab attained a VA of 20/40 or better, as compared with 11% of the sham group.

Anti-VEGF Antibody for the Treatment of Predominantly Classic Choroidal Neovascularization in Age-Related Macular Degeneration (ANCHOR) Study

Study Design

In the Anti-VEGF Antibody for the Treatment of Predominantly Classic Choroidal Neovascularization in age-related macular degeneration (Study FVF2587g) (ANCHOR) Study, patients are randomized 1:1:1 to receive 24 monthly ranibizumab 300 or 500 μg intravitreal injections with sham PDT or a sham injection with standard PDT. Patients were eligible to receive additional sham or standard PDT treatment every 3 months if they show leakage from CNV on fluorescein angiography.

Primary Outcome

Proportion of patients who lose <15 letters at month 12 compared with the baseline in the best-corrected VA score.

Major Inclusion Criteria

- Age ≥50
- Predominantly classic subfoveal CNV due to AMD
- ETDRS BCVA (Snellen equivalent) between 20/40 to 20/320 in study eye.
- Lesion eligible for PDT (<9 MPS DA)
- No prior laser treatment involving the center of the fovea
- No prior PDT or experimental treatments for AMD.

Results

Approximately 94% of patients treated with 0.3 mg of ranibizumab and 96% of those treated with 0.5 mg of ranibizumab maintained or improved vision (defined as a loss of <15 letters in VA) as compared to approximately 64% of those treated with verteporfin (Visudyne) PDT (*p* <0.0001) during the first year of the two-year study (Kaiser PK, Macula 2006, New York, NY, 2006). The ranibizumab treatment groups further demonstrated a statistically significant difference from the control arm in an important secondary end point: Mean change in VA from the baseline to month 12. On average, patients treated with ranibizumab improved, while patients treated with PDT declined.

Anecortave Acetate (RETAANE, Alcon Pharmaceuticals)

Anecortave Acetate (RETAANE, Alcon Pharmaceuticals) is an angiostatic agent administered by posterior juxtascleral depot administration (see Figure 7.12). The drug is being clinically evaluated for the treatment of wet AMD, and for the prevention of wet AMD in patients with high-risk dry AMD, and wet AMD in the fellow eye.

Anecortave acetate is one of a new class of steroids ("angiostatic" steroids) introduced in 1985[28] that inhibits angiogenesis, yet has little glucocorticoid (anti-inflammatory) or mineralocorticoid (salt-retaining) activity. Anecortave acetate inhibits angiogenesis further downstream from VEGF, and therefore has the potential to inhibit angiogenesis driven by multiple stimuli.[29]

Anecortave acetate is a white depot suspension preparation, available in a 15 mg dose (0.5 mL of 30 mg/mL) and a 30 mg dose (0.5 mL of 60 mg/mL). It is administered by the posterior juxtascleral route, using a specifically designed protocol and cannula.

Phase III Clinical Trials

The C-01-99 Study
Study Design

Prospective, randomized, multicenter, phase III comparison of Anecortave Acetate 15 mg for Depot Suspension (RETAANE 15 mg Depot, Alcon Research, Ltd.) to verteporfin (Visudyne, Novartis) PDT for the treatment of predominantly classic, subfoveal CNV due to AMD.

Major Inclusion Criteria

- Age ≥50 years
- Subfoveal predominantly classic CNV due to AMD
- Lesions had to be <5,400 μm in the greatest linear dimension
- ETDRS BCVA (Snellen equivalent) between 20/40 to 20/400

Primary Outcome

Primary outcome was the percentage of patients with <3 lines of VA loss. The goal was to demonstrate the noninferiority of anecortave acetate to verteporfin PDT at month 12 after the start of treatment within a 95% confidence interval defined as 7%.

Results

Of the 511 patients enrolled in the study, 255 received treatment with anecortave acetate 15 mg every 6 months with a corresponding sham PDT treatment every 3 months, whereas 256 patients received PDT every 3 months if there was any leakage, according to the standard PDT guidelines, with corresponding sham juxtascleral depot administration. There was a 10% or less dropout rate over the 12-month time frame in the two groups of patients; results of 214 patients in the anecortave acetate group and 220 patients in the PDT group were analyzed.

The primary statistical objective was to demonstrate that anecortave acetate 15 mg is non-inferior to PDT in patients eligible for initial treatment with PDT using the per protocol data set. Using the predefined 7 percentage points confidence interval, the

Posterior juxtascleral depot
administration

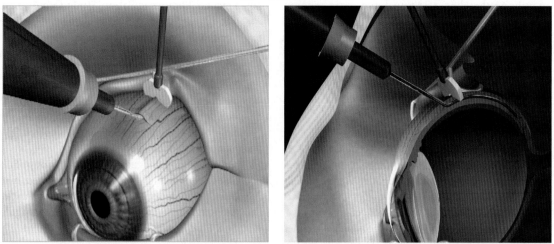

FIGURE 7.12 ☐ Retaane is delivered by posterior juxtascleral depot administration using a specially designed blunt tipped cannula that delivers the drug in a depot over the macula.

primary efficacy end point of statistical noninferiority of anecortave acetate 15 mg to PDT was not met in this study. However, if the more relevant 14 percentage points confidence interval for predominantly classic lesions had been used, this end point would have been met. Indeed, there was no clinically relevant difference in efficacy between the two groups (45% responders for anecortave acetate 15 mg vs. 49% for PDT, $p = 0.4305$). Reflux of study drug and treatment interval between drug administrations were two potentially controllable factors that had an effect on the outcome in the anecortave acetate 15 mg group. Future trials are being designed with this in mind.

C-02-60 Trial (Anecortave Acetate Risk Reduction Trial)

Trial C-02-60 is a 48-month study of anecortave acetate, 15 or 30 mg, or sham (1:1:1) administered every 6 months, to determine whether anecortave acetate reduces the risk of CNV developing in eyes with dry AMD. Approximately 2,596 patients with exudative CNV in the nonstudy eye were enrolled, with the following characteristics in the study eye: Five or more intermediate or larger soft drusen, and/or confluent drusen within 3,000 μm of the foveal center, and hyperpigmentation. Best-corrected ETDRS logMAR VA must be 0.5 (20/62.5 Snellen) in the study eye.

Primary Outcome

Development of sight-threatening CNV is defined as any CNV within 2,500 μm of the center of the fovea. The greatest linear diameter (GLD) of classic CNV must be 100 μm or more, and if occult, 500 μm or greater, unless associated with subretinal hemorrhage or lipid, in which case 100 μm meets the criteria. Subretinal hemorrhage >500 μm GLD is also considered sight-threatening CNV.

Future Horizons

Other compounds currently under clinical testing include intravitreal SIRNA-027, a small interfering RNA molecule that targets the VEGF receptor 1 (SIRNA Therapeutics and Allergan), intravitreal Cand5, a small interfering RNA molecule that targets VEGF (Acuity Pharmaceuticals), intravenous squalamine lactate (Evizon, Genarea Corporation), intravenous Combretastatin A4 Prodrug (CA4P) (Oxigene, Inc), intravitreal AdPEDF (GenVec, Inc), intravitreal bevacizumab (Avastin, Genentech), oral tyrosine kinase inhibitor PTK787 (Novartis), and intravitreal VEGF-TRAP, a VEGF receptor decoy (Regeneron).

In addition, clinical trials are also focusing on preventing the progression of dry to wet AMD. The Multicenter Investigation of Rheopheresis for AMD (MIRA-1 trial) did not demonstrate a statistically significant difference in the mean change of ETDRS BCVA between the treated and placebo groups at 12 months postbaseline. Additional studies are ongoing. The age-related eye disease study (AREDS) II trial is underway to assess the effect of 10 mg of lutein and 2 mg of zeaxanthin a day and/or 1 g of omega-3 long-chain polyunsaturated fatty acids on the risk of progression of AMD.

References

1. Ferris FL 3rd, Fine SL, Hyman L. Age-related macular degeneration and blindness due to neovascular maculopathy. *Arch Ophthal.* 1984;102(11):1640–1642.
2. Klein R, Klein BE, Jensen SC, et al. The five-year incidence and progression of age-related maculopathy: The Beaver Dam Eye Study. *Ophthalmologica.* 1997;104(1):7–21.
3. Macular Photocoagulation Study Group. Argon laser photocoagulation for senile macular degeneration. Results of a randomized clinical trial. *Arch Ophthalmol.* 1982;100:912–918.
4. Macular Photocoagulation Study Group. Argon laser photocoagulation for neovascular maculopathy: Three-year results from randomized clinical trials. *Arch Ophthalmol.* 1986;104:694–701.
5. Macular Photocoagulation Study Group. Argon laser photocoagulation for neovascular maculopathy. Five-year results from randomized clinical trials. *Arch Ophthalmol.* 1991;109:1109–1114.
6. Macular Photocoagulation Study Group. Krypton laser photocoagulation for neovascular lesions of age-related macular degeneration. Results of a randomized clinical trial. *Arch Ophthalmol.* 1990;108:816–824.
7. Macular Photocoagulation Study Group. Persistent and recurrent neovascularization after krypton laser photocoagulation for neovascular lesions of age-related macular degeneration. *Arch Ophthalmol.* 1990;108:825–831.
8. Macular Photocoagulation Study Group. Laser photocoagulation for juxtafoveal choroidal neovascularization: Five-year results from randomized clinical trials. *Arch Ophthalmol.* 1994;112:500–509.
9. Macular Photocoagulation Study Group. Laser photocoagulation of subfoveal neovascular lesions in age-related macular degeneration: Results of a randomized clinical trial. *Arch Ophthalmol.* 1991;109:1220–1231.
10. Macular Photocoagulation Study Group. Laser photocoagulation of subfoveal neovascular lesions of age-related macular degeneration: Updated findings from two clinical trials. *Arch Ophthalmol.* 1993;111:1200–1209.
11. Macular Photocoagulation Study Group. Laser photocoagulation of subfoveal neovascular lesions in age-related macular degeneration. Results of a randomized clinical trial. *Arch Ophthal.* 1991;109(9):1220–1231.
12. Macular Photocoagulation Study Group. Subfoveal neovascular lesions in age-related macular degeneration: Guidelines for evaluation and treatment in the Macular Photocoagulation Study. *Arch Ophthalmol.* 1991;109:1220–1231.
13. Macular Photocoagulation Study Group. Laser photocoagulation of subfoveal recurrent neovascular lesions in age-related macular degeneration. Results of a randomized clinical trial. *Arch Ophthalmol.* 1991;109:1232–1241.
14. Macular Photocoagulation Study Group. Persistent and recurrent neovascularization after laser photocoagulation for subfoveal choroidal neovascularization of age-related macular degeneration. *Arch Ophthalmol.* 1994;112:489–499.
15. Schmidt-Erfurth U, Hasan T, Gragoudas E, et al. Vascular targeting in photodynamic occlusion of subretinal vessels. *Ophthalmologica.* 1994;101(12):1953–1961.
16. Moshfeghi DM, Kaiser PK, Grossniklaus HE, et al. Clinicopathologic study after submacular removal of choroidal neovascular membranes treated with verteporfin ocular photodynamic therapy. *Am J Ophthalmol.* 2003;135(3):343–350.
17. Treatment of Age-Related Macular Degeneration with Photodynamic Therapy (TAP) Study Group. Photodynamic therapy of subfoveal choroidal neovascularization in age-related macular degeneration with verteporfin: One-year results of 2 randomized clinical trials—TAP report. *Arch Ophthal.* 1999;117(10):1329–1345; Erratum in: *Arch Ophthalmol.* 2000;118(4):488.
18. Bressler NM. Treatment of Age-Related Macular Degeneration with Photodynamic Therapy (TAP) Study Group. Photodynamic Therapy of Subfoveal Choroidal Neovascularization in Age-Related Macular Degeneration with Verteporfin:

Two-Year Results of 2 Randomized Clinical Trials-Tap Report 2. *Arch Ophthalmol.* 2001; 119:198–207.

19. Blumenkranz MS, Bressler NM, Bressler SB, et al. Treatment of Age-Related Macular Degeneration with Photodynamic Therapy (TAP) Study Group. Verteporfin therapy for subfoveal choroidal neovascularization in age-related macular degeneration: Three-year results of an open-label extension of 2 randomized clinical trials--TAP Report no. 5. *Arch Ophthal.* 2002;120(10):1307–1314.

20. Bressler NM, Bressler SB, Kaiser PK, et al. Verteporfin therapy for subfoveal choroidal neovascularization in age-related macular degeneration: Four-year results of an open-label extension of 2 randomized clinical trials: TAP Report No. 7. *Arch Ophthalmol.* 2005;123(9):1283–1285.

21. Blinder KJ, Bradley S, Bressler NM, et al. Treatment of Age-related Macular Degeneration with Photodynamic Therapy Study Group; Verteporfin in Photodynamic Therapy Study Group. Effect of lesion size, visual acuity, and lesion composition on visual acuity change with and without verteporfin therapy for choroidal neovascularization secondary to age-related macular degeneration: TAP and VIP report no. 1. *Am J Ophthalmol.* 2003;136(3): 407–418.

22. Kvanta A, Algvere PV, Berglin L, et al. Subfoveal fibrovascular membranes in age-related macular degeneration express vascular endothelial growth factor. *Invest Ophthalmol Vis Sci.* 1996;37(9):1929–1934.

23. Lopez PF, Sippy BD, Lambert HM, et al. Trans-differentiated retinal pigment epithelial cells are immunoreactive for vascular endothelial growth factor in surgically excised age-related macular degeneration-related choroidal neovascular membranes. *Invest Ophthalmol Vis Sci.* 1996;37(5):855–868.

24. Aiello LP, Avery RL, Arrigg PG, et al. Vascular endothelial growth factor in ocular fluid of patients with diabetic retinopathy and other retinal disorders. *N Engl J Med.* 1994; 331(22):1480–1487.

25. Gragoudas ES, Adamis AP, Cunningham ET, et al. VEGF inhibition study in ocular neovascularization clinical trial group. Pegaptanib for neovascular age-related macular degeneration. *N Engl J Med.* 2004;351:2805–2816.

26. Mordenti J, Cuthbertson RA, Ferrara N, et al. Comparisons of the intraocular tissue distribution, pharmacokinetics, and safety of 125I-labeled full-length and Fab antibodies in rhesus monkeys following intravitreal administration. *Toxicol Pathol.* 1999;27(5):536–544.

27. Gaudreault J, Escandon E, Maruoka M, et al. Vitreal Pharmacokinetics of rhuFab V2 in Rabbits Using a Non-invasive Method. Association for Research in Vision and Ophthalmology; 2002, Abstract 2801.

28. Crum R, Szabo S, Folkman J. A new class of steroids inhibits angiogenesis in the presence of heparin or a heparin fragment. *Science.* 1985; 230:1375–1378.

29. Casey R, Li WW. Factors controlling ocular angiogenesis. *Am J Ophthalmol.* 1997;124(4): 521–529.

Treatment of Central Retinal Vein Occlusion: Lessons from Clinical Trials

Henry Tseng, MD, PhD and Sharon Fekrat, MD, FACS

Various systemic diseases, such as hypertension, diabetes mellitus, cardiovascular disease, or peripheral vascular disease can contribute to the development of an occlusion in the central retinal vein.[1] In eyes with a central retinal vein occlusion (CRVO), a thrombus is suspected at the level of the lamina cribrosa. This generally results in the sudden unilateral decrease of visual acuity (VA) associated with the four quadrants of dilated tortuous retinal veins, intraretinal hemorrhages, optic disc swelling and hyperemia, and cystoid macular edema (CME) in most eyes. Long-term sequelae may include persistent CME and neovascularization of the iris (NVI), angle, disc, or retina. Persistent visual loss and the development of neovascular glaucoma present a tremendous challenge to the ophthalmologist when confronted with an eye with a CRVO.

The Central Vein Occlusion Study

The Central Vein Occlusion Study (CVOS) was a multicenter, prospective, controlled clinical trial conducted between 1988 and 1992.[2–5] The CVOS sought to understand the natural history of perfused CRVO, determine the role of grid-pattern laser photocoagulation in the treatment of macular edema, and ascertain when to treat an eye with a CRVO using panretinal photocoagulation (PRP) to prevent complications associated with NVI or neovascularization of the angle (NVA). Before the CVOS, it was already generally accepted that standard of care was to treat eyes with NVI or NVA with PRP, but it was unknown

whether early PRP treatment, before the development of NVI or NVA, was helpful in preventing NVI/NVA.

In the CVOS, eyes were categorized according to perfusion status on fluorescein angiography into three groups: Perfused, nonperfused, or indeterminate. A perfused CRVO was defined as the presence of capillary nonperfusion of <10 disc areas in size on fluorescein angiography. The onset of the CRVO had to be within the preceding 12 months. Eyes were excluded from the CVOS if they had previous laser photocoagulation for any retinal vascular disease in the affected eye, presence of diabetic retinopathy, new or old branch arterial/venous occlusion, retinal neovascularization, vitreous hemorrhage, peripheral anterior synechiae, or concurrent eye disease that decreased VA.

In addition to the CVOS, various smaller studies also contributed to our understanding of CRVO and to the search for developing alternative treatment modalities. These studies will also be discussed in this chapter.

Natural History

The characteristics of the patients enrolled in the CVOS are summarized in Table 8A.1. Over the course of the CVOS, nine clinical centers participated and enrolled 714 eyes of 711 patients. The number of males was slightly more than that of female patients, and over 50% of the patients were 65 years or older. Sixty-one percent of the patients had some evidence of hypertension. Five hundred and forty-six eyes were classified as perfused on angiography during the

TABLE 8A.1 □ Summary of Patient Characteristics of the Central Vein Occlusion Study

Characteristic (n = 711 eyes)	Number of Patients (%)
Male	375 (53)
Older than 65 years	406 (57)
Caucasian	665 (94)
Diagnosed with hypertension	435 (61)
Diabetic	52 (7)
Visual acuity >20/50	209 (29)
Visual acuity <20/200	201 (28)

initial visit. Once a patient developed a CRVO in one eye, it was also determined in the CVOS that there was an annual risk of 0.9% per year of developing a CRVO in the fellow eye.[2–5]

Improvement in VA was associated strongly with the initial baseline VA.[2] VA outcomes were studied in the CVOS without distinguishing the perfusion status of the CRVO. At study entry, the VA varied: 29% were 20/40 or better, 43% were between 20/50 and 20/200, and 28% were 20/200 or worse. Of the eyes with an initial VA of 20/40 or better, 65% retained VA at this level, while the remaining worsened. Similarly, 19% with an initial VA between 20/50 and 20/200 maintained the same level at the final follow-up visit. Eyes with an initial VA of worse than 20/200 had an 80% chance of staying at that level.

The CVOS demonstrated that eyes with a non-perfused CRVO had a higher risk of developing NVI/NVA.[2] One third of the study eyes were nonper-fused by 3 years after the initial diagnosis of CRVO. Thirty-five percent of the nonperfused eyes (61 of 176 eyes) developed NVI/NVA, compared to 10% (56 of 538) of perfused eyes. Of the 117 (16%) eyes that developed NVI/NVA during the CVOS, 56 were previously classified as perfused, 42 as nonperfused, and 19 as indeterminate. The median time to the development of NVI/NVA in nonperfused eyes was 61 days (range, 6 days to 8 months) after the eye was enrolled in the study. The CVOS found that instances of NVI/NVA were more likely in males, and eyes with a VA worse than 20/200 that had at least 30 disc areas of nonperfusion, had moderate-to-severe venous tor-tuosity and retinal hemorrhage, or had the CRVO for a duration of <1 month.

In the CVOS, of the eyes that were initially classified as perfused, 34% (185 of 547 eyes) converted to a nonperfused status by 3 years.[2] This progression was found to be strongly associated with a duration of CRVO <1 month, VA worse than 20/200, and the presence of 5 to 9 disc areas of nonperfusion on the baseline fluorescein angiogram.

The natural history of CRVO was also described in other studies. A retrospective study by Quinlan et al. chronicled VA in perfused and nonperfused eyes separately.[6] Fifteen percent of perfused eyes gained three or more lines, while 31% lost three or more lines on VA testing. Within the nonperfused group, 28% gained three or more lines, while 24% lost the same amount. Therefore, the study demonstrates a lack of visual stability in untreated eyes with CRVO. More-over, another study analyzed 144 eyes with perfused CRVO and found significant visual improvement fol-lowing the resolution of the retinopathy. Sixty-five percent of all eyes in this study had a VA between 20/15 and 20/40 following resolution.[7]

Medical Treatment

There is currently no proven medical intervention to improve VA for eyes with CRVO.[8] The CVOS was not designed to address the medical management of CRVO. Various interventions have been attempted, including systemic anticoagulation with medications such as aspirin, heparin, and warfarin. These agents have not been shown to prevent or alter the course of eyes with a CRVO.[9–11]

Topical aqueous suppressants have been utilized to prevent the development of CRVO and to treat the same. Altering intraocular pressure (IOP) may have a secondary effect on the position of the lamina cribrosa and, in turn, on any associated compression of the central retinal vein. However, little clinical data exist to demonstrate whether lowering normal IOP in eyes without glaucoma prevents or alters the course of the CRVO.

One therapeutic agent under investigation is the synthetic xanthine derivative, pentoxifylline, which has been found to enhance pulsatile flow in nonoc-cluded retinal veins, decrease blood viscosity, and promote vasodilation. A dose-dependent effect was found with a maximum benefit being achieved 150 to 180 minutes after the start of the pentoxifylline infusion in 10 healthy volunteers.[12] However, the drug's ability to prevent or alter the course of CRVO was not specifically studied and is hence unknown.

Since increased blood viscosity has been positively correlated with CRVOs,[13] reduction of blood hyperviscosity has been investigated as a possible therapeutic approach. Two small studies found hemodilution to improve VA.[14,15] A prospective, randomized, single-masked clinical trial combining both hemodilution and pentoxifylline administration found a significant improvement in the mean VA at one year.[16] Patients who were treated with this combination approach had an increase in VA of 1.5 lines compared to control patients who demonstrated a decrease of 1.5 lines in the affected eye. This was shown to be the result of improved blood flow subsequent to decreased blood viscosity. However, no statistically significant difference was observed between the treated and untreated groups with respect to progression from a perfused to a non-perfused status.

Grid-Pattern Laser Photocoagulation

Macular edema is commonly present in eyes with CRVO and may result in significant visual loss. The CVOS demonstrated that macular grid-pattern laser treatment did not significantly improve the VA of CRVO eyes when compared to untreated eyes.[17] Laser photocoagulation was performed in a grid pattern within two disc diameters of the foveal center but outside of the foveal avascular zone. Initial median visual acuities of 20/125 (untreated) and 20/160 (treated) were comparable to final median visual acuities of 20/160 (untreated) and 20/200 (treated).

There was a clinical trend suggesting that photocoagulation may be more effective in eyes of patients under the age of 65. Seventeen treated eyes (23%) had an improvement of two or more lines of VA, and 11 of those were persons who were <60 years old. The results, however, were not statistically significant.

Although laser photocoagulation did not improve the VA in CRVO eyes, treatment resulted in less macular edema on fluorescein angiography. In 21 of 68 treated eyes (31%), there was no angiographic macular edema one year posttreatment compared to 6 of 78 (8%) untreated eyes ($p < 0.0001$). It is uncertain why grid laser photocoagulation improves macular edema angiographically without a clinical improvement in VA.

The CVOS concluded that grid laser photocoagulation in eyes with CRVO-associated macular edema was not beneficial and therefore not indicated. Further evaluation is warranted to determine if any benefits may result from an age-based treatment approach.[17]

Panretinal Photocoagulation

Despite any definitive clinical trial data, prophylactic PRP was widely accepted for the prevention of NVI/NVA in ischemic CRVO at the time that the CVOS was conducted. But the timing of the PRP treatment was not clear. Therefore, the CVOS examined whether PRP treatment should be initiated immediately following the diagnosis of CRVO or delayed until the development of any iris or angle neovascularization. While prophylactic PRP decreased the rate of developing NVI/NVA (18 treated eyes out of 90; 20%) when compared with untreated eyes (32 of 91; 35%), the difference was not statistically significant. Furthermore, once NVI/NVA has developed, additional PRP was four times less effective in eyes that had received prophylactic PRP (4 of 18 eyes; 22%) than control eyes (18 of 32 eyes; 56%) in inducing the regression of neovascularization; thus, data from CVOS does not support prophylactic PRP treatment.[18]

The CVOS showed that not all eyes with CRVO develop anterior segment neovascularization. As such, many eyes would be subjected to unnecessary PRP treatment and the associated risks of PRP if such a treatment were given prophylactically.[18] Furthermore, there was no statistically significant effect of PRP on VA outcome. Approximately one third of the PRP-treated eyes had no change in VA, another third lost two or more lines, and the final third gained two or more lines.[18] Therefore, the CVOS concluded that PRP should only be implemented after a diagnosis of neovascularization to prevent unnecessary photocoagulation. Prophylactic PRP may be considered when close follow-up is impossible or unlikely.

If PRP is appropriately initiated following first identification of any neovascularization, post-procedural follow-up is recommended at 2 to 4 weeks to ensure that there is no progression; if progression is noted at that time, then additional PRP is indicated to prevent the development of neovascular glaucoma.

Intravitreal Triamcinolone Acetonide

A novel treatment for CRVO-associated macular edema is the intravitreal injection of triamcinolone (Kenalog; Bristol-Myer Squibb). More recent data indicates that intravitreal triamcinolone treatment can decrease macular edema and improve VA in eyes with CRVO. Before the publication of two retrospective case series, there were only scattered case reports showing that eyes with macular edema secondary to a CRVO responded to intravitreal triamcinolone injection.[19–21] One study that included 10 eyes showed that the administration of (4 mg in 0.1 mL) intravitreal triamcinolone in eyes with CRVO resulted in a mean VA increase of 20 letters and a mean improvement in volumetric optical coherence tomography (OCT) measurements by 1.6 mm^3 after an average follow-up of 5 months.[22] Another study with eight eyes reported a mean VA gain of two or more lines at 3 months in four out of eight eyes associated with the resolution of macular edema on clinical examination and OCT.[23]

Subsequently, numerous studies have confirmed that CRVO-associated macular edema responds to intravitreal injections of triamcinolone.[21,23–30] These reports demonstrated that while intravitreal triamcinolone effectively reduced macular edema initially, the effect did not persist and often wore off in 4 to 6 months.

Although intravitreal triamcinolone is emerging as an effective short-term treatment for CRVO-associated macular edema, its use may be tempered by the well-known side-effect profile of intraocular steroids, as well as the need for intravitreal delivery of the drug. Such side effects include steroid-induced cataract formation, steroid-induced IOP elevation,[31] retinal detachment, and endophthalmitis.

With data strongly suggesting that intravitreal triamcinolone may effectively treat CRVO-associated macular edema, a clinical trial is warranted to fully evaluate this emerging treatment modality.[32] There is currently an ongoing multicenter, randomized phase III clinical trial, sponsored by the National Eye Institute, called The Standard of Care versus Corticosteroid for Retinal Vein Occlusion (SCORE) Study.[33] The study is expected to enroll 1,260 study participants: 630 with CRVO and 630 with branch retinal vein occlusion (BRVO). The SCORE study will randomize eyes with macular edema secondary to CRVO into three treatment groups. One group will receive the standard of care (observation), a second group will receive 4 mg of intravitreal triamcinolone, and a third group will receive 1 mg of intravitreal triamcinolone (see Fig. 8A.1). Recruitment of patients began in October 2004 and these groups will be followed every 4 months for a total of 36 months. The primary efficacy will be measured by an improvement of 15 or more letters in VA at the 12-month visit. The SCORE study will evaluate the safety profile of triamcinolone by monitoring cataract formation, IOP changes, and injection-related events such as endophthalmitis, vitreous hemorrhage, and retinal detachment.

Sustained Drug Release Devices

An alternative method of delivering intraocular steroids is through a sustained-release device that is implanted through a pars plana incision into the vitreous cavity. One such device that is currently being evaluated in eyes with macular edema in the setting of CRVO is the fluocinolone acetonide implant (Retisert, Bausch and Lomb). Retisert is non-biodegradable and is secured in the vitreous cavity with scleral sutures. The device is designed to release 0.5 mcg of fluocinolone, a synthetic steroid, per day for 3 years. This device is currently being evaluated for the treatment of other retinal diseases, including macular edema associated with diabetic retinopathy, and choroidal neovascularization, and is now

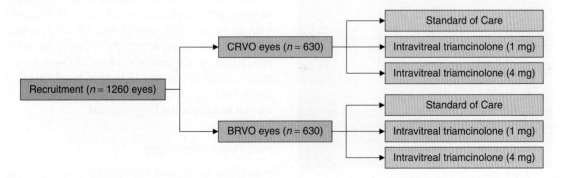

FIGURE 8A.1 ☐ Randomization schema for the Standard of Care versus Corticosteroid for Retinal Vein Occlusion (SCORE) study. CRVO, central retinal vein occlusion; BRVO, branch retinal vein occlusion.

approved by the U.S. Food and Drug Administration (FDA) for the treatment of uveitis.[34,35]

Proposed advantages of this device include constant drug levels and sustained duration of treatment appropriately tailored to the disease for long-term treatment.[34,36,37] One disadvantage of Retisert is the need for vitreoretinal surgery for implantation. This is associated with a higher risk of complications than a single intravitreal injection. Furthermore, increased IOP and cataract progression may occur with increased frequency in these eyes. Most cases of elevated IOP can be satisfactorily treated with drops, but surgical intervention may be required.

Laser Chorioretinal Venous Anastomosis

A chorioretinal anastomosis (CRA) bypasses the occluded retinal venous system by creating an anastomotic outflow channel from the high resistance retinal venous system to the low resistance choroidal circulation (see Fig. 8A.2). The creation of an outflow channel may reduce macular edema and result in improved VA in eyes with a perfused CRVO. Enhanced outflow may also halt the conversion of a perfused CRVO to a nonperfused status.[38–42]

The most common method for creating a CRA is by using the argon laser, with high power—as high as 6 watts, as found in some reports. Typically, a CRA is performed by directing a 50 μm spot of argon green laser of variable duration at an area adjacent to a branch retinal vein nasal to the optic nerve head. The goal is to rupture Bruch's membrane at this location; a "bubble" is usually visualized upon successful rupture. The adjacent branch vein is then treated to rupture the wall of the vein. It is preferable to find a branch vein without any intervening branchings

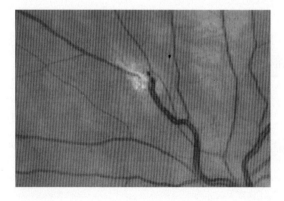

FIGURE 8A.2 ◻ Color photograph of a successful laser chorioretinal venous anastomosis.

from the optic nerve head. Alternatively, a CRA bypass can be created surgically through a transretinal venipuncture technique.[38]

A retrospective study by McAllister and Constable demonstrated a 33% success rate as measured by a functioning anastomosis.[39] VA improved in six out of the eight eyes with successful anastomoses. In the other two eyes, the acuity remained stable. The authors showed an association between anastomotic success and the following fundoscopic signs: Retinal venous hemorrhage and choroidal vacuole. These findings probably indicate rupture of venous vessels and Bruch's membrane, respectively; however, these findings were not always associated with a successful anastomosis in follow-up studies.

Browning and Antoszyk performed laser CRA on eight eyes with CRVO and had less encouraging results.[41] Only 2 anastomoses (out of 20 attempts) were created, and they were not of the same appearance as those created by McAllister and Constable. Complications such as vitreous hemorrhage, rubeosis, retinal neovascularization, retinal detachment, and neovascular glaucoma were reported. The authors concluded that the risks of CRA outweighed the therapeutic benefits in their study.

Fekrat et al. performed CRA on 24 eyes in their series and achieved successful anastomoses in 9. Visual improvement of 6 or more lines in 2 (8%) of 24 eyes, 1 to 3 lines in 5 (21%), and no improvement in 2 (8%) were reported two months post-CRA.[42] Neovascular complications as well as retinal fibrosis and detachment were reported.

Even with the creation of a successful CRA, complications may occur and visual recovery may be hampered by the development of pigment abnormalities, thrombosis of the treated vein, progressive retinal ischemia, and neovascular membrane formation.[40,42] Leonard et al. reported a modified CRA technique to minimize complications, and achieved successful CRA in 19 out of 19 nonischemic CRVO eyes with moderate visual improvement.[43] Given the other emerging treatment modalities for CRVO and in view of the complications due to laser-induced CRA and the lack of a reproducible effect, the early enthusiasm for this technique has largely waned.

Pars Plana Vitrectomy

Pars plana vitrectomy (PPV) with removal of the posterior hyaloid may be utilized to treat visual loss associated with CME, vitreous hemorrhage, or fibrovascular proliferation in eyes with CRVO. Data from a retrospective study by Hikichi et al. demonstrate that there was an association between the presence of vitreomacular attachment and the development of macular edema in eyes with CRVO.[44] In their study, 76% of perfused eyes with macular edema either possessed no posterior vitreous detachment (PVD) or only a partial PVD with vitreomacular detachment. In contrast, only 25% of the perfused group without macular edema had no PVD or partial PVD. The authors speculated that a complete PVD prevents the development of neovascularization and that vitreomacular attachment may be the etiology of persistent macular edema in eyes with a CRVO.

An improvement in macular edema in CRVO eyes after PPV with peeling of the internal limiting membrane (ILM) was reported in a separate study involving 14 eyes. Within 6 weeks of the surgery, 79% of the patients showed an improvement in macular edema and VA.[45] They speculated that simultaneous removal of the ILM would promote the movement of fluid out of the inner retinal layers, resulting in decreased macular edema. This speculation is also supported by a limited case series of five eyes that demonstrated an average improvement of 311 μm with OCT imaging within two weeks of PPV.[46] This was associated with an improvement in VA by two or more lines in three of five eyes.[46]

These studies suggest that there may be a role for PPV with or without ILM peeling in the reduction of macular edema secondary to CRVO and improvement of VA. However, larger scale, randomized trials are needed for further evaluation.

Vitreous hemorrhage occurs from retinal hemorrhages breaking through the ILM or from neovascularization of the retina or disc. Nonclearing vitreous hemorrhage can be cleared using standard vitreoretinal surgical techniques.[47] Additionally, at the time of the vitrectomy, the source of the hemorrhage and stimulus for neovascularization can be reduced with transcleral cryotherapy[48] or PRP using an endolaser. Removal of any epiretinal membrane or fibrovascular proliferation resulting from the CRVO can also be performed concurrently with the PPV. VA outcome is typically limited by the initial insult to the macula from the CRVO.[47]

Recombinant Tissue Plasminogen Activator

Because CRVO is caused presumably by a thrombus in the central retinal vein, the dissolution of thrombus would theoretically restore proper retinal blood circulation with reperfusion of the central retinal vein. Thrombolytic agents have thus been proposed as a possible treatment for CRVO. One such thrombolytic agent that has been under investigation is recombinant tissue plasminogen activator (rt-PA). It is a synthetic fibrinolytic agent that facilitates the conversion of plasminogen to plasmin in the presence of fibrin, thereby reducing the size of the intravascular clot and permitting reperfusion of the central retinal vein.

The delivery of rt-PA has been investigated through several routes that include systemic, intravitreal, and intraoperative endovascular cannulation of retinal vessels. Systemic administration of rt-PA has been reported in a pilot study of 89 CRVO eyes,[49] in which 42% of the eyes reportedly gained 3 or more lines of vision, while 37% remained stable. Another study reported that 10 out of 14 eyes (7 CRVO, 3 BRVO) had 1 line or more of improvement in VA, associated with a reduction of areas of capillary nonperfusion in 8 (6 CRVO, 2 BRVO) of those eyes after systemic rt-PA administration.[50] Other studies reported improvements in VA from 34.8% (8 of 23 eyes)[51] to 44% of their study eyes (10 out of 23 patients) after systemic rt-PA.[52] Although intravenous administration of rt-PA revealed promising results, serious complications were described. Three patients developed intraocular bleeding while one died from a hemorrhagic stroke.

Because of the risk of mortality and other serious complications from systemic rt-PA, alternative routes of administration have been investigated. Intravitreal injections of rt-PA improved visual acuities in 28 to 44% of eyes described in several small studies.[53–55] However, intravitreal rt-PA was not associated with improvement of the final perfusion status.

Alternatively, rt-PA can be directly delivered to the thrombus in the occluded vein.[56,57] This endovascular approach involves performing a PPV followed by the cannulation of the retinal vein and subsequent rt-PA infusion into the occluded vein. It is technically more challenging and requires sophisticated vitreoretinal surgical techniques that are still being refined. A pilot study by Weiss and Bynoe reported that up to 54% (15 out of 28) gained three or more lines of acuity within 6 months following the injection of rt-PA, with seven eyes developing a vitreous hemorrhage and one eye developing a retinal detachment. Furthermore, endovascular delivery of rt-PA can be combined with intravitreal injections of triamcinolone acetonide to result in an improvement of 8 to 11 lines of VA, as described in 2 young patients with CRVO.[58]

Antivascular Endothelial Growth Factor (anti-VEGF) Agents

Pegaptanib sodium (Macugen) is an aptamer that selectively inhibits one human isoform of vascular endothelial growth factor[59] and has been recently approved for the treatment of choroidal neovascularization in eyes with age-related macular degeneration. Its ability to reduce macular edema in eyes with CRVO is currently under study and it may subsequently be evaluated in eyes with BRVO. Macugen itself is associated with a few adverse effects; however, the intravitreal injection itself may rarely result in endophthalmitis or retinal detachment.

Another anti-VEGF agent is bevacizumab (Avastin), which is also currently being investigated as another agent that might reduce macular edema associated with CRVO. A recent case report demonstrated that an intravitreal injection of 1.0 mg bevacizumab resulted in the resolution of CME[60] for at least 4 weeks. It was reported that within 1 week of the bevacizumab injection, VA improved from 20/200 to 20/50. Resolution of the CME was demonstrated on OCT. While being encouraging, the results warrant further investigation.

Surgical Decompression of the Central Retinal Vein

Optic Nerve Sheath Decompression

Because the etiology of CRVO may be related to compression of the retinal vein by its corresponding retinal artery with subsequent thrombus formation, decompression of the occluded vein can theoretically reestablish perfusion. Decompression of the central retinal artery and vein is performed by cutting the posterior scleral ring and creating fenestrations in the optic nerve sheath,[61–63] using an orbital approach similar to that performed in the treatment of optic nerve swelling in pseudotumor cerebri patients. Sonographic reduction in the caliber of the central retinal vein has been observed in eyes following optic nerve sheath decompression (ONSD),[64] suggesting indirect resolution of venous congestion.

Early retrospective studies of ONSD for CRVO noted improved VA in up to 39% of patients.[61,63] Dev and Buckley performed ONSD in eight eyes with CRVO and found VA to improve postoperatively in three-fourths of the study eyes. The mean preoperative VA of 20/160 improved to 20/70 at an average postoperative follow-up of 1 year. There was a documented decrease or resolution of optic disc edema in all cases. No complications were noted.[62] Small study numbers limit the validation of an orbital approach to nerve sheath decompression in treating CRVO.

Radial Optic Neurotomy

This surgical procedure may improve venous outflow in eyes with CRVO by relieving pressure on the occluded vein as it crosses the cribriform plate and scleral outlet.[65] Radial optic neurotomy (RON) may relieve the "compartment syndrome" caused by the compression of the central retinal vein. The procedure consists of a PPV followed by the use of a 20-gauge microvitreoretinal (MVR) blade to relax the scleral ring, cribriform plate, and adjacent sclera of the optic disc by radially cutting the scleral ring and its adjacent sclera transvitreally (see Fig. 8A.3). The posterior hyaloid should also be separated from the retina and removed in all eyes.

In a retrospective pilot study, Opremcak et al. demonstrated visual improvement in 8 out of 11 eyes that underwent RON. All eyes had an initial acuity <20/400, and five eyes were perfused. With a mean follow-up time of 9 months, 73% had mean visual improvement of five lines, with a final overall mean VA of >20/70.[65]

Two subsequent case series yielded more modest results. A study of four eyes with CRVO and one with hemiretinal vein occlusion resulted in only modest improvement in VA, from a mean preoperative VA of 4/200 to a mean postoperative VA of 20/400 after 4.5 months.[66] A second study of 14 patients with CRVO (with initial VA less than 20/125) showed six eyes (43%) improving by two or more lines.[67] However, chorioretinal anastomoses formed at the RON site in six eyes showed better median VA (20/60) than those without anastomoses (20/110).

A recent interventional case series of 15 eyes with CRVO using indocyanine green (ICG) videoangiography and computer-assisted image analysis evaluated whether RON actually improved retinal circulation.[68] The study showed improved blood circulation in 53% of eyes receiving RON. But consistent with the result of Garcia-Arumi et al., the authors also found that the development of chorioretinal

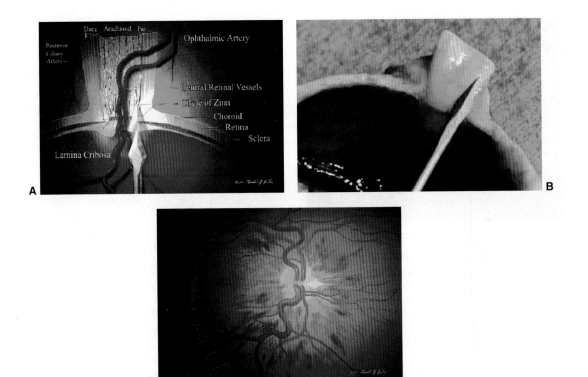

FIGURE 8A.3 ☐ Radial optic neurotomy. Cutting the scleral ring around the optic nerve and adjacent sclera relieves compression of the central retinal vein (**A**). This is shown in a cadaveric eye with a microvitreal blade over the optic nerve (**B**). A fundus photograph from a patient after surgery illustrates the RON incision performed temporal to the optic nerve (**C**). Please note that the major blood vessels are not perforated and that the scleral ring is relaxed. (From Opremcak EM, et al. Radial optic neurotomy for central retinal vein occlusion: A retrospective pilot study of 11 consecutive cases. *Retina.* 2001;21(5):408–415.)

anastomoses at the RON site (see Fig. 8A.4) correlated with improved circulation and improved VA. This suggests the possibility that collaterals may contribute to any treatment effects yielded by RON rather than an actual decompression of the central retinal vein.

The efficacy and safety of RON remains controversial. The development of retinociliary collaterals is common in the natural history of CRVO, and it may be incorrect to attribute their presence to the RON.[69] Improvements in VA so far have been fairly modest with significant postoperative complications such as neovascularization of the anterior segment or at the neurotomy site, vitreous hemorrhage, and retinal detachment.[66,70] Difficulty in standardizing the surgical technique also results in variable efficacy. Standardization of incision lengths in the optic disc may be difficult because of variations in the size of the disc and cup, especially in eyes with tilted discs. This

problem is augmented in the glaucomatous eye when enlarged cups and shifted vessels leave little space for the radial incision.[71] Finally, more studies of RON's effect on visual fields are needed since the cutting of optic nerve fibers and nearby vessels can result in significant visual field defects.[69] A histologic study of porcine eyes following RON showed marked axonal nerve fiber loss distal to the surgical site as well as focal hemorrhages and interstitial edema of the optic nerve.[72] Because of these complications and modest VA improvement, RON remains to be validated as a treatment option for eyes with CRVO.

Conclusion

CRVO remains an important cause of visual loss, and remains difficult to treat effectively. Recovery from the initial ischemic insult is further complicated by sequelae such as the development of macular

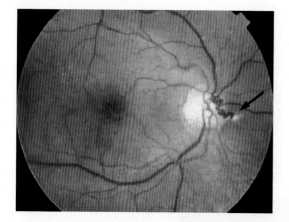

FIGURE 8A.4 ☐ Development of a chorioretinal anastomoses at the radial optic neurotomy site temporal to the optic disk. (Courtesy of Jose Garcia-Arumi, Professor of Ophthalmology, Universidad Autónoma de Barcelona, Instituto de Microcirugia Ocular [IMO].)

edema and neovascular glaucoma. Data from the CVOS have contributed to our knowledge of the natural history of CRVO, the importance of perfusion status, as well as our understanding of when and how to use laser photocoagulation to treat CRVO complications. PRP remains the widely accepted treatment to prevent neovascular complications in ischemic CRVO eyes. No effective medical or surgical treatments have yet been developed. Excitement about both laser chorioretinal venous anastomosis formation and RON has been tempered by modest improvement in VA and complications. However, new treatments are being investigated, including anti-VEGF agents. Intravitreal triamcinolone injection as a treatment modality for CRVO-associated macular edema appears promising, at least in the short-term. The SCORE study is currently recruiting.

References

1. The Eye Disease Case-Control Study Group. Risk factors for central retinal vein occlusion. *Arch Ophthalmol.* 1996;114(5):545–554.
2. The Central Vein Occlusion Study Group. Natural history and clinical management of central retinal vein occlusion. *Arch Ophthalmol.* 1997; 115(4):486–491.
3. Central Vein Occlusion Study Group. Central vein occlusion study of photocoagulation therapy. Baseline findings. *Online J Curr Clin Trials.* 1993; **Doc No 95.**
4. The Central Vein Occlusion Study. Baseline and early natural history report. *Arch Ophthalmol.* 1993;111(8):1087–1095.
5. Central Vein Occlusion Study Group. Central vein occlusion study of photocoagulation. Manual of operations. *Online J Curr Clin Trials.* 1993; **Doc No 92.**
6. Quinlan PM, Elman MJ, Bhatt AK, et al. The natural course of central retinal vein occlusion. *Am J Ophthalmol.* 1990;110(2): 118–123.
7. Hayreh SS. Retinal vein occlusion. *Indian J Ophthalmol.* 1994;42(3):109–132.
8. Parodi MB. Medical treatment of retinal vein occlusions. *Semin Ophthalmol.* 2004;19(1–2): 43–48.
9. Browning DJ, Fraser CM. Retinal vein occlusions in patients taking warfarin. *Ophthalmology.* 2004;111(6):1196–1200.
10. Hayreh SS. Prevalent misconceptions about acute retinal vascular occlusive disorders. *Prog Retin Eye Res.* 2005;24(4):493–519.
11. Mruthyunjaya P, Chandrashekar R, Stinnett S, et al. Central retinal vein occlusion in patients on long term Coumadin anticoagulation. *Retina.* 2005; **(in press).**
12. Schmetterer L, Kemmler D, Breiteneder H, et al. A randomized, placebo-controlled, double-blind crossover study of the effect of pentoxifylline on ocular fundus pulsations. *Am J Ophthalmol.* 1996;121(2):169–176.
13. Ring CP, Pearson TC, Sanders MD, et al. Viscosity and retinal vein thrombosis. *Br J Ophthalmol.* 1976;60(6):397–410.
14. Hansen LL, Danisevskis P Arntz HR et al. A randomised prospective study on treatment of central retinal vein occlusion by isovolaemic haemodilution and photocoagulation. *Br J Ophthalmol.* 1985;69(2):108–116.
15. Hansen LL, Wiek J, Wiederholt M. A randomised prospective study of treatment of non-ischaemic central retinal vein occlusion by isovolaemic haemodilution. *Br J Ophthalmol.* 1989;73(11):895–899.
16. Wolf S, Arend O, Bertram B, et al. Hemodilution therapy in central retinal vein occlusion. One-year results of a prospective randomized study. *Graefes Arch Clin Exp Ophthalmol.* 1994;232(1):33–39.

17. The Central Vein Occlusion Study Group M Report. Evaluation of grid pattern photocoagulation for macular edema in central vein occlusion. *Ophthalmology.* 1995;102(10):1425–1433.

18. The Central Vein Occlusion Study Group N Report. A randomized clinical trial of early panretinal photocoagulation for ischemic central vein occlusion. *Ophthalmology.* 1995;102(10):1434–1444.

19. Greenberg PB, Martidis A, Rogers AH, et al. Intravitreal triamcinolone acetonide for macular oedema due to central retinal vein occlusion. *Br J Ophthalmol.* 2002;86(2):247–248.

20. Jonas JB, Kreissig I, Degenring RF. Intravitreal triamcinolone acetonide as treatment of macular edema in central retinal vein occlusion. *Graefes Arch Clin Exp Ophthalmol.* 2002; 240(9):782–783.

21. Degenring RF, Kamppeter B, Kreissig I, et al. Morphological and functional changes after intravitreal triamcinolone acetonide for retinal vein occlusion. *Acta Ophthalmol Scand.* 2003;81(4):399–401.

22. Park CH, Jaffe GJ, Fekrat S. Intravitreal triamcinolone acetonide in eyes with cystoid macular edema associated with central retinal vein occlusion. *Am J Ophthalmol.* 2003; 136(3):419–425.

23. Ip MS, Gottlieb JL, Kahana A, et al. Intravitreal triamcinolone for the treatment of macular edema associated with central retinal vein occlusion. *Arch Ophthalmol.* 2004;122(8):1131–1136.

24. Williamson TH, O'Donnell A. Intravitreal triamcinolone acetonide for cystoid macular edema in nonischemic central retinal vein occlusion. *Am J Ophthalmol.* 2005;139(5):860–866.

25. Krepler K, Ergun E, Sacu S, et al. Intravitreal triamcinolone acetonide in patients with macular oedema due to central retinal vein occlusion. *Acta Ophthalmol Scand.* 2005;83(1):71–75.

26. Flynn HW Jr, Scott IU. Intravitreal triamcinolone acetonide for macular edema associated with diabetic retinopathy and venous occlusive disease: It's time for clinical trials. *Arch Ophthalmol.* 2005;123(2):258–259.

27. Soto-Pedre E, Hernaez-Ortega MC. Intravitreal triamcinolone acetonide in eyes with cystoid macular edema associated with central retinal vein occlusion. *Am J Ophthalmol.* 2004; 137(3):596; author reply 596–7.

28. Lee WF, Yang CM. Intravitreal triamcinolone injection for macular edema secondary to increased retinal vascular permeability. *J Formos Med Assoc.* 2004;103(9):692–700.

29. Kwong YY, Lai WW, Lam DS. Intravitreal triamcinolone acetonide in eyes with cystoid macular edema associated with central retinal vein occlusion. *Am J Ophthalmol.* 2004;137(3):593–594; author reply 594.

30. Bashshur ZF, Ma'luf RN, Allam S, et al. Intravitreal triamcinolone for the management of macular edema due to nonischemic central retinal vein occlusion. *Arch Ophthalmol.* 2004;122(8):1137–1140.

31. Kaushik S, Gupta V, Gupta A, et al. Intractable glaucoma following intravitreal triamcinolone in central retinal vein occlusion. *Am J Ophthalmol.* 2004;137(4):758–760.

32. Scott IU, Ip MS. It's time for a clinical trial to investigate intravitreal triamcinolone for macular edema due to retinal vein occlusion: The SCORE study. *Arch Ophthalmol.* 2005; 123(4):581–582.

33. (NEI), N.E.I. The standard care vs. Corticosteroid for retinal vein occlusion (SCORE) Study: Two randomized trials to compare the efficacy and safety of intravitreal injection(s) of triamcinolone acetonide with standard care to treat macular edema. 2005.

34. Jaffe GJ, Ben-Num J, Guo H, et al. Fluocinolone acetonide sustained drug delivery device to treat severe uveitis. *Ophthalmology.* 2000;107(11):2024–2033.

35. Holekamp NM, Thomas MA, Pearson A. The safety profile of long-term, high-dose intraocular corticosteroid delivery. *Am J Ophthalmol.* 2005;139(3):421–428.

36. Jaffe GJ, Yang CH, Guo H, et al. Safety and pharmacokinetics of an intraocular fluocinolone acetonide sustained delivery device. *Invest Ophthalmol Vis Sci.* 2000;41(11):3569–3575.

37. Perkins SL, Gallemore RP, Yang CH, et al. Pharmacokinetics of the fluocinolone/5-fluorouracil codrug in the gas-filled eye. *Retina.* 2000;20(5):514–519.

38. Fekrat S, de Juan E Jr. Chorioretinal venous anastomosis for central retinal vein occlusion: Transvitreal venipuncture. *Ophthalmic Surg Lasers.* 1999;30(1):52–55.

39. McAllister IL, Douglas JP, Constable IJ, Constable IJ. Laser-induced chorioretinal venous

anastomosis for treatment of nonischemic central retinal vein occlusion. *Arch Ophthalmol.* 1995;113(4):456–462.

40. McAllister IL, et al. Laser-induced chorioretinal venous anastomosis for nonischemic central retinal vein occlusion: Evaluation of the complications and their risk factors. *Am J Ophthalmol.* 1998;126(2):219–229.

41. Browning DJ, Antoszyk AN. Laser chorioretinal venous anastomosis for nonischemic central retinal vein occlusion. *Ophthalmology.* 1998; 105(4):670–677; discussion 677–9.

42. Fekrat S, Goldberg MF, Finkelstein D. Laser-induced chorioretinal venous anastomosis for nonischemic central or branch retinal vein occlusion. *Arch Ophthalmol.* 1998;116(1): 43–52.

43. Leonard BC, Coupland SG, Kertes PJ, et al. Long-term follow-up of a modified technique for laser-induced chorioretinal venous anastomosis in nonischemic central retinal vein occlusion. *Ophthalmology.* 2003;110(5):948–954; discussion 955.

44. Hikichi T, Konno S, Trempe CL. Role of the vitreous in central retinal vein occlusion. *Retina.* 1995;15(1):29–33.

45. Mandelcorn MS, Nrusimhadevara RK. Internal limiting membrane peeling for decompression of macular edema in retinal vein occlusion: A report of 14 cases. *Retina.* 2004;24(3): 348–355.

46. Sekiryu T, Yamauchi T, Enaida H, et al. Retina tomography after vitrectomy for macular edema of central retinal vein occlusion. *Ophthalmic Surg Lasers.* 2000;31(3):198–202.

47. Yeshaya A, Treister G. Pars plana vitrectomy for vitreous hemorrhage and retinal vein occlusion. *Ann Ophthalmol.* 1983;15(7):615–617.

48. Stefaniotou M, Paschides CA, Psilas K. Panretinal cryopexy for the management of neovascularization of the iris. *Ophthalmologica.* 1995;209(3):141–144.

49. Elman MJ. Thrombolytic therapy for central retinal vein occlusion: Results of a pilot study. *Trans Am Ophthalmol Soc.* 1996;94: 471–504.

50. Hattenbach LO, Steinkamp G, Scharrer I, et al. Fibrinolytic therapy with low-dose recombinant tissue plasminogen activator in retinal vein occlusion. *Ophthalmologica.* 1998;212(6): 394–398.

51. Lahey JM, Fong DS, Kearney J. Intravitreal tissue plasminogen activator for acute central retinal vein occlusion. *Ophthalmic Surg Lasers.* 1999;30(6):427–434.

52. Hattenbach LO, Wellermann G, Steinkamp GM, et al. Visual outcome after treatment with low-dose recombinant tissue plasminogen activator or hemodilution in ischemic central retinal vein occlusion. *Ophthalmologica.* 1999;213(6):360–366.

53. Elman MJ, Raden RZ, Carrigan A. Intravitreal injection of tissue plasminogen activator for central retinal vein occlusion. *Trans Am Ophthalmol Soc.* 2001;99:219–221; discussion 222–3.

54. Glacet-Bernard A, Kuhn D, Vine AK, et al. Treatment of recent onset central retinal vein occlusion with intravitreal tissue plasminogen activator: A pilot study. *Br J Ophthalmol.* 2000;84(6):609–613.

55. Ghazi NG, Noureddine B, Haddad RS, et al. Intravitreal tissue plasminogen activator in the management of central retinal vein occlusion. *Retina.* 2003;23(6):780–784.

56. Weiss JN. Treatment of central retinal vein occlusion by injection of tissue plasminogen activator into a retinal vein. *Am J Ophthalmol.* 1998;126(1):142–144.

57. Weizer JS, Fekrat S. Intravitreal tissue plasminogen activator for the treatment of central retinal vein occlusion. *Ophthalmic Surg Lasers Imaging.* 2003;34(4):350–352.

58. Bynoe LA, Weiss JN. Retinal endovascular surgery and intravitreal triamcinolone acetonide for central vein occlusion in young adults. *Am J Ophthalmol.* 2003;135(3):382–384.

59. Vinores SA. Technology evaluation: Pegaptanib, Eyetech/Pfizer. *Curr Opin Mol Ther.* 2003;5(6):673–679.

60. Rosenfeld PJ, Fung AE, Puliafito CA. Optical coherence tomography findings after an intravitreal injection of bevacizumab (Avastin®) for macular edema from central retinal vein occlusion. *Ophthalmic Surg Lasers Imaging.* 2005; 36(4):336–339.

61. Vasco-Posada J. Modification of the circulation in the posterior pole of the eye. *Ann Ophthalmol.* 1972;4(1):48–59.

62. Dev S, Buckley EG. Optic nerve sheath decompression for progressive central retinal vein occlusion. *Ophthalmic Surg Lasers.* 1999; 30(3):181–184.

63. Arciniegas A. Treatment of the occlusion of the central retinal vein by section of the posterior ring. *Ann Ophthalmol.* 1984;16(11):1081–1086.

64. Lee SY, Shin DH, Spoor TC, et al. Bilateral retinal venous caliber decrease following unilateral optic nerve sheath decompression. *Ophthalmic Surg.* 1995;26(1):25–28.

65. Opremcak EM, Bruce RA, Lomeo MD, et al. Radial optic neurotomy for central retinal vein occlusion: A retrospective pilot study of 11 consecutive cases. *Retina.* 2001;21(5):408–415.

66. Weizer JS, Stinnett SS, Fekrat S. Radial optic neurotomy as treatment for central retinal vein occlusion. *Am J Ophthalmol.* 2003;136(5): 814–819.

67. Garcia-Arumii J, Boixadera A, Martinez-Castillo V, et al. Chorioretinal anastomosis after radial optic neurotomy for central retinal vein occlusion. *Arch Ophthalmol.* 2003;121(10):1385–1391.

68. Nomoto H, Shiraga F, Yamaji H, et al. Evaluation of radial optic neurotomy for central retinal vein occlusion by indocyanine green videoangiography and image analysis. *Am J Ophthalmol.* 2004; 138(4):612–619.

69. Hayreh SS. Radial optic neurotomy for non-ischemic central retinal vein occlusion. *Arch Ophthalmol.* 2004;122(10):1572–1573.

70. Samuel MA, Desai UR, Gandolfo CB. Peri-papillary retinal detachment after radial optic neurotomy for central retinal vein occlusion. *Retina.* 2003;23(4):580–583.

71. Shukla D. Radial optic neurotomy as treatment for central retinal vein occlusion. *Am J Ophthalmol.* 2004;137(6):1161; author reply 1161–2.

72. Czajka MP, Cummings TJ, McCuen BW, et al. Radial optic neurotomy in the porcine eye without retinal vein occlusion. *Arch Ophthalmol.* 2004;122(8):1185–1189.

Treatment of Branch Retinal Vein Occlusion: Lessons from Clinical Trials

Henry Tseng, MD, PhD and Sharon Fekrat, MD

A branch retinal vein occlusion (BRVO) results from a blockage of blood flow in a branch of the central retinal vein. This blockage typically occurs where the branch vein crosses over a branch of the central retinal artery, resulting in visual loss secondary to the accumulation of fluid in the retina (macular edema) and blood (intraretinal hemorrhage), particularly in the fovea (foveal hemorrhage). Secondary neovascular complications can lead to vitreous hemorrhage and traction retinal detachment.

The mechanism of a BRVO is multifactorial and is suggested by the associated risk factors. Although BRVO occurs equally in males and females between the ages of 60 and 70, the risk of developing a BRVO is increased with systemic arterial disease, such as hypertension, diabetes, hyperlipidemia, atherosclerosis, increased body mass index, and smoking.[1] Actual thrombus formation at the point of venous occlusion has also been reported.[2]

The majority of current treatment options focus on treating sequelae of the occluded venous branch, such as macular edema[3] and vitreous hemorrhage or traction retinal detachment from neovascularization.[4] Visual loss persists in approximately two-thirds of eyes without treatment.[3] Visual gain is minimal even with laser treatment. More effective treatment options are necessary to improve visual outcome.

Diagnosis and Classification of BRVO

An eye with a BRVO usually displays characteristic ophthalmoscopic findings.[5] Extending from an arteriovenous crossing in a triangular, wedge-shaped distribution, variable amounts of superficial and deep intraretinal hemorrhages are seen, with some in the foveal center, depending on the branch retinal vein involved. This is often accompanied by venous tortuosity and dilation, retinal edema, and cotton-wool spots. A BRVO that affects visual acuity (VA) is almost always associated with macular edema, a common complication that can cause permanently decreased VA.[3] Some eyes with chronic macular edema may develop subfoveal retinal pigment epithelial hyper- or hypopigmentation. Sclerosis and sheathing of the retinal vasculature in the distribution of the occlusion may also be seen with time. Optic disc or retinal neovascularization may occur and may be associated with preretinal or vitreous hemorrhage, and/or traction retinal detachment.[4]

The diagnosis of a BRVO is usually straightforward unless there are several BRVOs in one eye, the affected segment is small, or if another retinal vascular disease (such as diabetic retinopathy) coexists. The diagnosis may also be challenging if the BRVO has been present for >6 months because the intraretinal hemorrhage may have been reabsorbed, leaving retinal vascular abnormalities, such as capillary dilation, capillary nonperfusion, microaneurysms, and collateral vessel formation as the only clues to indicate a BRVO. In these cases, fluorescein angiography may facilitate the diagnosis by delineating the segmental retinal capillary abnormalities better.

It may be useful to determine whether the BRVO is *perfused (nonischemic)* or *nonperfused (ischemic)* by fluorescein angiography. If capillary nonperfusion in the affected distribution occupies a retinal area whose greater linear dimension is *less* than five disc diameters on fluorescein angiography, the occlusion is classified as perfused (nonischemic).[4] If capillary nonperfusion in the affected distribution occupies a retinal area whose greatest linear dimension is five or *more* disc diameters on fluorescein angiography, the occlusion is classified as nonperfused (ischemic).[4]

Angiographic identification of retinal capillary nonperfusion may not be feasible in eyes with a significant amount of intraretinal hemorrhage, since the hemorrhage may block underlying patches of retinal capillary nonperfusion throughout the affected distribution and the fluorescein outline of the parafoveal vascular network. As a result, fluorescein angiography may not be very useful to determine perfusion status until the hemorrhage reabsorbs sufficiently to permit visualization of the underlying capillary architecture. Intraretinal hemorrhages may take months to resolve in some eyes.

Natural History

A BRVO is three times more common than a central retinal vein occlusion (CRVO) and second only to diabetic retinopathy as the most common retinal vascular cause of visual loss.[3,4,6] In a report on the use of eye care services based on the 1991 claims from a representative 5% sample of Medicare beneficiaries, the case incidence of all venous occlusive disease (both BRVO and CRVO) was about 75,000, which led to almost 150,000 visits to an ophthalmologist.[7] The natural history of eyes with a BRVO had not been documented until the Branch Vein Occlusion Study (BVOS). This was a multicenter, prospective, randomized controlled trial (RCT) for the treatment

of BRVO sequelae sponsored by the National Eye Institute.[3] The BVOS was originally designed to study patients from 1977 to 1984 to determine whether peripheral argon laser photocoagulation can prevent the development of neovascularization and/or vitreous hemorrhage, and whether grid-pattern laser photocoagulation can improve VA in eyes with macular edema.

In the BVOS, eyes with a BRVO were placed into four groups (see Fig. 8B.1). Group I eyes had a BRVO without neovascularization, but had involvement of an area that is at least five disc diameters, which presumably places these eyes at high risk for developing neovascularization. Eyes in this group were randomized to no laser treatment or sector panretinal photocoagulation (PRP) to determine whether PRP treatment prevented the development of neovascularization. Group II eyes had a BRVO with neovascularization on the disc or within one-disc diameter of the disc and were at risk for the development of vitreous hemorrhage. The eyes were randomized to sector PRP or no laser treatment to determine whether PRP could prevent vitreous hemorrhage. Group III eyes had a BRVO with macular edema and reduced vision to 20/40 or less. Randomization of group III eyes to no laser treatment or grid-pattern laser photocoagulation was designed to determine if such treatment can improve the VA in these eyes. Finally, the inclusion criteria of Group X eyes are similar to Group I eyes. However, these eyes were recruited only after Group I recruitment was closed and were followed up primarily for natural history information.

It is difficult to determine the natural history of eyes with a BRVO precisely from the BVOS. All eyes with BRVO for 3 to 18 months before entry into

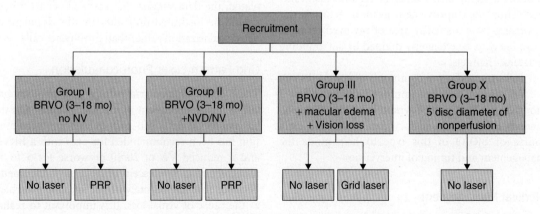

FIGURE 8B.1 ■ Randomization schema of the Branch Vein Occlusion Study. BRVO, branch retinal vein occlusion; PRP, panretinal photocoagulation; NV, neovascularization; NVD, neovascularization of the disc.

the study were grouped together. It is not possible to obtain adequate natural history information from such a variable duration of BRVO before entry into the study. Moreover, no patient was entered into the BVOS until 3 months after the occlusion because of a clinical impression that spontaneous improvement occurred often during that period. The change in VA and natural history of untreated BRVO eyes from the onset until 3 months after the occlusion cannot be extracted from the BVOS. Also, only eyes with perfused macular edema were evaluated in the BVOS (group III). Groups I, II, and X were not utilized to study the natural history or effect of laser photocoagulation on macular edema.

Spontaneous VA improvement in BRVO eyes has been reported in smaller studies.[8,9] For example, in a retrospective study, Finkelstein found that in 23 untreated BRVO eyes with macular capillary nonperfusion and macular edema, there was a greater likelihood of spontaneous improvement than in untreated eyes with intact macular capillaries.[8] In fact, 91% of BRVO eyes with nonperfused macular edema improved without treatment as compared to 29% with perfused macular edema. The time to best VA ranged from 3 to 64 months (median, 14 months). Median initial VA was 20/80, and median final VA was 20/30.

In a 1999 report by Battaglia-Parodi et al. all 99 eyes with a *macular* BRVO of <2 weeks duration upon entry into the study had statistically significant spontaneous improvement in mean logMAR (logarithm of the inverse of the Snellen fraction) VA values at 3 months as compared with the baseline.[10] However, only macular BRVO, a subgroup of BRVO in which the occlusion is limited to a small vessel draining a sector of the macular region, was evaluated. Thus, the improvement in mean acuity is not surprising since a smaller area of involved retina is more likely to be efficiently drained by surrounding collateral channels.

In larger and more commonly observed BRVO, the VA may or may not improve within the first 3 months after the onset of symptoms. Unfortunately, there is little natural history data about the early course of BRVO of this type to help guide the management and timing of intervention.

Medical Management

Currently, there is no proven medical treatment for an eye with BRVO. The use of systemic anticoagulation may result in adverse effects, such as increased intraretinal hemorrhage and systemic bleeding sequelae, and is therefore not recommended for this indication alone.[11] The utility of troxerutin in BRVO has been investigated but awaits more formal evaluation with a large-scale trial.[11,12]

Scatter Argon Laser Photocoagulation

The data from both BVOS groups I and II demonstrated that scatter laser photocoagulation in the affected distribution effectively reduces the development of retinal neovascularization and vitreous hemorrhage when compared to eyes in the untreated group. In group I, it was found that 35 of 159 untreated eyes (22%) developed retinal neovascularization when compared to 19 of 160 treated eyes (12%). In group II, 29% of 41 treated eyes developed a vitreous hemorrhage as compared to 61% of 41 untreated eyes. Thus it was concluded that scatter laser effectively decreases the likelihood of developing neovascularization and/or vitreous hemorrhage.[3,4]

Should scatter laser be performed before or after the development of neovascularization in ischemic eyes? While the BVOS did not directly address this question, data from both groups I and II suggest a trend. Of the 19 laser-treated eyes in group I that later developed retinal neovascularization, 12 (63%) developed vitreous hemorrhage. In group II, 31% of the untreated eyes developed neovascularization, whereas 29% of the treated eyes developed vitreous hemorrhage. This suggests that 31% of the 29% (9%) of patients who were treated only after the development of neovascularization can expect to develop vitreous hemorrhage (vs. 63% seen in group I).[4] The results are summarized in Table 8B.1. When extrapolated, the data suggest that scatter laser treatment should be instituted only after the development of neovascularization rather than prophylactically.

Grid-Pattern Laser Photocoagulation

The BVOS evaluated grid-pattern laser photocoagulation for the treatment of macular edema.[3] On the basis of BVOS data, grid-pattern laser photocoagulation has been recommended for eyes with a BRVO and a reduced VA of 20/40 or worse for 3 to 18 months and if fluorescein angiography documents perfused macular edema without foveal hemorrhage as the cause of visual loss. It is important to realize that the eyes in the BVOS were not rigorously divided into categories of macular perfusion (i.e., perfused

TABLE 8B.1 □ BVOS Results: Reduction in the Development of Retinal Neovascularization and Vitreous Hemorrhages with Panretinal Photocoagulation

		No. of Patients Who Developed Neovascularization (%)	No. of Patients Who Developed Vitreous Hemorrhage (%)
Group I	Treated	19/160 (12)	12 of 19 with NV (63)
	Untreated	35/159 (22)	
Group II	Treated		12/41(29)
	Untreated		25/41 (61)

NV, neovascularization.

vs. nonperfused macular edema) because the quality of the fluorescein angiograms was generally not high enough.[13] However, patients with "distinct" areas of capillary nonperfusion in the macula were excluded. Although the BVOS is the largest randomized trial evaluating laser treatment for macular edema, 139 eyes were enrolled in the macular edema arm, 71 treated and 68 not treated; however, the reported 3-year data were only from 78 eyes, 43 treated and 35 not treated.[3] These small numbers and lack of precise angiographic differentiation of macular edema make the results more difficult to interpret.

Nevertheless, the BVOS demonstrated a benefit of grid-pattern laser photocoagulation treatment for macular edema that met the criteria defined in the preceding text (results summarized in Table 8B.2).[3] At 3 years, 65% of 43 treated individuals gained at least two lines of vision as compared to 37% of the 35 eyes in the untreated, control group. A higher percentage of treated eyes had a VA of 20/40 or better at 3 years (60% vs. 34%). The mean number of lines of vision gained was 1.33 in the treated group and 0.23 in the control group at 3 years. While the improved outcome of treated eyes was statistically significant,

it offers little hope to those with poor acuity. A 1.33 line improvement in a patient with 20/100 or worse VA does not provide vision that meets the legal driving limit in that eye in most states in the United States, which typically requires around 20/40 vision to obtain an unrestricted license. These results indicate that the natural course of this retinal vascular disease is relatively static at 3 years with only an average 0.23 line improvement in untreated eyes. Since eyes with foveal hemorrhage or macular nonperfusion were excluded from the BVOS, currently there is no recommended treatment for these subgroups.

VA improvement in BRVO eyes after grid-pattern laser photocoagulation has also been reported elsewhere. In a small, retrospective, uncontrolled study, 11 of 12 eyes with macular edema from BRVO had improved VA after grid-pattern laser photocoagulation treatment administered per the BVOS guidelines, and all of the 12 eyes had improvement or disappearance of the macular edema.[14] VA measurements were not standardized or masked. The angiographic type of macular edema was not mentioned nor was concurrent foveal hemorrhage noted.

TABLE 8B.2 □ Summary of BVOS Results on the Effect of Grid-Pattern Laser Photocoagulation on the Treatment of Macular Edema at the 3-year Follow-up Visit

	Control (n = 35 eyes) (%)	Treated (n = 43 eyes) (%)	p value
Gained at least 2 lines	37	65	$p = 0.014$
VA of 20/40 or better	34	60	$p = 0.021$
Average number of lines gained	0.23	1.33	$p < 0.0001$
Average VA	20/70	20/40–20/50	$p < 0.0001$

VA, visual acuity.

Some studies have suggested that grid-pattern laser photocoagulation may *not* be effective in improving VA in eyes with BRVO. In another study by Parodi et al., 99 eyes with a macular BRVO and equivalent numbers of both nonischemic and ischemic macular edema in all groups were prospectively studied.[15] Eyes were randomized to observation or laser treatment (early at 3 months or later at 6 to 18 months). No statistically significant difference was found in VA or the reduction of angiographic leakage between the treated and control groups. Similarly, Shilling and Jones demonstrated that eyes receiving grid-pattern laser photocoagulation did not have vision that was significantly better than that of untreated eyes, even though the macular edema decreased in treated eyes.[16] Shilling and Jones evaluated two groups of eyes with a BRVO.[16] One group consisted of 22 eyes with a BRVO of 3 months duration or less and nonperfused macular edema (13 eyes received grid-pattern laser treatment to areas of angiographic capillary leakage at 3 months and 9 eyes were untreated). Treated eyes did not have VA that was significantly better than that of untreated eyes at both the 1- and 2-year follow-up visits. The second group consisted of 25 eyes with a BRVO >1 year in duration (15 eyes that received grid-pattern laser photocoagulation treatment and 10 that did not). Treated eyes did not have VA that was significantly better than that of untreated eyes. Within the treated and untreated groups, those with perfused macular edema had a significantly better visual prognosis than those with macular nonperfusion.

Finally, Barbazetto and Schmidt-Erfurth evaluated functional defects in BRVO before and after grid-pattern laser photocoagulation treatment per the BVOS using scanning laser perimetry (see Figs. 8B.2 and 8B.3).[17] Of 39 treated eyes with BRVO, the central scotoma remained unchanged or encroached on foveal fixation in 67% of eyes. In addition, the total scotoma size increased in 50% of eyes after laser treatment. Treated eyes had worse mean VA 3 months after laser treatment as compared to untreated eyes, although the numbers were small.

Although the BVOS showed that laser photocoagulation in perfused macular edema may be beneficial, it is important to keep in mind that the number of study eyes in the BVOS was small, and the improvement in VA was also small. A recent study reported that multiple grid-pattern laser photocoagulation treatments might be needed to see a significant improvement in macular edema or VA.[18] Furthermore, conflicting data regarding grid-pattern laser photocoagulation treatment have been reported by other studies. It is therefore important to reevaluate conventional grid-pattern laser treatment and to consider novel treatment modalities for macular edema in eyes with BRVO.

Intravitreal Triamcinolone Acetonide

Intravitreal triamcinolone (Kenalog, Bristol-Myer Squibb) has been documented in numerous recent studies to improve macular edema and VA in eyes with a BRVO; however, these studies are preliminary and involve small numbers of eyes.[19–25] Furthermore, the effect of intravitreal triamcinolone is transient, and its use may lead to steroid-induced cataract

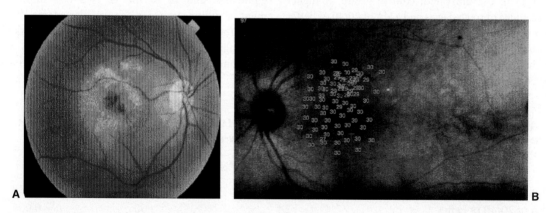

FIGURE 8B.2 □ A branch retinal vein occlusion eye with significant macular edema **(A)** reflecting a small central scotoma as detected by scanning laser perimetry **(B)**. Red numbers on the perimetry overlaid on the photograph result indicate decreased sensitivity to the projected stimuli. (From Barbazetto IA, Schmidt-Erfurth UM. Evaluation of functional defects in branch retinal vein occlusion before and after laser treatment with scanning laser perimetry. *Ophthalmology.* 2000;107(6):1089–1098.)

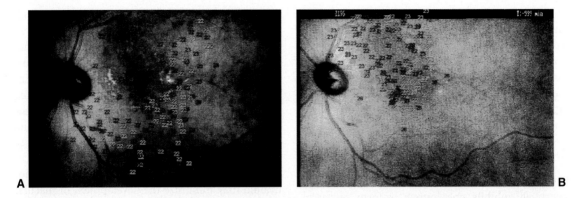

FIGURE 8B.3 ◻ Microperimetry of a branch retinal vein occlusion eye with macular edema before **(A)** and after **(B)** treatment with grid-pattern laser photocoagulation. The laser treatment resulted in the decrease of macular edema and an improvement in microperimetry sensitivity. (From Barbazetto IA, Schmidt-Erfurth UM. Evaluation of functional defects in branch retinal vein occlusion before and after laser treatment with scanning laser perimetry *Ophthalmology.* 2000;107(6):1089–1098.)

formation and steroid-induced intraocular pressure (IOP) elevation. There is currently a multicenter, RCT in progress called the Standard of Care versus Corticosteroid for Retinal Vein Occlusion (SCORE) Study.[26] The SCORE study will randomize eyes with macular edema secondary to BRVO into three treatment groups (see Fig. 8B.4). One group will receive the standard of care (observation or grid-pattern laser photocoagulation per the BVOS criteria), a second group will receive 4 mg of intravitreal triamcinolone, and a third group will receive 1 mg of intravitreal triamcinolone. In total, these groups will be followed up for 36 months. The primary efficacy will be measured by an improvement of 15 or more letters in VA at the 12-month visit. The SCORE study will evaluate the safety profile of triamcinolone by monitoring cataract formation, IOP changes, and injection-related events such as endophthalmitis, vitreous hemorrhage, and retinal detachment. Enrollment for the SCORE study is still ongoing.

Sustained Drug Release Devices

Intraocular devices that provide sustained release of medication have been used in several posterior segment diseases. Proposed advantages include constant drug levels and duration of treatment tailored to the appropriate disease. Two such devices, the fluocinolone acetonide implant (Retisert)[27] and dexamethasone implant (Posurdex),[28] have been used to treat diabetic macular edema. Retisert is currently being evaluated in eyes with retinal vein occlusion.

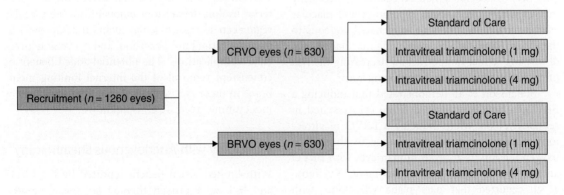

FIGURE 8B.4 ◻ Randomization schema for the Standard of Care versus Corticosteroid for Retinal Vein Occlusion (SCORE) study. CRVO, central retinal vein occlusion; BRVO, branch retinal vein occlusion.

Retisert is nonbiodegradable and is secured intravitreally with a scleral suture. The device is designed to release 0.5 μg of fluocinolone per day for 3 years. Adverse effects, such as increased IOP and cataract progression, were seen in eyes that received the implant. Most patients with elevated IOP were satisfactorily treated with drops. Eight eyes required trabeculectomy. The study is currently ongoing.

Antivascular Endothelial Growth Factor Agents

Pegaptanib sodium (Macugen) is an aptamer that selectively inhibits one human isoform of vascular endothelial growth factor (VEGF)[29] and has been recently approved by the U.S. Food and Drug Administration (FDA) for the treatment of choroidal neovascularization in eyes with age-related macular degeneration. Macugen itself is associated with few adverse effects; however, the intravitreal injection itself may rarely result in endophthalmitis or retinal detachment. Another anti-VEGF agent is bevacizumab (Avastin), which has not yet received FDA approval for use in the eye. These agents are currently being investigated as possible treatments for BRVO-related macular edema.

Pars Plana Vitrectomy

An increased risk of BRVO formation is present in eyes with decreased axial length and hyperopia,[30–33] possibly because of a higher likelihood of vitreomacular attachment or vitreous compression in these shorter eyes. An attached hyaloid may similarly compress a susceptible arteriovenous crossing, resulting in BRVO formation in addition to or irrespective of the adventitial sheath. Eyes with vitreomacular separation may be less likely to develop a BRVO or have BRVO-associated macular edema.[34] Vitrectomy in eyes with vitreomacular separation and macular edema may allow access of oxygenated aqueous to the inner retina, thereby improving macular edema, decreasing retinal nonperfusion, decreasing the risk of neovascularization, and improving VA.[28]

Stefansson et al. demonstrated that inducing a BRVO in nonvitrectomized feline eyes resulted in retinal hypoxia, while inducing a BRVO in vitrectomized eyes produced no change in the retinal oxygen tension.[35] In seven human eyes with BRVO and no posterior vitreous detachment, Kurimoto et al. reported that pars plana vitrectomy with intraoperative posterior hyaloid separation/removal

improved VA and decreased macular edema, both angiographically and by retinal thickness analysis in seven eyes 1-month postoperatively.[36] In another series of 16 eyes with nonperfused macular edema from BRVO, vitrectomy with intraoperative detachment and removal of the hyaloid resulted in improved VA in 12 of 16 eyes (75%) and no change in the remaining 4.[37] In these eyes, there was new vessel and collateral vessel growth in the previously nonperfused areas postoperatively.

Recent data also suggest that a detached posterior hyaloid may minimize the development of macular edema in eyes with a BRVO. Studies by Avunduk et al. [38] and Takahashi et al. [39] demonstrated that eyes with BRVO and separation of the vitreous from the macula had a significantly lower rate of macular edema. Takahashi et al. further suggested that the status of the vitreomacular interface might affect macular edema associated with BRVO. Of 58 eyes that were retrospectively studied, the incidence of macular edema was significantly lower in eyes with vitreomacular separation (41%) than vitreomacular attachment (93%).[39]

However, eyes with vitreomacular separation may still develop cystoid macular edema.[39] In these cases, the remaining vitreous, although detached from the retinal surface, may prevent access of oxygenated aqueous to the deprived inner retinal surface.[28] Trempe et al. reported no significant correlation between the status of the hyaloid (separated in only 8 of 28 eyes with macular edema) and the development of macular edema, despite acknowledging that the vitreous may have influenced the evolution of BRVO in 50 eyes with BRVO when compared to age-matched controls.[40] The number of eyes in this study was too small for definitive conclusions.

These studies suggest that vitrectomy and posterior hyaloid separation/removal from the macular region can decrease macular edema and improve VA, improve retinal nonperfusion, and decrease neovascular complications. The potential added benefit of concurrent removal of the internal limiting membrane in these eyes with or without the assistance of indocyanine green (ICG) is unknown.

Vitrectomy with Arteriovenous Sheathotomy

With limited visual benefit reported by the BVOS and lack of a proven therapy for the remaining eyes with BVO, there has been widespread interest in developing alternative therapeutic approaches to the current standard of care to improve vision and prevent visual loss from BVO. Pars plana vitrectomy and posterior hyaloid separation/removal with sectioning of the adventitial sheath (sheathotomy) at the etiologic arteriovenous crossing has been performed as a treatment for BRVO. Preliminary studies have been reported in the ophthalmologic literature demonstrating[41–51] that vitrectomy with sheathotomy can result in retinal reperfusion, decreased macular edema, and visual improvement with a favorable safety profile.

The rationale behind this procedure is the surgical restoration of venous outflow by sectioning the adventitial sheath at the etiologic arteriovenous intersection with separation of the artery from the vein. If a thrombus is not present, is small, or has not yet formed,[2] theoretically, this procedure should improve venous outflow and lead to improved VA by lessening macular edema. Moreover, it may prevent conversion of a perfused BRVO to a nonperfused BRVO, reperfuse previously closed vasculature in the affected distribution,[37,44] and decrease the risk of neovascularization and its associated complications.[37]

Osterloh and Charles initially reported significant visual improvement after sheathotomy in a 54-year-old woman with a 3-week history of a BRVO.[43] The perfusion status of the vein occlusion, status of the posterior hyaloid, and amount of macular edema was not indicated. Preoperatively, the VA was 20/200, and this gradually improved to 20/40 by 3 months and 20/25 by 8 months postoperatively. No changes were noted in the caliber of the affected vein intraoperatively. At 8 months, intraretinal hemorrhages had reabsorbed, which may also be due to the natural history of the BRVO alone.

In a prospective, nonrandomized series, Oprem-cak and Bruce reported equal or improved VA in 12 of 15 eyes (80%).[41] Ten (67%) eyes had improved postoperative visual acuities, with a mean gain of four lines. Three eyes had a mean decline in acuity of two lines. VA examiners in this small series were not masked to treatment, potentially biasing the results. All eyes had marked resolution of intraretinal hemorrhage and edema over a mean follow-up of 5 months. The duration of visual symptoms ranged from 1 to 12 months, with a mean of 3.3 months.

Improvement in VA has been reported in other smaller studies. In a retrospective study of 13 eyes undergoing arteriovenous sheathotomy, Brantley reported visual improvement in 7 (54%) of 13 eyes of one or more lines, with a mean of four lines, after a mean follow-up of 8 months.[52] Shah et al. reported four of five eyes with visual improvement after arteriovenous sheathotomy in another retrospective, uncontrolled series.[42] All five had a preoperative VA of 20/200 or worse, which improved to 20/30 to 20/70 over a mean follow-up of 6.5 years in four eyes. In a prospective, uncontrolled study, Mester and Dillinger reported improved VA in all 12 eyes following sheathotomy and 25% of eyes gained >4 lines in the few weeks postoperatively.[53] The perfusion status of the BRVO was not disclosed.

Arteriovenous sheathotomy has been compared to grid-pattern laser photocoagulation. Five of 14 (36%) eyes that underwent sheathotomy in a retrospective case–control study of 24 eyes, and 6 of 14 (43%) eyes that underwent grid-pattern laser photocoagulation improved two or more lines ($p = 1.00$) at a mean follow-up of 7.8 months.[46] There were no intraoperative complications. There was progression of nuclear sclerotic cataract in 50% of those eyes that underwent sheathotomy and this was not observed in those eyes that received laser. The cataract may have lessened any beneficial effect on VA from the sheathotomy procedure in this series.

The application of recombinant tissue plasminogen activator (rt-PA) at the venous occlusion site following sheathotomy has also been used to achieve additional fibrinolysis during arteriovenous sheathotomy. A recent study by Garcia-Arumi et al. demonstrated that sheathotomy with intraoperative rt-PA dripped onto the crossing site resulted in a 40% postoperative reduction in macular thickness in 31 of 40 eyes. VA also increased by three or more lines in 70% of treated eyes.[54]

Visual improvement following sheathotomy may not be the direct result of intervention. VA may improve because of the natural history, or perhaps the visual improvement is the direct result of the vitrectomy alone and *not* the sheathotomy portion of the procedure. Moreover, if indeed a thrombus is present in the branch vein at the etiologic arteriovenous crossing,[55,56] relieving the obstruction may not remove the organized thrombus, rendering the sheathotomy portion of the surgery ineffective in some cases. Thus, if arteriovenous sheathotomy is to be effective in eyes with an organized thrombus at the crossing, the procedure may have to be performed early in the course of the BRVO for a better chance of visual improvement. Which eyes form an organized thrombus and which do not, cannot currently be predicted preoperatively.

Conclusion

Visual loss from a BRVO varies and is usually due to macular edema, macular ischemia, vitreous hemorrhage, and neovascular complications. Spontaneous improvement in VA may occur in some eyes. Treatment for eyes with BRVO remains a challenge for the ophthalmologist. As in CRVO, no effective medical treatment has been developed. Grid-pattern laser photocoagulation remains the only proven treatment for the macular edema. Intravitreal injection of triamcinolone is used to treat BRVO-associated macular edema without significant short- or long-term data and is currently being investigated in the ongoing NEI-sponsored SCORE clinical trial. Anti-VEGF agents are a new venue being explored for these eyes. Pars plana vitrectomy with arteriovenous sheathotomy has been investigated as a surgical approach in many small studies; however, whether its benefits outweigh potential surgical complications has been controversial and remains to be determined. The role of vitrectomy alone in the management of these eyes is still unclear.

References

1. The Eye Disease Case-control Study Group. Risk factors for branch retinal vein occlusion. *Am J Ophthalmol.* 1993;116(3):286–296.
2. Seitz R. *The retinal vessels: Comparative ophthalmoscopic and histologic studies of healthy and diseased eyes.* St. Louis: Mosby; 1964.
3. The Branch Vein Occlusion Study Group. Argon laser photocoagulation for macular edema in branch vein occlusion. *Am J Ophthalmol.* 1984;98(3):271–282.
4. Branch Vein Occlusion Study Group. Argon laser scatter photocoagulation for prevention of neovascularization and vitreous hemorrhage in branch vein occlusion. A randomized clinical trial. *Arch Ophthalmol.* 1986;104(1):34–41.
5. Fekrat SFD. Branch retinal vein occlusion. In: Franunfelder FTHR, ed. *Current ocular therapy,* 5th ed. Philadelphia, PA: WB Sauders; 2000: 600–604.
6. Orth DH, Patz A. Retinal branch vein occlusion. *Surv Ophthalmol.* 1978;22(6):357–376.
7. Ellwein LB, Friedlin V, McBean AM, et al. Use of eye care services among the 1991 medicare population. *Ophthalmology.* 1996;103(11):1732–1743.
8. Finkelstein D. Ischemic macular edema. Recognition and favorable natural history in branch vein occlusion. *Arch Ophthalmol.* 1992;110(10):1427–1434.
9. Clemett RS, Kohner EM, Hamilton AM. The visual prognosis in retinal branch vein occlusion. *Trans Ophthalmol Soc U K.* 1973;93:523–535.
10. Battaglia Parodi M, Saviano S, Ravalico G. Grid laser treatment in macular branch retinal vein occlusion. *Graefes Arch Clin Exp Ophthalmol.* 1999;237(12):1024–1027.
11. Parodi MB. Medical treatment of retinal vein occlusions. *Semin Ophthalmol.* 2004;19(1–2): 43–48.
12. Glacet-Bernard A, Coscas G, Chabanel A, et al. A randomized, double-masked study on the treatment of retinal vein occlusion with troxerutin. *Am J Ophthalmol.* 1994;118(4):421–429.
13. Finkelstein D. Laser treatment of macular edema resulting from branch vein occlusion. *Semin Ophthalmol.* 1994;9(1):23–28.
14. Arnarsson A, Stefansson E. Laser treatment and the mechanism of edema reduction in branch retinal vein occlusion. *Invest Ophthalmol Vis Sci.* 2000;41(3):877–879.
15. Battaglia Parodi M, Saviano S, Bergamini L, et al. Grid laser treatment of macular edema in macular branch retinal vein occlusion. *Doc Ophthalmol.* 1999;97(3–4):427–431.
16. Shilling JS, Jones CA. Retinal branch vein occlusion: A study of argon laser photocoagulation in the treatment of macular oedema. *Br J Ophthalmol.* 1984;68(3):196–198.
17. Barbazetto IA, Schmidt-Erfurth UM. Evaluation of functional defects in branch retinal vein occlusion before and after laser treatment with scanning laser perimetry. *Ophthalmology.* 2000;107(6):1089–1098.
18. Esrick E, Subramanian ML, Heier JS, et al. Multiple laser treatments for macular edema attributable to branch retinal vein occlusion. *Am J Ophthalmol.* 2005;139(4):653–657.
19. Lee H, Shah GK. Intravitreal triamcinolone as primary treatment of cystoid macular edema

secondary to branch retinal vein occlusion. *Retina*. 2005;25(5):551–555.

20. Kaiser PK. Steroids for branch retinal vein occlusion. *Am J Ophthalmol*. 2005;139(6):1095–1096.

21. Hayashi K, Hayashi H. Intravitreal versus retrobulbar injections of triamcinolone for macular edema associated with branch retinal vein occlusion. *Am J Ophthalmol*. 2005;139(6):972–982.

22. Ozkiris A, Evereklioglu C, Erkilic K, et al. The efficacy of intravitreal triamcinolone acetonide on macular edema in branch retinal vein occlusion. *Eur J Ophthalmol*. 2005;15(1):96–101.

23. Ozkiris A, Evereklioglu C, Erkilic K, et al. Intravitreal triamcinolone acetonide for treatment of persistent macular oedema in branch retinal vein occlusion. *Eye*. 2006;20(1):13–17.

24. Yepremyan M, Wertz FD, Tivnan T, et al. Early treatment of cystoid macular edema secondary to branch retinal vein occlusion with intravitreal triamcinolone acetonide. *Ophthalmic Surg Lasers Imaging*. 2005;36(1):30–36.

25. Jonas JB, Akkoyun I, Kamppeter B, et al. Branch retinal vein occlusion treated by intravitreal triamcinolone acetonide. *Eye*. 2005;19(1):65–71.

26. NEI NEI. The Standard Care vs. Corticosteroid for Retinal Vein Occlusion (SCORE) Study: Two Randomized Trials to Compare the Efficacy and Safety of Intravitreal Injection(s) of Triamcinolone Acetonide with Standard Care to Treat Macular Edema. 2005.

27. Adis International Limited. Fluocinolone acetonide ophthalmic--Bausch & Lomb: Fluocinolone acetonide envision TD implant. *Drugs R D*. 2005;6(2):116–119.

28. Bayes M, Rabasseda X, Prous JR. Gateways to clinical trials. *Methods Find Exp Clin Pharmacol*. 2004;26(2):129–161.

29. Vinores SA. Technology evaluation: Pegaptanib, Eyetech/Pfizer. *Curr Opin Mol Ther*. 2003; 5(6):673–679.

30. Goldstein M, Leibovitch I, Varssano D, et al. Axial length, refractive error, and keratometry in patients with branch retinal vein occlusion. *Eur J Ophthalmol*. 2004;14(1):37–39.

31. Majji AB, Janarthanan M, Naduvilath TJ. Significance of refractive status in branch retinal vein occlusion. A case-control study. *Retina*. 1997;17(3):200–204.

32. Bandello F, Tavola A, Pierro L, et al. Axial length and refraction in retinal vein occlusions. *Ophthalmologica*. 1998;212(2):133–135.

33. Timmerman EA, de Lavalette VW, van den Brom HJ. Axial length as a risk factor to branch retinal vein occlusion. *Retina*. 1997;17(3):196–199.

34. Thompson JT. What is the role of vitrectomy for macular edema from branch retinal vein occlusion? *Am J Ophthalmol*. 2004;138(6):1037–1038.

35. Stefansson E, Novack RL, Hatchell DL. Vitrectomy prevents retinal hypoxia in branch retinal vein occlusion. *Invest Ophthalmol Vis Sci*. 1990;31(2):284–289.

36. Kurimoto MTH, Suzuma K, Oh H, et al. Vitrectomy for macular edema secondary to retinal vein occlusion: Evaluation by retinal thickness analyzer. *Jpn J Ophthalmol*. 1999;53:717–720.

37. Ando N. Vitrectomy for ischemic maculopathy associated with retinal vein occlusion. *Vail Vitrectomy Meeting*, Vail, CO; 2000.

38. Avunduk AM, Cetinkaya K, Kapicioglu Z, et al. The effect of posterior vitreous detachment on the prognosis of branch retinal vein occlusion. *Acta Ophthalmol Scand*. 1997;75(4):441–442.

39. Takahashi MK, Hikichi T, Akiba J, Role of the vitreous and macular edema in branch retinal vein occlusion. *Ophthalmic Surg Lasers*. 1997;28(4):294–299.

40. Trempe CL, Takahashi M, Topilow HW. Vitreous changes in retinal branch vein occlusion. *Ophthalmology*. 1981;88(7):681–687.

41. Opremcak EM, Bruce RA. Surgical decompression of branch retinal vein occlusion via arteriovenous crossing sheathotomy: A prospective review of 15 cases. *Retina*. 1999;19(1):1–5.

42. Shah GK, Sharma S, Fineman MS, et al. Arteriovenous adventitial sheathotomy for the treatment of macular edema associated with branch retinal vein occlusion. *Am J Ophthalmol*. 2000;129(1):104–106.

43. Osterloh MD, Charles S. Surgical decompression of branch retinal vein occlusions. *Arch Ophthalmol*. 1988;106(10):1469–1471.

44. Mester U, Dillinger P. Vitrectomy with decompression in branch retinal vein occlusion. *XXIInd Meeting of the Club Jules Gonin*, Taormina, Italy; 2000.

45. Opremcak EMBR. AV crossing sheathotomy for BRVO (RVS-BRVO). *Invest Ophthalmol Vis Sci*. 2001;42:S718.

46. Lee W-HTJ, Sjaarda RN. Visual acuity results in arteriovenous sheathotomy versus grid laser photocoagulation in branch retinal vein occlusion. *Invest Ophthalmol Vis Sci.* 2001;42: S718.

47. Yamamoto S, Saito W, Yagi F, et al. Vitrectomy with or without arteriovenous adventitial sheathotomy for macular edema associated with branch retinal vein occlusion. *Am J Ophthalmol.* 2004;138(6):907–914.

48. Mason J 3rd, Feist R, White M Jr, et al. Sheathotomy to decompress branch retinal vein occlusion: A matched control study. *Ophthalmology.* 2004;111(3):540–545.

49. Kroll P, Meyer CH, Mester U, et al. Sheathotomy to decompress BRVO. *Ophthalmology.* 2005;112(3):528–529.

50. Horio N, Horiguchi M. Effect of arteriovenous sheathotomy on retinal blood flow and macular edema in patients with branch retinal vein occlusion. *Am J Ophthalmol.* 2005;139(4): 739–740.

51. Yamaji H, Shiraga F, Tsuchida Y, et al. Evaluation of arteriovenous crossing sheathotomy for branch retinal vein occlusion by fluorescein videoangiography and image analysis. *Am J Ophthalmol.* 2004;137(5):834–841.

52. Brantley MA, Holekamp NM, Shah GK, et al. Increased retinal perfusion after arteriovenous sheathotomy for branch retinal vein occlusion. *Annual Meeting of the American Academy of Ophthalmology*, New Orleans; 2001.

53. Mester U, Dillinger P. Vitrectomy with arteriovenous decompression and internal limiting membrane dissection in branch retinal vein occlusion. *Retina.* 2002;22(6):740–746.

54. Garcia-Arumi J, Martinez-Castillo V, Boixadera A, et al. Management of macular edema in branch retinal vein occlusion with sheathotomy and recombinant tissue plasminogen activator. *Retina.* 2004;24(4):530–540.

55. Frangieh GT, Green WR, Barraquer-Somers E, et al. Histopathologic study of nine branch retinal vein occlusions. *Arch Ophthalmol.* 1982;100(7): 1132–1140.

56. Kumar B, Yu DY, Morgan WH, et al. The distribution of angioarchitectural changes within the vicinity of the arteriovenous crossing in branch retinal vein occlusion. *Ophthalmology.* 1998;105(3):424–427.

CHAPTER 9

Retinal Detachment and Proliferative Vitreoretinopathy

Amani A. Fawzi, MD , Jay M. Stewart, MD , and Michael A. Samuel, MD

The management of rhegmatogenous retinal detachment (RD) has evolved over the last century as a result of advances made in surgical techniques and surgical instruments, and of the advent of vitreous substitutes.

The "Custodis" method of segmental scleral buckle to seal the retinal break, without drainage of subretinal fluid (SRF), allowing for spontaneous resorption of SRF, the earliest technique, was only suitable for isolated small tears. Encircling scleral buckles offered a more effective, though more invasive, alternative for more extensive detachments and breaks. With the introduction of pneumatic retinopexy by Dominguez,[1] followed by the popularization of pars plana vitrectomy by Machemer, the strategies for tackling RDs have become more sophisticated, especially with the advent of vitreous substitutes, the use of long-acting gases, and more recently wide-angle viewing systems and high-speed state-of-the-art vitreous cutters. Despite the significant advances in techniques, proliferative vitreoretinopathy (PVR) remains the most common cause of failure for primary rhegmatogenous RD.

Randomized controlled trials (RCTs) have been designed to ask several important questions regarding RD management. The question of pneumatic retinopexy as a safe and effective alternative to scleral buckle was addressed by the RD Study group. The Silicone Oil study was designed to test the hypothesis that silicone oil offered an advantage over the various gas tamponades in the management of advanced PVR. The question of vitrectomy versus scleral buckle in primary uncomplicated RD

remains to be answered in a large multicenter RCT, which is currently underway in Europe. Randomized trials have been conducted to address this question in a group of patients with pseudophakic and aphakic RD.

Pneumatic Retinopexy versus Scleral Buckle: The Retinal Detachment Study Group

Pneumatic retinopexy was first introduced by Dominguez in 1984 and popularized by Hilton and Grizzard in 1985 for a nonincisional repair of RD.[1,2] Pneumatic retinopexy is based on the principle that an inert long-acting gas, when injected into the vitreous cavity, is capable of sealing a retinal break by positioning the gas bubble against the retinal tear to create an internal tamponade. The surface tension of the gas prevents continued ingress of liquid vitreous, thereby allowing the SRF to be naturally absorbed by the RPE pump. Typically, the fluid that has accumulated under the retina will be reabsorbed within 1 to 2 days depending on the chronicity and extent of SRF. Given the fact that gas will disappear from the eye within 1.5 to 6 weeks, it is necessary to create a more permanent seal surrounding the retinal tear.[2] Alternatives in performing retinopexy include laser and cryopexy. Transconjunctival cryopexy can be performed before the injection of the gas bubble or on a subsequent day after resolution of the SRF. Laser photocoagulation requires attached retina and hence reabsorption of the SRF in the area of the break and is therefore performed following gas injection.

Sulfur hexafluoride (SF_6) and perfluoropropane (C_3F_8) are the gases most frequently used in pneumatic retinopexy. Sterile room air can also be used.[3] The type of gas selected is based on the preference of the surgeon, the size of the retinal breaks, the number of breaks, the chronicity of detachment, the ability of patient to position properly, and the duration of tamponade required. A gas bubble of 0.3 mL covers more than 45 degrees of arc of the retina. To cover 80 to 90 degrees, a bubble of 1.2 mL is required.[4] Generally, 1.0 mL is sufficient to cover all breaks simultaneously or alternately. This requires an injection of 0.5 mL of pure SF_6, 0.3 mL of pure C_3F_8, and if sterile room air is injected, 0.6 to 0.8 mL is recommended. Sterile air, because of the requisite large volume of gas injected will require a large volume paracentesis or multiple paracenteses to normalize intraocular pressure following injection.

Patient selection and compliance are essential for success with pneumatic retinopexy. Patients with back or neck problems may not be ideal candidates. The location of the retinal breaks will determine the position that must be maintained. Breaks between the 11 and 1 o'clock positions are the easiest to target. Generally, the break should have a tamponade maintained for 3 to 5 days[5] to allow for the resolution of the SRF and maturation of the chorioretinal adhesion. Restrictions that must be adhered to while the gas is present in the eye include no travel above 4,000 feet and no air travel because of decreases in atmospheric pressure leading to bubble expansion and an unsafe rise in intraocular pressure. In addition, patients should not have anaesthesia that requires the use of nitrous oxide. Nitrous oxide is more soluble in blood and rapidly diffuses into the vitreous gas bubble, also leading to an unsafe rise in intraocular pressure. Phakic patients should also be instructed not to lie flat on their back until the bubble dissipates to avoid prolonged contact with the lens.

Before pneumatic retinopexy the primary operation for repair of RD had been scleral buckling (SB) with single surgery success rates between 75% and 88%.[6,7] However, there had been no randomized controlled clinical trial to compare the two procedures. The controversy concerning the safety, efficacy, and indications for pneumatic retinopexy led to the conduction of the Pneumatic Retinopexy Study.

Study Objectives

The Pneumatic Retinopexy Study was conducted to determine the efficacy of pneumatic retinopexy in comparison with SB for selected RDs.

Inclusion/Exclusion Criteria

Patients were eligible for the study if they had:

1. A single break that is no larger than 1 clock hour located in the superior 8 clock hours, or a group of small breaks within 1 clock hour of each other
2. Media sufficiently clear to rule out other retinal breaks that determine macular attachment and not significantly reduce visual acuity
3. Availability for follow-up for at least 6 months
4. History of good vision before RD
5. Macula-on eyes with corrected visual acuity of 20/50 or better
6. Macula-off eyes with corrected visual acuity of 20/50 or worse
7. Shortest diameter of detachment of at least 6DD

Exclusion criteria included the following:

1. PVR, grade C or D
2. Uncontrolled glaucoma or cup-disc ratio exceeding 0.6
3. Retinal breaks in inferior 4 clock hours
4. Inability to maintain the required postoperative head position

Treatment Groups/Trial Design

Before randomization, RDs were stratified into two separate groups:

1. Macula on
2. Macula off

Outcome Measures

The primary outcome measures were anatomic and functional success following surgical intervention. Single operation success was strictly defined as retinal reattachment at 6 months after one surgical intervention or injection of gas with one laser and/or cryotherapy performed immediately or within 72 hours.

Important Methodologic Aspects

Pneumatic Retinopexy

Pneumatic retinopexy was performed in accordance with a specific protocol (see following text). The type and volume of gas injected, the number of cryopexy or laser photocoagulation applications, paracentesis, and IOP at 5, 10, 20, 30, and 60 minutes were noted. The patients were not randomized to the type of gas used for the procedure.

Summary of Protocol

1. Transconjunctival cryotherapy of retinal break
2. Eyelid Speculum
3. Topical Betadine solution with equal parts balanced salt solution, followed by a 3- minute wait
4. Dry injection site 3- to 4-mm posterior to limbus with cotton-tipped applicator
5. Briskly inject sterile (Millipore filter) C_3F_8 (0.3 mL) or SF_6 (0.6 mL) with a 30-gauge needle in the uppermost pars plana (supine patient with head turned 45 degrees to side)[7a] (see Table 9.1)
6. Conjunctival perforation covered with sterile cotton-tipped applicator as the needle is withdrawn and the head turned to move the gas bubble away from the injection site
7. Observing the central retinal artery: A 10-minute wait if the artery is closed; if artery does not pulsate, use of paracentesis or vitreous aspiration
8. "Steamroller maneuver" done at this time, if indicated
9. Monitoring of IOP and central retinal artery for 60 minutes
10. Topical antibiotics and eye pad
11. Diamox (250 mg four times daily for 3 days) if patient will drive to a higher altitude not exceeding 4,000 feet

Scleral Buckling

When SB was used, the surgeons were asked to perform the surgery using their usual and customary techniques. The surgeon recorded the type of buckling material, number of cryopexy applications, drainage of SRF, paracentesis, the type and volume of gas injected.

Follow-up

Follow-up was done on days 1,3,7,14,30,60,120, and 180. Visual acuity was obtained using an Early Treatment Diabetic Retinopathy Study (ETDRS) chart in a masked manner. Refractions were performed at 1 and 6 months after surgery. The macula was examined for holes, pucker, and edema. The peripheral retina was examined for new tears, SRF or blood, PVR, and choroidal detachment.

Summary of Major Results

Major results obtained with scleral buckling and pneumatic retinopexy are summarized in the subsequent text (see Table 9.2).

1. A total of 198 eyes were followed up for a minimum of 6 months, 145 (81%) were followed up for 1 year.
2. In the scleral buckle group, most cases were managed with the drainage of SRF and an encircling buckle. In one third of the cases, gas was injected.
3. In the pneumatic group, most cases were managed with C_3F_8, and approximately one-quarter required paracentesis.
4. Average cryotherapy applications were similar in both groups.
5. With one operation, retinal reattachment was slightly higher in the SB group (82% with scleral buckle versus 73% with pneumatic retinopexy), but the difference was not statistically significant. The addition of postoperative laser photocoagulation or cryotherapy resulted in similar reattachment rates (84% with scleral buckle and 81% with pneumatic retinopexy).
6. With reoperations, the final reattachment rate was 98% in the SB group and 99% in the pneumatic retinopexy group.
7. If the detachment did not include the macula, the 6-month final visual acuity was similar for both groups.
8. If the detachment included the macula for 14 days or less, final visual acuity was significantly better in the pneumatic retinopexy group ($p = 0.01$). Of the cases treated with pneumatic

TABLE 9.1 □ Expansion and Duration of Intraocular Gases

Gas	Final Volume	Time to Final Volume (h)	Duration of Effective Size	Duration of Bubble
Air	Injected volume	Immediate	1–3 d	1 wk
SF_6	Doubles	36	7–10 d	10–12 d
C_3F_8	Quadruples	72	4–5 wk	6 wk

Lincoff H, Haft D, Ligget P, et al. Intravitreal expansion of perfluorcarbon bubbles. *Arch Ophthalmol.* 1980;98:1646.

TABLE 9.2 □ Summary of the Pneumatic Retinopexy Study

Outcome	Scleral Buckle	Pneumatic Retinopexy
Reattachment with 1 operation	82%	73%
Reattachment with 1 operation and postoperative laser/cryo	84%	81%
Final attachment	98%	99%
VA better than 20/50 with preop macular detachment	56%	80%

VA, visual acuity.

retinopexy, 80% had better than 20/50 visual acuity as compared with 56% with scleral buckle.

9. Phakic eyes had similar cure rate when treated by either procedure. Aphakic/pseudophakic eyes also had similar success rates with both the procedures. However, as a group, aphakic/pseudophakic eyes have a lower cure rate than phakic eyes, regardless of the procedure used.

10. New/missed retinal breaks occurred with significantly greater frequency in the pneumatic retinopexy group.

11. PVR developed in 5% of the SB group and 3% of the pneumatic retinopexy group. This difference was not statistically significant.

12. Complications were similar in both groups.

Interpretation of Results and Implications for Clinical Practice

Multiple methods exist to successfully repair RDs. The success of surgery is measured by the anatomic reattachment and the final visual outcome. Pneumatic retinopexy, due to its relatively noninvasive nature, is less likely to be associated with complications including anisometropia and diplopia as compared to scleral buckle. Pneumatic retinopexy can restore vision more quickly with lower morbidity than other retinal operations, therefore, in selected patients it offers certain advantages over other more invasive techniques of RD repair. The Pneumatic Retinopexy Study demonstrated that patients with a preoperative macular detachment of <2 weeks duration had a significantly better chance of achieving 20/50 or better visual acuity, when treated with pneumatic retinopexy as compared to that with scleral buckle.[5] This finding has not been found in other retrospective, comparative series, where no difference in final visual acuity was noted between scleral buckle and pneumatic retinopexy.[8,9]

Although the success of single operation pneumatic retinopexy is desirable because it is associated with the highest level of visual acuity return, the evidence suggests that a failed pneumatic attempt does not disadvantage ultimate anatomic correction of the RD. In the Pneumatic Retinopexy Study the single-procedure success rate was lower with pneumatic retinopexy as compared with that with scleral buckle; however, the final anatomic success rate was similar.[5] Similar findings have been observed in retrospective, comparative studies of pneumatic retinopexy versus scleral buckle.[8,9] Higher single-procedure failure rates with pneumatic retinopexy are ascribed to reopening of the original break, missed retinal breaks, and new retinal breaks.

Success with pneumatic retinopexy depends upon case selection and surgical technique. The most favorable cases include phakic eyes with less extensive detachment, secondary to a superior retinal break less than 1 clock hour in size, and no PVR. Retrospective series of pneumatic retinopexy suggest that patients with a single retinal break and an RD in the superior two thirds of the fundus have a single-procedure success rate that is as high as 97%.[10] Factors negatively influencing single operation anatomic success include pseudophakia, an increased number of retinal breaks, and a greater area of detached retina. Factors not influencing the outcome include the presence of lattice degeneration (less than 3 clock hours), the type of retinal break, the type or volume of gas used, the type of retinopexy (laser or cryotherapy), the sequence of gas insertion versus retinopexy application, the status of the posterior capsule, and gender.

With increased attention to health care costs, the ability to treat RDs with a minimally invasive, office-based procedure may make pneumatic retinopexy increasingly important in management. Estimates have suggested that pneumatic retinopexy may cost 25% to 50% less than scleral buckle when operating room and anesthesia costs are considered.[10]

Controversies and Future Use of Pneumatic Retinopexy:

Increased familiarity and comfort with pneumatic retinopexy has led to expanded usage of this technique in the management of RD. Technique modifications have been suggested to improve the outcomes of pneumatic retinopexy.

Inferior RD was initially considered to be an exclusion for treatment with pneumatic retinopexy.[5] Inverted positioning required to tamponade the inferior retinal breaks was considered to be impractical. In addition, concerns have arisen regarding the practicality of prolonged inverted positioning required to achieve adequate reabsorption of SRF and chorioretinal adhesion. Inverted pneumatic retinopexy had been previously used to successfully reattach the retina following recurrent RD after scleral buckle.[11] Recent case series have revisited and expanded the role of inverted pneumatic retinopexy. In one series of recurrent inferior RD following encircling scleral buckle, 17 patients underwent inverted positioning.[12] Positioning was achieved with 10 degree Trendelenberg, 10 degree neck extension and 10 degree ocular supraduction. Tamponade was achieved with injection of 0.3 to 0.8 mL of intraocular gas. Patients maintained the position strictly for 48 hours and over part of the time for 1 week. Eighty-eight percent of patients achieved lasting retinal reattachment with a median follow-up of 1.3 years (0.1 to 11.5 years). A second case series of 11 patients, including 5 primary inferior RDs, achieved an 82% single-procedure success rate with inverted pneumatic retinopexy.[13] Patients were positioned with their head dependent in a prone position for 8 hours. No further positioning was required. This series suggests that limited positioning in selected patients may allow inferior retinal reattachment. No comparative trials exist to determine the true efficacy of inverted pneumatic retinopexy versus scleral buckle in a larger population.

The lower single-procedure success rate observed with pneumatic retinopexy has been ascribed to the frequent development of new retinal breaks. Most of these breaks occur within 1 month of the procedure.[5] The majority will occur in the superior fundus, often in relative proximity to the initial retinal break. It is postulated that the gas bubble may shift the vitreous leading to new areas of vitreoretinal traction. One attempt to reduce the rate of new retinal breaks is the application of 360-degree laser retinopexy. In one retrospective case series, prophylactic laser treatment was suggested to reduce the rate of new retinal breaks.[10] These findings have not been validated in prospective studies nor have the potential complications of extensive laser been fully explored.

The popularity and comfort of surgeons with pars plana vitrectomy has prompted many to treat primary uncomplicated RD with primary vitrectomy. A randomized controlled clinical trial to compare pneumatic retinopexy to primary pars plana vitrectomy (PPPV) would help answer these questions further, and elucidate whether the risk of an operating room procedure with its added cost is justified by the potential benefits of earlier rehabilitation, enhanced primary success, and faster and more complete visual recovery.

Vitrectomy Versus Scleral Buckle for Primary Rhegmatogenous Retinal Detachment

Introduction

The choice of surgical treatment for patients with primary RD uncomplicated by PVR remains controversial. Traditionally, the initial management of RD has been with scleral buckle. Increased experience with vitrectomy, improvements in surgical instrumentation, the advent of high-speed cutters and the introduction of wide-field viewing systems have led to an increased utilization of vitrectomy in the management of primary RD. Potential advantages of primary vitrectomy include removal of vitreous opacities and capsular remnants, possibly faster, and increased rate of foveal reattachment in macula-off RDs and the avoidance of complications associated with SB including refractive shifts, extraocular muscle imbalance, and buckle extrusion.[14,15]

Data published to date suggest that vitrectomy compares favorably with SB. The two primary outcome measures of success in RD repair cited in most studies are anatomic retinal reattachment and visual acuity. The overall retinal reattachment rate for PPV in a recent review was 85%, compared with the 71% to 95% reattachment rate achieved in retrospective reports of SB procedures.[16,17]

Evaluation of the literature to determine the true efficacy of primary vitrectomy compared with SB is difficult for several reasons. There is a lack of uniform inclusion criteria in the studies, including different configurations of RD, duration of detachment and preoperative lens status, that could significantly influence the results.[18,19] While the bulk of the literature on the primary repair of RD is composed of case series, there are several comparative trials; however, not in all of these studies were the subjects truly randomized and therefore selection bias may influence the stated results.[20] In addition, many randomized studies lack an *a priori* sample size calculation and therefore it is difficult to determine whether the study enrollment had adequate power to detect a true difference in treatment efficacy. Duration of follow-up varies between studies. In some cases, a lack of long-term follow-up makes the results of the studies difficult to compare.

In general, vitrectomy has been compared to SB in two separate groups: Pseudophakic/aphakic RD and phakic RD. In addition, some literature has examined the role of primary vitrectomy as compared with combination vitrectomy/scleral buckle.

Primary Vitrectomy versus Scleral Buckle in Primary Pseudophakic and Aphakic Retinal Detachment

Capsular opacities, poor dilation, vitreous debris, and the presence of small retinal breaks have been cited as the reasons for failure of primary scleral buckle in cases of pseudophakic and aphakic retinal detachment (PARD). Primary vitrectomy has become increasingly popular in the management of these cases because of the ease of improving visualization of small retinal breaks and the lack of induced myopia secondary to the presence of a scleral buckle. In addition, these cases are not subject to the primary complication of vitrectomy, cataract.

Several case series have been conducted examining the role of primary vitrectomy alone in the management of PARD.[21–24] These series report a primary retinal reattachment success rate ranging from 88% to 94% and a final reattachment rate of 96% to 100%. There is a 69% to 79% rate of final visual acuity better than 20/50.

Nonrandomized, comparative series have studied vitrectomy versus scleral buckle in patients with pseudophakic RD.[20] Similar primary and final retinal reattachment rates as well as visual acuities were reported.

Two RCTs have compared primary vitrectomy with scleral buckle in the management of pseudophakic RD.[25,26] One study was a single-center trial conducted with a single surgeon.[25] The other was conducted as a multicenter trial.[26] Both studies benefited from clear inclusion and exclusion criteria, *a priori* sample size calculations to ensure adequate statistical power, and a defined randomization schedule.

In the single-center RCT 150 patients with pseudophakic RD were randomized to an encircling silicone scleral band (240 style, 2.5 mm) versus a conventional 20-gauge three-port vitrectomy, retinal reattachment with perfluoro-n-octane (PFO) and gas tamponade with 20% SF_6.[25] Results from this study indicated that vitrectomy was associated with a significantly higher single-procedure anatomic reattachment rate (94% with PPV vs. 83% with SB). Operative time was significantly shortened with vitrectomy. The number of unidentifiable retinal breaks was significantly higher in the scleral buckle group, which partially accounted for the better single-procedure success rate of vitrectomy that was observed. Final retinal reattachment rates were similar in both groups (95% in SB group vs. 99% in PPV group). No difference in final visual acuity was observed. Axial length was significantly increased in the scleral buckle group postoperatively.

The PARD study group recently reported their 6-month results comparing vitrectomy to SB in the management of primary aphakic or pseudophakic RD.[26] PARD is a multicenter, prospective randomized controlled clinical trial. Eligible patients had RD following cataract extraction with or without intraocular lens. A total of 225 eyes in 225 patients were enrolled in 6 centers, of which 64% were pseudophakic. Patients who were eligible for the study were randomized to one of the following treatment groups:

Scleral buckle group (SB)

- Meridional sponge with encircling 240 band was used if fishmouthing was anticipated or if encircling was not feasible.
- If there is no identifiable break:
  - Encircling 276 tire was used for patients with total RD with 240 band.
  - Localized 276 tire was used to cover detached quadrants with encircling 240 band in cases with incomplete RD.
- If breaks were identified, cryotherapy was applied; otherwise 360-degree laser treatment was applied on the buckle within 1 week postoperatively.
- Drainage of SRF was performed unless the RD was shallow with scant SRF.

PPPV group

- Three-port pars plana vitrectomy were done without debulking of the vitreous base.
- Perfluorocarbon liquid was used to assist drainage of SRF.

- Endolaser was applied to identifiable breaks; otherwise 2 to 3 rows of laser were applied postoperatively to the vitreous base.
- Air-fluid exchange was followed by SF_6 20%.
- Prone positioning was maintained for 5 days.

The findings of the PARD demonstrated a comparable single procedure, anatomic reattachment rate (68% in the SB group and 62.6% in the PPPV group). The final success rate was similar in both groups (85% in the SB and 92% in the PPPV group). The percentage of patients achieving 20/40 or better acuity at 6 months was equivalent in both groups (12.8% in the SB group and 11.3% in the PPV group). Myopia was associated with a significantly higher redetachment rate at 6 months in both groups ($p = 0.04$). No statistically significant difference in the incidence of complications was observed between the two groups.

The differences between the results of these two RCTs likely reflect differences in the populations studied. The PARD group at enrollment had 84% of eligible eyes with hand motions or light perception visual acuity as compared with a 40% to 45% rate of eyes with baseline acuity <20/400 in the single-center study. Thus, the lower single-procedure success rate and lower rates of visual recovery observed in the PARD group reflect the presence of more extensive RD, and possibly detachments of longer duration.

The choice between scleral buckle and vitrectomy for the management of primary RD in pseudophakic eyes continues to be determined by surgeon preference. Improvements in vitrectomy technology, increased emphasis on refractive outcomes in vitreoretinal surgery, and attention to cost issues including operative time will likely lead to continued increases in the popularity of vitrectomy as the initial choice for the management of these RDs.

Primary Vitrectomy versus Scleral Buckle in Phakic Patients

One potential concern with the use of vitrectomy as a method of primary repair of RD in phakic patients is the high rate of cataract formation. Improvements in cataract surgery techniques have made lens extraction a commonplace outpatient surgical procedure. Therefore, cataract formation as a complication of RD repair has been viewed by some surgeons as a minor problem that does not create a significant disadvantage to vitrectomy. This is particularly true when the complications of vitrectomy are weighed against the potential complications of SB such as anisometropia and diplopia.

Several retrospective case series have examined the role of vitrectomy in the repair of primary RD in phakic patients.[18,19,27] Many of these series did not specifically include only phakic patients. In the series that contained both phakic and pseudophakic patients, the anatomic reattachment rates were not separated by preoperative lens status. It is, therefore, difficult to clearly answer the question of whether preoperative lens status significantly affects the outcome of vitrectomy.

The primary anatomic reattachment rate ranged from 64% to 89% with final reattachment rates ranging from 92% to 100%. Final visual acuity better than 20/50 was reported in 41% to 76% of cases, though the rate of preoperative macula-off RD varied significantly between the series making interpretation of the visual acuity data difficult.

The SPR Study is a randomized trial of vitrectomy versus SB in the management of primary RD.[28] The study consists of two parallel trials stratified by preoperative lens status.

Inclusion criterion:

1. Phakic RD with well demonstrated pathologic retinal breaks

   Exclusion criteria:

1. Posterior retinal breaks or breaks that cannot be supported by a scleral buckle
2. Greater than Grade B proliferative vitreoretinopathy
3. Other ocular diseases that would influence final visual outcome
4. Myopia >7 diopters
5. Previous intraocular surgery

   Primary outcome measures:

1. Retinal reattachment posterior to the equator
2. Change in visual acuity
3. Development of cataract based on LOCS III grading system
4. Development of proliferative vitreoretinopathy

   The study randomizes patients to:

1. Scleral buckle performed in the preferred technique of the operating surgeon
2. Vitrectomy with removal of traction on the retinal tear, retinopexy and gas tamponade

Encircling scleral buckle may be included at the surgeon's discretion.

To date, no data has been reported by the SPR Study group. It is hoped that this investigation will provide further evidence for clinicians regarding the role of vitrectomy in the management of primary RD in phakic patients.

Combination Primary Scleral Buckle and Vitrectomy versus Primary Vitrectomy Alone

SB has been combined with vitrectomy in cases of unrelieved vitreoretinal traction such as proliferative vitreoretinopathy. In addition, encircling bands were once popular during vitrectomy to provide support to the vitreous base and possibly avoid postoperative retinal breaks resulting from vitreous incarceration in the sclerotomies. The advent of wide-field viewing systems has led to a decline in the use of encircling bands in vitrectomy cases. Some authors have suggested adding an encircling scleral band to vitrectomy in the management of primary RD, particularly pseudophakic RD.[29–31] The case for scleral buckle in addition to vitrectomy has been traditionally made in cases of inferior retinal breaks where the buckle may provide support in areas that are difficult to tamponade with intraocular gas.[32,33] The single-procedure success rate reported in these studies ranges from 92% to 100%. The final reattachment rates were 93% to 100%.

No randomized trials have been conducted to compare these interventions. Two nonrandomized, comparative studies have been conducted.[33,34] In both studies, the single-procedure and final reattachment rates observed were similar between the two groups. Final visual outcomes were similar between the two groups. As one would expect, the addition of a scleral buckle increases the rate of postoperative myopia significantly.

Overall, the value of the addition of a scleral buckle to vitrectomy in the primary management of RD remains unclear. Evidence from nonrandomized series leads to the question whether the buckle adds significant benefit to vitrectomy in the age of wide-field viewing systems.

Vitreous Substitutes: Silicone Oil

Silicone Study

Introduction

PVR is the leading cause of failure in RD surgery. The development of preretinal membranes results in progressive traction on the retina, leading to redetachment. PVR is observed in 5% to 10 % of cases of RD[7] and is characterized by the growth of cellular membranes composed of metaplastic retinal pigment epithelial cells and glial cells. These membranes adhere to the retina and subsequent contraction prevents complete retinal reattachment.[35]

The management of PVR requires the removal of the vitreous, dissection of preretinal membranes to relieve retinal traction, application of retinopexy to close the pathologic retinal breaks, and maintenance of retinal reattachment to allow maturation of the chorioretinal adhesion. In cases of severe retinal contracture, creation of a relaxing retinotomy or retinectomy may be required to achieve retinal reattachment.

Intraocular tamponade at the end of surgery is a crucial component in achieving long-term attachment. Tamponade may be achieved with long-acting gas or silicone oil. Long-acting gases provide temporary tamponade but are ultimately reabsorbed. Silicone oil provides long-term tamponade and generally must be surgically removed in a separate procedure. Before the Silicone Oil Study, the prevailing attitude was that the anatomic results of vitrectomy in cases of severe PVR would be better with silicone oil than with gas, but that the complications associated with this modality would jeopardize the visual outcomes. The concerns about the safety and efficacy of the various methods of long-term tamponade were the primary impetus for the study.

Study Objectives

1. To compare the anatomic and visual outcomes in cases of severe PVR treated with long-acting gas versus silicone oil
2. To compare the frequency of complications between silicone oil and long-acting gas

Inclusion/Exclusion Criteria

1. Patients 18 years and older
2. PVR at least Grade C3 or higher by the Retina Society Classification (see Table 9.3)[35]
3. Sufficient retinal contracture to warrant intraocular dissection
4. Visual acuity better than light perception
5. No concomitant eye disease including giant retinal tears and proliferative diabetic retinopathy
6. No prior penetrating trauma
7. No blunt trauma within 3 months of enrollment

TABLE 9.3 □ Retina Society Classification of Proliferative Vitreo Retinopathy[35]

Grade	Name	Clinical Features
A	Minimal	Vitreous haze and pigment
B	Moderate	Wrinkling of the inner retinal surface, rolled edge to retinal break, retinal stiffness, vessel tortuosity
C	Marked	Full thickness fixed folds
C1		One quadrant
C2		Two quadrants
C3		Three quadrants
D	Massive	Fixed folds in four quadrants
D1		Wide funnel RD
D2		Narrow funnel RD
D3		Closed funnel RD

RD, retinal detachment.

Study Conduct

A total of 404 eyes were included in the study. At randomization, patients were stratified into two groups: Group 1 had no previous vitrectomy; Group 2 had at least one prior unsuccessful vitrectomy with gas tamponade. From 1985 to 1987, eyes were randomized to receive either silicone oil or 20% SF_6 gas. From 1987 to 1990, eyes were randomized to receive either silicone oil or 14% C_3F_8 gas.

All eyes underwent vitrectomy with removal of epiretinal membranes and intraoperative reattachment of the retina before administration of the tamponade. Retinal breaks were treated with laser or cryopexy. An encircling scleral buckle was placed at the discretion of the surgeon. Lensectomy was performed as needed.

Outcome Measures

1. Anatomic reattachment was defined as continuous attachment of the macula (with or without attachment of the retina posterior to the encircling scleral buckle).
2. Functional success was measured by visual acuity of 5/200 or better.
3. Complications measured were as follows:
   a. Elevation of intraocular pressure >25 mm Hg
   b. Hypotony (IOP <5 mm Hg)
   c. Keratopathy including edema, localized opacity, or band keratopathy

Results

Phase 1 of the silicone study compared 20% SF_6 tamponade to silicone oil. (see Table 9.4) Eyes treated with silicone oil had a higher rate of anatomic success and better functional outcome. In eyes treated with SF_6, 50% had total retinal attachment at 36 months and 60% had macular reattachment. In the silicone oil group, 60% to 70% achieved total reattachment and 80% had macular reattachment. Correspondingly, visual acuity results were better in the silicone

TABLE 9.4 □ Phase 1 Silicone Study Results

Group	VA >5/200 (%)	P	Retinal Attachment (%)	P	Hypotony (%)	Keratopathy (%)
Group1						
SF_6	30–40		Macula 60		Macula-on <5	Macula-on 25–30
			Total 50		Macula-off 40–50	Macula-off 55–60
Silicone oil	50–60	<0.05	Macula 80	<0.05	Macula-on <5	Macula-on 10–15
					Macula-off 25–30	Macula-off 55–60
			Total 60–70			
Group 2						
SF_6	31		46		20	23
Silicone oil	64		71		20	41

VA, visual acuity.

TABLE 9.5 ☐ **Phase 2 Silicone Study Results**

Group	Visual Acuity >5/200 (%)	p	Retinal Attachment (%)	p	Hypotony (%)	p	Keratopathy (%)
Group 1							
C_3F_8	43		Macula 81	NS	30	<0.05	33
			Total 73	<0.05			
Silicone oil	45	NS	Macula 78		16		30
Group 2			Total 64				
C_3F_8	38		Macula 76	NS	42	<0.05	45
			Total 73				
Silicone oil	33	NS	Macula 77		22		43
			Total 62				

NS, not significant.

oil group with 50% to 60% achieving better than 5/200 compared with 30% to 40% in the SF_6 group. Additional surgery was required in 35% to 40% of eyes without prior vitrectomy (group 1). In eyes with macular reattachment, keratopathy was more common in SF_6 eyes while no difference was observed in cases with persistent macular detachment. Hypotony was infrequent in both groups with macular reattachment. Hypotony was more common in eyes with persistent macular detachment treated with SF_6.[36]

Phase 2 of the study compared the outcomes in eyes treated with 14% C_3F_8 and those treated with silicone oil. No statistically significant difference was found in the anatomic or functional outcomes between the two groups[36a] (see Table 9.5). Total reattachment was achieved in 73% in both groups treated with C_3F_8 and 64% of group 1 eyes and 61% of group 2 eyes treated with silicone oil. Macular attachment rates were similar. Accordingly, visual acuity results were similar (81% of C_3F_8 eyes and 78% of silicone oil eyes in group 1 achieving better than 5/200 and 38% of C_3F_8 eyes and 33% of silicone

oil eyes in group 2). Reoperation was required in 30% to 35% of eyes. No difference in the rate of keratopathy was observed. Hypotony was statistically more frequent in eyes treated with C_3F_8.

Analysis of all group 1 eyes compared to group 2 eyes treated with silicone oil or C_3F_8 (SF_6 eyes were excluded from this analysis) demonstrated no difference in the rates of complete retinal reattachment (67% group 1 vs. 67% group 2), macular attachment (78% vs. 77%) and visual acuity better than 5/200 (44% vs. 39%) (see Table 9.6).[37] No differences in the rates of hypotony were noted; however, keratopathy was more common in group 2 eyes. Eyes requiring more than one surgery were less likely to regain visual acuity better than 5/200.

Postoperative elevations of intraocular pressure occurred in 5% of eyes. It was more common in silicone oil eyes (8% silicone oil vs. 2% C_3F_8). Hypotony occurred in 24% of eyes. It was more prevalent in C_3F_8 eyes (31%) compared with silicone oil eyes (18%). Eyes were more likely to have chronic hypotony with a persistent macular detachment

TABLE 9.6 ☐ **Outcomes of Group 1 and 2 Silicone Study Results**

Group	Visual Acuity >5/200 (%)	Retinal Attachment (%)	Hypotony (%)	Keratopathy (%)
1	44	Macula 78	20	29
		Total 67		
2	39	Macula 77	19	46
		Total 67		

(48% with macular RD vs. 16%). This was true in both the silicone oil (42% vs. 10%) and C_3F_8 groups (54% vs. 21%). Preoperative predictors of hypotony included preoperative hypotony, chronic retinal contraction anterior to the equator, rubeosis, and large retinal breaks. Chronic hypotony was associated with poor visual acuity, persistent RD, corneal opacity, and abnormal anterior chamber depth.[38]

Corneal abnormalities occurred in 27% of eyes postoperatively. No difference in the rate of corneal abnormality was observed between the treatment groups. The predictors of corneal abnormalities were preoperative rubeosis, preoperative aphakia or pseudophakia, postoperative aqueous flare, and reoperations. Corneal abnormalities were associated with poor visual acuity and hypotony.[39]

Macular pucker was present in 64% of eyes at baseline. At 6-month follow-up, 15% of eyes had evidence of macular pucker. Of these 31% were new. No difference in the rate of macular pucker was observed in the treatment groups. Preoperative predictors of macular pucker formation were preoperative aphakia or pseudophakia, absence of focal posterior or intravitreal contraction, and larger-sized retinal breaks (>2 disc diameters). Functional success, with visual acuity better than 5/200, was more common in eyes without macular pucker.[40]

Retinotomies are performed in cases of severe retinal contracture not relieved by removal of the preretinal membranes. Relaxing retinotomy was performed in 29% of eyes. It was required more commonly in group 2 eyes (42%) compared with group 1 eyes (20%). Relaxing retinotomy was required more frequently in eyes with diffuse anterior contraction, anterior retinal displacement, and subretinal membranes, reflecting more severe anterior retinal traction. Eyes not requiring relaxing retinotomies were significantly more likely to achieve posterior retinal reattachment (69% vs. 50% in group 1 and 75% vs. 48% in group 2), visual acuity better than 5/200 (60% vs. 32% in group 1 and 63% vs. 20% in group 2) and less hypotony (35% vs. 17%). Silicone oil reduced the rate of hypotony in group 1 eyes but not in group 2.[41]

Silicone oil may be removed in some eyes. In the silicone study, 45% of eyes randomized to silicone oil had the oil removed at a median time of 6 months postoperatively. Eyes from which the oil was removed were more likely to have an attached retina, a successful visual outcome and no hypotony. Eyes with the oil removed were more likely to experience visual improvement; however, they were also more likely to experience recurrent RD.[42]

The study also included the creation of a new grading system for PVR that included both anterior and posterior contraction. The prior Retinal Society classification emphasized pathology posterior to the equator. The silicone oil grading system described six patterns of retinal contracture and their location relative to the equator (see Table 9.7)[43].

Implications for Clinical Practice

The Silicone Study demonstrated that silicone oil and C_3F_8 are equivalent methods of achieving retinal tamponade following surgery for severe PVR. Silicone oil and C_3F_8 offered similar visual and anatomic outcomes, with a slightly higher rate of hypotony associated with C_3F_8. Both are superior to SF_6 in the treatment of RD and PVR. This observation is likely the result of the shorter duration of tamponade offered by SF_6.

The Silicone Study achieved macular reattachment in approximately 80% of cases. Improvements in surgical experience, technique, and instrumentation have led to continued improvement in the success of PVR surgery. The primary goal of surgery in these cases continues to be anatomic success with a single procedure. The Silicone Study confirmed that, regardless of the tamponade used, a single procedure offers the best results.

Given the equivalence of C_3F_8 to silicone oil demonstrated by the Silicone Study, the choice of tamponade rests upon the surgeon's clinical decision. Factors that may favor silicone oil include preoperative hypotony, anterior PVR, intraoperative retinotomy, need for rapid visual recovery, or inability to position postoperatively.

Inferior PVR remains one area of continued difficulty for surgeons. The silicone oil that is currently available has a specific gravity less than water and therefore floats. It is exceptionally difficult to achieve a 100% oil fill and therefore the inferior retina cannot be adequately tamponaded with standard silicone oil. Fluorinated silicone oil with a specific gravity more than that of water has been developed, but its widespread use has been limited by complications. Perfluorocarbon liquids also possess a higher specific gravity than water. While these have become useful intraoperative tools, concern about retinal toxicity has limited their use in long-term retinal tamponade. Newer, partially fluorinated alkanes may provide a safer, heavier-than-water tamponade. Early series

TABLE 9.7 □ Silicone Study Proliferative Vitreoretinopathy Classification[44]

Type Number	Type of Contraction	Location	Clinical Signs
1	Focal	Posterior	Starfold
2	Diffuse	Posterior	Confluent irregular retinal folds in the posterior retina; remainder of retina drawn posterior; optic nerve may not be visible
3	Subretinal	Posterior	"Napkin ring" around the disc or "clothes line" elevation of the retina
4	Circumferential	Anterior	Irregular folds in the anterior retina; series of radial folds more posterior; peripheral retina within vitreous base stretched inward
5	Perpendicular	Anterior	Smooth circumferential fold of retina at the insertion of posterior hyaloid
6	Anterior	Anterior	Circumferential fold of retina at the insertion of posterior hyaloid pulled forward; trough of peripheral retina anteriorly; ciliary processes stretched with possible hypotony; iris retraction

Grade	Clinical Signs
A	Vitreous haze and vitreous pigment
B	Inner retinal wrinkling, rolled edge to break
P	Starfold and/or diffuse contraction in posterior retina and/or subretinal membrane
P1: One quadrant	
P2: Two quadrants	
P3: Three quadrants	
P4: Four quadrants	
A	Circumferential and/or perpendicular and/or anterior traction in anterior retina
A1: One quadrant	
A2: Two quadrant	
A3: Three quadrant	
A4: Four quadrant	

utilizing a mixture of 30% perfluorohexyloctane and 70% polydimethylsiloxane 1000 (silicone oil) demonstrated efficacy in providing inferior retinal tamponade without significant complications such as ocular hypertension and keratopathy.[44a] Future investigations will be required to establish the efficacy and safety of these alternative tamponade agents.

Pharmacologic Prevention of Proliferative Vitreoretinopathy

Proliferative vitreoretinopathy results in the development of contractile membranes on the retinal surface leading to recurrent RD. Numerous agents including dexamethasone, retinoic acid, colchicine, danorubicin, low molecular weight heparin, and 5 fluorouracil (5-FU) have been suggested as possible pharmacologic agents capable of reducing the formation and contracture of PVR membranes. To date, few of these agents are routinely used in clinical practice.

5-FU is a pyrimidine analog that inhibits DNA synthesis. Its effects are found predominantly in proliferative cells. It has been shown to inhibit fibroblast activity and PVR formation in animal models.[45] Studies of retinal morphology and electroretinogram (ERG) in animal models have not shown evidence of toxicity with single and multiple injections.[46] Studies of single injections of 5-FU in cases of human RD have not been shown to improve the outcomes of surgery.[47] It has been hypothesized that prolonged exposure to 5-FU is necessary to achieve the inhibition of fibroblasts.

A prospective controlled trial of 5-FU has been conducted in cases of RD at a high risk of PVR.[48] In this study, adjuvant low molecular weight heparin (5 IU per mL) was combined with 5-FU (200 μg per mL). Low molecular weight heparin may reduce fibrin formation and act synergistically with 5-FU. Patients enrolled in the study underwent vitrectomy for repair of RD and were considered at a high risk of PVR. High-risk patients had uveitis, aphakia, previous cryotherapy, more extensive RD, vitreous hemorrhage, and preoperative PVR. The risk factors used were based on a previous risk factor study conducted at the same institution.[49] Patients enrolled could have had prior therapy for peripheral retinal pathology including retinopexy and scleral buckle in 11% to 15% of cases. Patients were randomized to saline infusion during vitrectomy versus an infusion fluid containing low molecular weight heparin and 5-FU. A total of 174 patients were enrolled in the study and had a similar distribution of PVR risk factors at baseline. The primary outcome measure was PVR of grade CP1 or worse by the new Retina Society Classification system. The rate of proliferative vitreoretinopathy was significantly lower in the treated group (12.6% vs. 26.4%). Primary retinal reattachment was achieved with one procedure in 78% of treated patients and 71% of placebo patients (no significant difference). A trend toward higher reoperation rate for PVR was noted in the placebo group (18.4% vs. 10.3%) though this did not reach statistical significance. PVR was associated with a significantly poorer visual outcome. Ten patients developed postoperative hyphemas. No difference in hyphema rate was noted between the two groups. No other significant complications were noted.

5-FU has also been studied in the management of active PVR to prevent recurrent RD.[50] A total of 157 patients with grade C anterior or posterior PVR involving at least 1 clock hour were enrolled. Patients with giant retinal tears, penetrating trauma, and proliferative diabetic retinopathy were excluded. Patients were randomized to standard infusion or an infusion containing 200 μg per mL of 5-FU and 5 IU per mL of low molecular weight heparin. The study infusion was continued for 1 hour. In cases of longer duration, the infusion fluid was changed to the standard infusion solution. All patients underwent vitrectomy with

removal of epiretinal membranes. Relaxing retinotomies were performed as required. All patients had 1,000-centistoke silicone oil placed at the time of surgery with planned removal at 3 months. The primary outcome measure was stable attachment of the posterior pole without silicone oil at 6 months. Owing to improved anatomic outcomes with advances in vitreoretinal surgery the investigators sought a more rigorous measure of success to determine the utility of adjuvant pharmacologic therapy.[50]

At the 6-month follow-up, 84% of eyes achieved total retinal reattachment and 94% had attachment of the posterior pole. At the 6-month follow-up, there was no significant difference in the primary outcome measure (posterior retinal reattachment without silicone oil) between the treatment and control groups (56% vs. 51%). There was a trend toward a lower rate of macular pucker in the treated group; however, this did not have any statistical significance.[50]

The inclusion of 5-FU in the infusion solution for patients who undergo vitrectomy for RD and who are at a high risk of proliferative vitreoretinopathy may reduce the rate of PVR and recurrent RD. The drug is relatively inexpensive and may provide a significantly cost-effective intervention for the prevention of PVR. In general, its use has not been widely adopted because of concerns of potential toxicity and drug dosage errors at the time of infusion. In addition, clinical data supporting its usage remain limited. Nonetheless PVR remains the primary reason for failure of RD surgery. Future investigations will likely focus on adjuvant therapies that specifically target precise steps in the pathogenesis of PVR. Gene transfer has been studied in experimental PVR and may provide options for clinical disease.[51,52] Further investigations will be necessary to better understand the role of pharmacologic agents in the prevention of PVR.

Vitreous Substitutes: Perfluorocarbon Liquids

Perfluoron Multicenter Clinical Trial

Perfluorocarbon liquids have become an indispensable tool in the management of complex RDs. Their physical properties include a high specific gravity (1.76 for PFO) and immiscibility in water. These properties can be utilized to facilitate anterior displacement of SRF or blood, unfold giant retinal tears, and provide countertraction and retinal stabilization during membrane peeling in PVR. Unlike silicone oil, their low viscosity (0.69 for PFO at 25 C) makes their injection quite simple, without a need for pressurized systems. As discussed previously, the long-term use of PFCLs in inferior PVR remains controversial with conflicting reports of retinal toxicity in animals and humans.[53]

The utility and safety of heavy liquids in retinal surgery has been explored in two prospective, multicenter collaborative studies.[54,55]

Perfluorperhydrophenanthrene (Vitreon) was studied in 162 eyes with retinal tears of >90 degrees. Vitreon was used as a surgical adjunct to achieve intraoperative retinal reattachment. In 97.5% of cases, intraoperative retinal reattachment was achieved. Recurrent RD occurred in 49% of eyes with a final reattachment rate of 90%. Complications observed in the series included cataract, macular pucker, corneal decompensation, and hypotony. Complications were not felt to be the result of the usage of Vitreon intraoperatively. In 9.9% of cases, Vitreon was left in the eye to provide long-term tamponade with a mean duration of 87 days. Cases with prolonged Vitreon exposure had similar outcomes to the remainder of the cases.[54]

The Perfluoron Study group was a multicenter, nonrandomized study on the use of PFO as an intraoperative adjunct in cases of RD complicated by PVR. Eligible patients were aged 15 months or more and underwent surgery for RD with PVR using intraoperative Perfluoron. No attempts were made to define the indications for the use of Perfluoron other than the surgeon's preference. The study was undertaken before PFO was approved by the U.S. Food and Drug Administration (FDA), and sought to explore the visual and anatomical outcomes associated with its use, as well as the rate of complications.

The study included 555 patients, followed up for a median duration of 5.6 months, with PVR grade C3 or higher in 73%. Postoperative visual acuity was 20/200 or better in 25% of patients, as compared with 10% preoperatively. Overall, postoperative acuity improved in 60%, remained stable in 23% and worsened in 18% of patients. Preoperative characteristics that were associated with final acuity of 20/200 or better included preoperative acuity of 5/200 or better, no diabetes mellitus, no prior vitrectomy, prior SB, no silicone oil tamponade, and no relaxing retinotomy.

Complete retinal reattachment was achieved intraoperatively in 91% of eyes, and at the last follow-up in 77% of eyes. Recurrent RD was associated with significantly poorer visual outcome; 20/200

or better acuity was achieved in 12% of patients with recurrent RD, compared with 35% of patients without recurrence ($p<.001$). Operative characteristics significantly associated with recurrent RD in univariate and multivariate analysis included female gender, creation of a relaxing retinotomy, and the use of sulfur hexafluoride, air or no tamponade as compared with perfluoropropane or silicone oil tamponade.

Retention of PFO was noted in 7.4% of patients, corneal edema in 7%, elevated IOP in 2% and hypotony in 15%. Significant cataract or cataract surgery were noted in 92% of phakic eyes without significant cataract preoperatively.

In summary, perfluorocarbon liquids appear to be safe and useful adjuncts in vitrectomy for complicated RDs, with an acceptable complication profile and success rate. While the Vitreon collaborative group included a small number of patients with longer-term retinal tamponade, little information currently exists about longer-term tamponade using perfluorocarbon liquids. Future investigations will focus on the safety and efficacy of longer-term usage of perfluorocarbons.

References

1. Dominguez A. Cirugia precoz y ambulatoria del desprendimiento de retina. *Arch Soc Esp Oftalmol*. 1985;48:47.
2. Hilton GF, Grizzard WS. Pneumatic retinopexy: A two-step outpatient operation without conjunctival incision. *Ophthalmology*. 1986;93:626–641.
3. Sebag J, Tang M. Pneumatic retinopexy using only air. *Retina*. 1993;13:8–12.
4. Parver LM, Lincoff H. Geometry of intraocular gas used in retinal surgery. *Mod Probl Ophthalmol*. 1977;19:338–343.
5. Hilton GF, Tornambe PR, the Retina Detachment Study Group. Pneumatic retinopexy: A multicenter randomized controlled clinical trial comparing pneumatic retinopexy with scleral buckling. *Ophthalmology*. 1989;96:772
6. Lincoff H, Kreissig I, Goldbaum M. Reasons for failure in non-drainage operations. *Mod Probl Ophthalmol*. 1974;12:40–48.
7. Rachal WF, Burton TC. Changing concepts of failures after retinal detachment surgery. *Arch Ophthalmol*. 1979;97:480.
7a. Lincoff H, Haft D, Ligget P, et al. Intravitreal expansion of perfluorcarbon bubbles. *Arch Ophthalmol*. 1980;98:1646.

8. Han DP, Mohsin NC, Guse CE, et al. The Southeastern Wisconsin Pneumatic Retinopexy Study Group. Comparison of pneumatic retinopexy and scleral buckling in the management of primary rhegmatogenous retinal detachment. *Am J Ophthalmol.* 1998;126:658–668.

9. McAllister IL, Meyers SM, Zegarra H, et al. Comparison of pneumatic retinopexy with alternative surgical techniques. *Ophthalmol.* 1987; 105:913–916.

10. Tornambe PE. Pneumatic retinopexy: The evolution of case selection and surgical technique. A twelve year study of 302 eyes. *Trans Am Ophthalmol Soc.* 1997;95:551–578.

11. Friberg TR, Eller AW. Pneumatic repair of primary and secondary retinal detachments using a binocular indirect ophthalmoscope laser delivery system. *Ophthalmology.* 1988;95:187–193.

12. Mansour AM. Pneumatic retinopexy for inferior retinal breaks. *Ophthalmology.* 2005;112:1771–1776.

13. Chang TS, Pelzek CD, Nguyen RL, et al. Inverted pneumatic retinopexy: A method of treating retinal detachments associated with inferior retinal breaks. *Ophthalmology.* 2003;110(3): 589–594.

14. The SPR Study Group. View 2: The case for primary vitrectomy. *Br J Ophthomol.* 2003; 87:784–784.

15. Wolfensberger TJ. Foveal reattachment after macula-off retinal detachment occurs faster after vitrectomy than after buckle surgery. *Ophthalmology.* 2004;111(7):1340–1343.

16. Barrie T. Debate overview. Repair of a primary rhegmatogenous retinal detachment. *Br J Ophthalmol.* 2003;87(6):790.

17. Schwartz SG, Kuhl DP, McPherson AR, et al. Twenty-year follow-up for scleral buckling. *Arch Ophthalmol.* 2002;120(3):325–329.

18. Heimann H, Bornfeld N, Friedrichs W, et al. Primary vitrectomy without scleral buckling for rhegmatogenous retina detachment. *Graefes Arch Clin Exp Ophthalmol.* 1996;234: 561–568.

19. Escoffery RF, Olk RJ, Grand MG, et al. Vitrectomy without scleral buckling for primary rhegmatogenous retinal detachment. *Am J Ophththalmol.* 1985;99:275–281.

20. Le Rouic JF, Behar-Cohen F, Azan F, et al. Vitrectomy without scleral buckle versus ab-externo approach for pseudophakic retinal detachment: Comparative retrospective study. *J Fr Ophtalmol.* 2002;25:240–245.

21. Bartz-Schmidt KE, Kirchhof B, Heimann K. Primary vitrectomy for pseudophakic retinal detachment. *Br J Ophthalmol.* 1996;80:346–349.

22. Campo RV, Sipperly JO, Sneed SR, et al. Pars plana vitrectomy without scleral buckle for pseudophakic retinal detachment. *Ophthalmology.* 1999;19:103–109.

23. Speicher MA, FU AD, Martin JP, et al. Primary vitrectomy alone for repair of retinal detachments following cataract surgery. *Retina.* 2000;20:459–464.

24. Newman DK, Burton RL. Primary vitrectomy for pseudophakic and aphakic retinal detachment. *Eye.* 1999;13:635–639.

25. Brazitikos PD, Androudi S, Christen WG, et al. Primary pars plana vitrectomy versus scleral buckle surgery for the treatment of pseudophakic retinal detachment. A randomized clinical trial. *Retina.* 2005;25:957–964.

26. Ahmadieh H, Moradian S, Faghihi H, et al. Pseudophakic and Aphakic Retinal Detachment (PARD) Study Group. Anatomic and visual outcomes of scleral buckling versus primary vitrectomy in pseudophakic and aphakic retinal detachment: Six-month follow-up results of a single operation--report no. 1. *Ophthalmology.* 2005;112(8):1421–1429.

27. Tanner V, Miniham M, Williamson TH. Management of inferior retinal breaks during pars plana vitrectomy for retinal detachment. *Br J Ophthalmol.* 2001;85:480–482.

28. Heimann H, Hellmich M, Bornfeld N, et al. Scleral buckling versus primary vitrectomy in rhegmatogenous retinal detachment (SPR Study): Design issues and implications. SPR Study Group Report No.1. *Graefes Arch Clin Exp Ophthalmol.* 2001;239:567–674.

29. Desai UR, Strassman IB. Combined pars plana vitrectomy and scleral buckling for pseudophakic and aphakic retinal detachment in which a break is not seen preoperatively. *Ophthalmic Surg Lasers.* 1997;28:718–722.

30. Devenyi RG, de Carvalho R, Nakamura H. Combined scleral buckle and pars plana vitrectomy as a primary procedure for pseudophakic retinal detachment. *Ophthalmic Surg Lasers.* 1999;30:615–618.

31. Pournaras CJ, Kapetanios AD. Primary vitrectomy for pseudophakic retinal detachment: A

prospective non-randomized study. *Eur J Ophthalmol.* 2003;13:298–306.

32. Wickham L, Connor M, Aylward GW. Vitrectomy and gas for inferior break retinal detachment: Are the results comparable to vitrectomy, gas and scleral buckle? *Br J Ophthalmol.* 2005;88:1376–1379.

33. Sharma A, Grigoropoulos V, Williamson TH. Management of primary rhegmatogenous retinal detachment with inferior breaks. *Br J Ophthalmol.* 2004;88:1372–1375.

34. Stangos AN, Petropoulos IK, Brozou CG, et al. Pars plana vitrectomy alone versus vitrectomy with scleral buckling for primary rhegmatogenous pseudophakic retinal detachment. *Am J Ophthalmol.* 2004;138:952–958.

35. Machemer R, van Horn D, Aaberg TM. Pigment epithelial proliferation in human retinal detachment with massive periretinal proliferation. *Arch Ophthalmol.* 1978;85:181–191.

36. The Silicone Study Group. Vitrectomy with silicone oil or sulphur hexafluoride gas in eyes with severe proliferative vitreoretinopathy: Results of a randomized clinical trial. Silicone Study Group Report 1. *Arch Ophthalmol.* 1992;110:770–779.

36a. The Silicone Study Group. Vitrectomy with silicone oil or perfluoropropane gas in eyes with severe proliferative vitreoretinopathy: Results of a randomized clinical trial. Silicone Study Group Report 2. *Arch Ophthalmol.* 1992;110; 780–792.

37. McCuen BW, Azen SP, Stern W, et al. Vitrectomy with silicone oil or perfluoropropane gas in eyes with severe proliferative vitreoretinopathy. Silicone Study Report Number 3. *Retina.* 1993;13:279–284.

38. Barr CC, Lai MY, Lean JS, et al. Postoperative intraocular pressure abnormalities in the Silicone Study. Silicone Study Report Number 4. *Ophthalmol.* 1993;100:1629–1635.

39. Abrams GW, Azen SP, Barr CC, et al. The incidence of corneal abnormalities in the Silicone Study. Silicone Study Group Report Number 7. *Arch Ophthalmol.* 1995;113:764–769.

40. Cox MS, Azen SP, Barr CC, et al. Macular pucker after successful surgery for proliferative vitreoretinopathy. Silicone Study Report Number 8. *Ophthalmology.* 1995;102:1884–1891.

41. Blumenkranz MS, Azen SP, Aaberg TM, et al. Relaxing retinotomy with silicone oil or long-acting gas in eyes with severe proliferative vitreoretinopathy. Silicone Study Report Number 5. *Am J Ophthalmol.* 1993;116:557–564.

42. Hutton WL, Azen SP, Blumenkranz MS, et al. The effects of silicone oil removal. Silicone Study Report Number 6. *Arch Ophthalmol.* 1994; 112:778–785.

43. Lean JS, Stern WH, Irvine AR, et al. Classification of proliferative vitreoretinopathy used in the silicone study. *Ophthalmology.* 1989;96: 765–771.

44. Retina Society Terminology Committee. The classification of retinal detachment with proliferative vitreoretinopathy. *Ophthalmology.* 1983: 90;121–125.

44a. Tognetto D, Minutola D, Sanguinetti G, et al. Anatomical and functional outcomes after heavy silicone oil tamponade in vitreoretinal surgery for complicated retinal detachment: a pilot study. *Ophthalmology.* 2005;112(9):1574. 1997;104:1159–1165.

45. Blumenkranz MS, Ophir A, Claflin AJ, et al. Fluorouracil for the treatment of massive periretinal proliferation. *Am J Ophthalmol.* 1982;94: 458–467.

46. Blumenkranz M, Hernandez E, Ophir A, et al. 5-fluorouracil: New applications in complicated retinal detachment for an established antimetabolite. *Ophthalmology.* 1984;91: 122–130.

47. Blankenship GW. Evaluation of a single intravitreal injection of 5-fluorouracil in vitrectomy cases. *Graefes Arch Clin Exp Ophthalmol.* 1989;227:565–568.

48. Asaria RHY, Kon CH, Bunce C, et al. Adjuvant 5-fluorouracil and heparin prevents proliferative vitreoretinopathy. *Ophthalmology.* 2001;108:1179–1183.

49. Kon CH, Asaria RH, Occleston NL, et al. Risk factors for proliferative vitreoretinopathy after primary vitrectomy: A prospective study. *Br J Ophthalmol.* 2000;84:506–511.

50. Chateris DG, Aylward GW, Won D, et al. A randomized controlled trial of combined 5 fluorouracil and low molecular weight heparin in management of established proliferative vitreoretinopathy. *Ophthalmology.* 2004;111:2240–2245.

51. Sakamoto T, Kimura H, Scuric Z, et al. Inhibition of experimental proliferative vitreoretinopathy by retroviral vector mediated transfer of suicide gene. Can proliferative vitreoretinopathy

be a target of gene therapy. *Ophthalmology.* 1995;102:1417–1424.

52. Ikuno Y, Kazlauskas A. An in vivo gene therapy approach for experimental proliferative vitreoretinopathy using the truncated platelet-derived growth factor alpha receptor. *Invest Ophthalmol Vis Sci.* 2002;43:2406–2411.

53. Velikay M, Wedrich A, Stolba U, et al. Experimental longterm vitreous replacement with purified and non-purified perfluorodecalin. *Am J Ophthalmol.* 1993;116:565–570.

54. Kertes PJ, Wafapoor H, Peyman GA, et al. Vitreon Collaborative Study Group. The management of giant retinal tears using perfluorperhydrophenanthrene. A multicenter case series. *Ophthalmology..* 1999;106:1792–1798.

55. Scott IU, Flynn HW Jr, Murray TG, et al. Perfluoron study group. Outcomes of surgery for retinal detachment associated with proliferative vitreoretinopathy using perfluoro-n-octane: A multicenter study. *Am J Ophthalmol.* 2003;136(3):454–463.

Retinal Detachment Study Group Publications

1. Hilton GF, Tornambe PE, The Retinal Detachment Study Group. Pneumatic retinopexy. An analysis of intraoperative and postoperative complications. *Retina.* 1991;11:285–294.

2. Tornambe PE, Hilton GF, The Retinal Detachment Study Group. Pneumatic retinopexy. A multicenter randomized controlled clinical trial comparing pneumatic retinopexy with scleral buckling. *Ophthalmology.* 1989;96:772–783.

3. Tornambe PE, Hilton GF, The Pneumatic Retinopexy Study Group. Pneumatic retinopexy. A two-year follow-up study of the multicenter clinical trial comparing pneumatic retinopexy with scleral buckling. *Ophthalmology.* 1991;98:1115–1123.

Silicone Study Group Publications

1. Abrams GW, Azen SP, Barr CC, et al. The Silicone Study Group. The incidence of corneal abnormalities in the silicone study. Silicone Study Report 7. *Arch Ophthalmol.* 1995;113:764–769.

2. Abrams GW, Azen SP, McCuen BW II, et al. The Silicone Study Group. Vitrectomy with silicone oil or long-acting gas in eyes with severe proliferative vitreoretinopathy: Results of additional and long-term follow-up. Silicone Study Report 11. *Arch Ophthalmol.* 1997;115:335–344.

3. Barr CC, Lai MY, Lean JS, et al. the Silicone Study Group. Postoperative intraocular pressure abnormalities in the silicone study. Silicone study report 4. *Ophthalmol.* 1993;100:1629–1635.

4. Blumenkranz MS, Azen SP, Aaberg T, et al. the Silicone Study Group. Relaxing retinotomy with silicone oil or long-acting gas in eyes with severe proliferative vitreoretinopathy. Silicone Study Report 5. *Am J Ophthalmol.* 1993;116:557–564.

5. Cox MS, Azen SP, Barr CC, et al. The Silicone Study Group. Macular pucker after successful surgery for proliferative vitreoretinopathy. Silicone Study Report 8. *Ophthalmol.* 1995;102:1884–1891.

6. Diddie KR, Azen SP, Freeman HM, et al. The Silicone Study Group. Anterior proliferative vitreoretinopathy in the silicone study. Silicone Study Report 10. *Ophthalmol.* 1996;103:1092–1099.

7. Hutton WL, Azen SP, Blumenkranz MS, et al. The Silicone Study Group. The effects of silicone oil removal. Silicone Study Report 6. *Arch Ophthalmol.* 1994;112:778–785.

8. Lean J, Azen SP, Lopez PF, et al. The Silicone Study Group. The prognostic utility of the silicone study classification system. Silicone Study Report 9. *Arch Ophthalmol.* 1996;114:286–292.

9. McCuen BW II, Azen SP, Stern W, et al. The Silicone Study Group. Vitrectomy with silicone oil or perfluoropropane gas in eyes with severe proliferative vitreoretinopathy. Silicone study report 3. *Retina.* 1993;13:279–284.

10. Silicone Study Group. Vitrectomy with silicone oil or sulfur hexafluoride gas in eyes with severe proliferative vitreoretinopathy: Results of a randomized clinical trial. Silicone study report 1. *Arch Ophthalmol.* 1992a;110:770–779.

11. Silicone Study Group: Vitrectomy with silicone oil or perfluoropropane gas in eyes with severe proliferative vitreoretinopathy: Results of a randomized clinical trial. Silicone study report 2. *Arch Ophthalmol.* 1992b;110:780–792.

CHAPTER 10

Evidence-Based Medicine and the Treatment of Endophthalmitis

Seenu M. Hariprasad, MD and William F. Mieler, MD

In spite of significant advances in the management of endophthalmitis over the past two decades, numerous issues remain unresolved. There is no doubt that approximately 20 years ago, the advent of intravitreal antibiotics paved the way for notably improved visual and anatomic outcomes. In the mid-1990s, the Endophthalmitis Vitrectomy Study (EVS) readily addressed the role of vitrectomy versus vitreous tap in the treatment of postoperative endophthalmitis, and documented that patients with hand motion or better vision fared equally well with either a complete pars plana vitrectomy or a vitreous tap.[1] If visual acuity was light perception, then outcomes were better with a complete vitrectomy. Both procedures employed intravitreal antibiotics consisting of vancomycin and amikacin. This study provided ophthalmologists with evidence-based outcomes in the management of postoperative endophthalmitis for the first time.

The EVS also provided ophthalmologists with very important data regarding the pathogens that most commonly cause postoperative endophthalmitis (see Fig. 10.1). Additionally, the study determined that there was no apparent benefit from the use of intravenous antibiotics (cephalosporins and aminoglycosides).[1] The systemic antibiotics chosen in the EVS were the best available at the time; however, several studies following the completion of the EVS revealed that systemically administered cephalosporins and aminoglycosides do not readily achieve therapeutic intraocular concentrations in the vitreous cavity.[2,3]

Unfortunately, even within the confines of a well-conceived and thought-out multicenter, prospective clinical trial like the EVS, a number of pertinent issues remain unresolved or were not fully addressed in the original study. These include the choice of the intravitreal antibiotics (ceftazidime was not employed, and today it has virtually replaced intravitreal amikacin), the management of types of endophthalmitis not specifically studied in the EVS (filtering bleb–associated, posttraumatic, indolent, and fungal endophthalmitis), the role of intravitreal corticosteroids, and inpatient versus outpatient management of infection.

Additionally, since the completion of the EVS, new antibiotics such as the fourth-generation fluoroquinolones have been developed, and these agents will most likely play a key role in the treatment of proven infection or in the prophylaxis against infection in the near future (as will be described in the following text).

The Endophthalmitis Vitrectomy Study

In the late 1980s, the EVS group set out to determine the role of vitrectomy versus vitreous tap in the treatment of postoperative endophthalmitis, and to address the role of intravenous antibiotics versus no intravenous antibiotics in treating endophthalmitis. Vitrectomy was introduced in the 1970s and many surgeons began to employ it in conjunction with intravitreal antibiotics for treating endophthalmitis. There were several theoretical advantages to vitrectomy including the removal of the infecting organisms and their toxins, better distribution of antibiotics, clearing of tractional membranes that could lead to retinal detachment, clearing of opacities in the vitreous, and providing a good volume

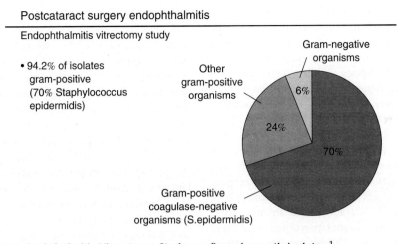

FIGURE 10.1 ☐ Endophthalmitis Vitrectomy Study confirmed growth isolates.[1]

of vitreous material for microbiologic culture. Before the EVS, small human studies were inconclusive regarding the benefits of vitrectomy and in previous studies it appeared that only the most advanced cases of endophthalmitis underwent vitrectomy. Therefore, visual outcomes were poor and it was uncertain if vitrectomy would yield superior outcomes in eyes with better presenting vision. In the late 1980s, the role of vitrectomy in the management of endophthalmitis remained quite controversial. During this time, the role and benefit of systemic intravenous antibiotics in the management of endophthalmitis was also uncertain. It was the "standard of care," yet it was questioned whether the theoretical benefit outweighed the systemic side effects of antibiotics used at the time. Additional factors included an analysis of the costs of the antibiotics and hospitalization for administration of these drugs. These unresolved issues served as the impetus for the largest prospective study on endophthalmitis management to date.[4]

Clinical centers in 25 US cities enrolled 420 patients over a 3½-year time frame. Entry criteria were stringent and were limited to patients who had a clinical diagnosis of endophthalmitis within 6 weeks of cataract extraction or secondary intraocular lens placement and had a vision worse than 20/50 but at least light perception. Additionally, patients were required to have a hypopyon and clouding of the anterior chamber or vitreous media sufficient to obscure clear visualization of second-order retinal arterioles. Patients who did not have a cornea and anterior chamber clear enough to visualize at least a portion of their iris were excluded. Furthermore,

the cornea needed to be clear enough to allow the possibility of pars plana vitrectomy.[4]

All eyes in the EVS underwent immediate cultures of the anterior chamber and vitreous. Intravitreal amikacin and vancomycin were administered, as were subconjunctival vancomycin and ceftazidime. Topical vancomycin, amikacin, and cycloplegics were administered in all patients as well.[1]

Patients were randomized to the following groups: (a) Three-port pars plana vitrectomy with intravenous antibiotics (ceftazidime and amikacin), (b) three-port pars plana vitrectomy without intravenous antibiotics, (c) vitreous tap with intravenous antibiotics, and (d) vitreous tap without intravenous antibiotics.[1] The vitreous tap could be performed with or without a cutting type instrument, with a tap defined as removal of <0.3 mL of vitreous fluid.

The EVS found no difference in outcomes between immediate three-port pars plana vitrectomy and vitreous tap/biopsy for patients with hand motion or better vision. For patients with a presenting visual acuity of only light perception, improved visual results occurred in the immediate three-port pars plana vitrectomy group as compared to the vitreous tap/biopsy group. These patients were three times more likely to achieve >20/40 vision (33% vs. 11%), two times more likely to achieve >20/100 vision (56% vs. 30%), and less likely to incur a vision <5/200 (20% vs. 47%). No difference in final visual acuity or media clarity was noted, whether or not systemic antibiotics were employed.[1]

Confirmed bacterial growth isolates were more likely to be positive in the vitreous compared to aqueous specimens. Figure 10.1 demonstrates that

94.2% of confirmed growth isolates were gram-positive organisms (the vast majority due to one organism alone *Staphylococcus epidermidis*—70%). Gram-negative organisms only comprised 5.9% of confirmed growth isolates. At the time of the EVS, all gram-positive organisms were sensitive to vancomycin. However, 2 of the 19 gram-negative organisms were resistant to both amikacin and ceftazidime.[5–8]

An analysis was performed to determine the causes of <20/40 vision after endophthalmitis. The following etiologies were found: Pigmentary degeneration of the macula (18%), macular edema (17%), unclear etiology (14%), and miscellaneous causes (10%). Epiretinal membranes, presumed optic nerve damage, corneal opacity, phthisis, posterior capsular opacity, retinal detachment, macular ischemia, and vitreous opacities each accounted for <10% of causes for <20/40 vision after endophthalmitis.[1]

A subset analysis of patients with diabetes included in the EVS resulted in two interesting findings. First, diabetes was associated with a higher yield of *Staphylococcus epidermidis*. Secondly, only 39% of patients with diabetes had a final visual outcome of >20/40 as compared with 55% of patients without diabetes. As a group, patients with diabetes fared worse and attained a less desirable visual outcome as compared with patients without diabetes.[1]

Retinal detachment occurred with an overall incidence of 8.3%. There was a minimal difference in the rates between the three-port vitrectomy group (7%) and the vitreous tap/biopsy group (9%). Retinal detachment repair was attempted in 66% of patients. The likelihood of obtaining a final visual outcome of >20/40 was 55% without a retinal detachment as compared with only 26% of patients who had a retinal detachment.[1]

The EVS answered some of the most controversial issues surrounding the management of endophthalmitis at the time. It was a well-designed study that utilized antibiotics that were the best available in the late 1980s. Additionally, the EVS taught us valuable information regarding the spectrum of causative organisms in postoperative endophthalmitis. The EVS clearly was a landmark study that provided ophthalmologists with evidence-based outcomes for managing postoperative endophthalmitis.

Potential New Treatment Regimens

Topical Fluoroquinolones

While topical antibiotics were not specifically studied in the EVS, they may soon play an increasingly important role in the management of and prophylaxis against ocular infection. In the early 1990s, topical ciprofloxacin was released as the first ophthalmic fluoroquinolone—this agent was embraced by corneal, cataract, and refractive surgeons as a powerful weapon against ocular infection. Other topical fluoroquinolones were subsequently released; however, some of our most powerful weapons have lost a portion of their effect because of increasing levels of resistant organisms each year, especially against the gram-positive organisms. A serious clinical problem could arise if current trends of resistance to older generation fluoroquinolones continue. The rise in resistant organisms has challenged empiric monotherapy, creating the need for newer topical antibiotics with a broader spectrum of coverage and less risk for resistance.

During the spring of 2003, topical gatifloxacin 0.3% (Zymar by Allergan Pharmaceuticals) and topical Moxifloxacin 0.5% (Vigamox by Alcon Laboratories) were released for clinical use (see Fig. 10.2). These fourth-generation fluoroquinolones have been engineered to be effective against a number of currently resistant organisms; thus, theoretically they should be able to delay the development of new resistant strains more effectively than their older-generation predecessors.

The structures of gatifloxacin and moxifloxacin give these drugs the capacity to delay resistance through a two-pronged approach that inhibits both the prokaryotic DNA gyrase and topoisomerase. The structure increases hydrophobicity, which decreases the resistance due to efflux pumps. Overall, the fourth-generation fluoroquinolones have enhanced gram-positive and atypical coverage while retaining gram-negative coverage, in a manner that is essentially identical to that of the older-generation flurorquinolones.[9]

Topical fourth-generation fluoroquinolones are poised to be a powerful weapon for the corneal, cataract, and refractive surgeon for various anterior segment indications. Unfortunately, there is limited data regarding the intraocular penetration of these new-generation agents in humans. Several prior studies of earlier-generation agents have demonstrated that topically administered agents do not achieve adequate intraocular concentrations to be effective against the pathogens most commonly responsible for bacterial endophthalmitis.[10]

We recently completed an investigation to determine the intraocular penetration of moxifloxacin

Fourth-generation fluoroquinolones

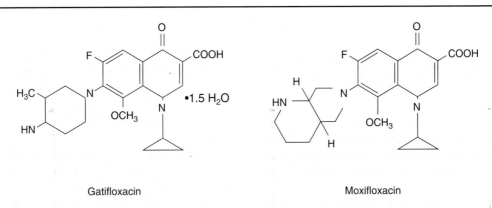

Gatifloxacin   Moxifloxacin

FIGURE 10.2 ☐ Graphic structures of gatifloxacin and moxifloxacin.

0.5% in humans to see if therapeutic concentrations of drug can be achieved in the aqueous and vitreous after topical administration.[11] In this study we obtained aqueous and vitreous samples in phakic, noninflamed eyes after topically administering moxifloxacin 0.5%, either every 2 hours (Q2H) or every 6 hours (Q6H), for 3 days before surgery. We found that mean moxifloxacin concentrations in the Q2H group for the aqueous ($n = 9$) and vitreous samples ($n = 10$) were 2.28 ± 1.23 μg per mL and 0.11 ± 0.05 μg per mL, respectively. Mean moxifloxacin concentrations in the Q6H group for the aqueous ($n = 10$) and vitreous ($n = 9$) samples were 0.88 ± 0.88 μg per mL and 0.06 ± 0.06 μg per mL, respectively (see Fig. 10.3). MIC_{90} levels (minimum inhibitory concentration of antibiotic required to kill 90% of isolates)

were far exceeded in the aqueous sample for a wide spectrum of key pathogens. Concentration of moxifloxacin in the vitreous did exceed the MIC_{90} for several organisms; however, the MIC_{50} (minimum inhibitory concentration of antibiotic required to kill 50% of isolates) was exceeded in the Q2H group for *S. epidermidis, Staphylococcus aureus, Streptococcus pneumoniae, Haemophilus influenzae, Bacillus cereus*, and other gram-negative organisms.

Further studies will determine the precise role of topically administered moxifloxacin 0.5% in the management and/or prophylaxis of intraocular infections. This data may be of significance when considering prophylaxis against the development of infection in such settings as an intravitreal injection of corticosteroids or antiproliferative agents.

Topical moxifloxacin 0.5%

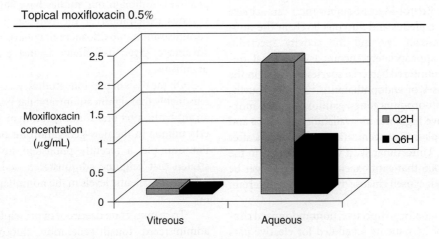

FIGURE 10.3 ☐ Intraocular concentrations of moxifloxacin after topical administration (Q2H = one drop every 2 hours for 3 days, Q6H = one drop every 6 hours for 3 days).[11]

Oral and Intravenous Antibiotics

While intravitreal antibiotic injections are clearly the most effective way to achieve therapeutic antibiotic levels in the vitreous, the use of certain orally administered antibiotics can be a potential alternative/adjunct as they have been shown to achieve vitreous concentrations exceeding the MIC_{90} level for the organisms most commonly involved in bacterial endophthalmitis. Hence, the use of oral antibiotics has important implications for the ophthalmologist, particularly in the prophylaxis and/or management of postoperative, posttraumatic, or bleb-associated bacterial endophthalmitis.

As previously noted, the EVS investigated the use of intravenous amikacin and ceftazidime in conjunction with intravitreal antibiotic injection for managing acute postoperative endophthalmitis and found no improved outcomes with the use of systemic antibiotics.[1] According to studies published later, amikacin and ceftazidime were found to have very limited intravitreal penetration.[2,3] Therefore, the only conclusion that can be inferred from the EVS data regarding systemic antibiotic use is that intravenous amikacin and ceftazidime specifically have no apparent role in managing postoperative endophthalmitis. Therefore, do EVS data still apply, given the recent advancements in the development of antimicrobials? The answer is, most likely, it does not.

Over the past 10 years there has been mounting evidence in the literature that agents in the fluoroquinolone class of antibiotics are able to achieve effective concentrations in the vitreous after oral administration (see Table 10.1).[12–14] Our group has reported that orally administered gatifloxacin (Tequin by Bristol-Myers Squibb, Inc.) can achieve therapeutic aqueous and vitreous levels in the noninflamed human eye and the activity spectrum appears to appropriately encompass the most frequently encountered bacterial species involved in the various causes of endophthalmitis.[12,13] The fourth-generation fluoroquinolones, gatifloxacin, and moxifloxacin have high oral bioavailability of >90% and reach peak plasma concentrations 1 to 2 hours after oral dosing. Unfortunately, it was announced in the spring of 2006 that gatifloxacin would no longer be marketed as it caused glucose dysregulation in certain patients.

We designed a prospective, nonrandomized clinical study of 24 patients scheduled for elective pars plana vitrectomy surgery to investigate the aqueous and vitreous concentration of gatifloxacin achieved after oral administration of two 400 mg tablets taken 12 hours apart before surgery. The percentages of plasma gatifloxacin concentration achieved in the vitreous and aqueous were 26.17% and 21.02%, respectively. Mean inhibitory vitreous and aqueous MIC_{90} levels were achieved against a wide spectrum of bacteria (e.g., the vitreous concentration of gatifloxacin achieved with this dosing regimen exceeded the MIC_{90} for *S. epidermidis* by >fivefold).

Garcia-Saenz et al. reported that orally administered moxifloxacin (Avelox by Bayer) can achieve therapeutic levels in the human aqueous; however, vitreous concentration data were not obtained in this study.[17] To address this, we designed a second prospective, nonrandomized clinical study of 15 patients scheduled for elective pars plana vitrectomy surgery to investigate the aqueous and vitreous concentration of moxifloxacin achieved after oral administration of two 400 mg tablets taken 12 hours apart before surgery. The percentages of plasma moxifloxacin concentration achieved in the vitreous and aqueous were 37.6% and 44.3%, respectively. Mean inhibitory vitreous and aqueous MIC_{90} levels were achieved against a wide spectrum of bacteria.[15]

Moxifloxacin has an inherent advantage over gatifloxacin for gram-positive organisms. Table 10.1 reviews the mean vitreous penetration of several fluoroquinolones along with their respective MIC_{90} levels for the organisms we are most concerned about in endophthalmitis. Upon reviewing this table, it is readily apparent that moxifloxacin has roughly 50% lower MIC_{90} levels compared to gatifloxacin for gram positives. Although our studies have shown similar vitreous penetration of the two agents after oral administration, moxifloxacin may have a theoretical advantage, given its activity against gram-positive organisms.

On the basis of previous studies, we can conclude reasonably that significant intraocular penetration of an antibiotic after oral administration may be a property unique to the new-generation fluroquinolones. For example, a recently published study demonstrated that cefipime administered orally does not achieve therapeutic levels in the noninflamed human eye.[18]

To demonstrate the proof of principle that orally administered fourth-generation fluoroquinolones could be used to treat intraocular infection in humans, we assessed the use of oral gatifloxacin

TABLE 10.1 ☐ *In vitro* **Susceptibilities of Moxifloxacin, Gatifloxacin, Levofloxacin, Ofloxacin, and Ciprofloxacin Showing Minimum Inhibitory Concentration at Which 90% of Isolates are Inhibited (μg/mL)**[a]

	Moxifloxacin[15]	Gatifloxacin[12]	Levofloxacin[14]	Ofloxacin[10]	Ciprofloxacin[16]
Mean vitreous penetration	1.34 ± 0.66	1.34 ± 0.34	2.39 ± 0.70	0.43 ± 0.47	0.56 ± 0.16
	μg/mL	μg/mL	μg/mL	μg/mL	μg/mL
Gram-positive organisms					
Staphylococcus epidermidis	0.13	0.25	0.50	0.50	1.00
Staphylococcus aureus (MSSA)	0.06	0.13	0.25	0.50	0.50
Streptococcus pneumoniae	0.25	0.50	2.00	2.00	2.00
Streptococcus pyogenes	0.25	0.50	1.00	2.00	1.00
Bacillus cereus	0.13[b]	0.25	–	0.50	–
Enterococcus faecalis	1.00	2.00	2.00	4.00	4.00
Gram-negative organisms					
Proteus mirabilis	0.25	0.25	0.25	0.125	0.06
Pseudomonas aeruginosa	32.0	32.0	32.0	4.00	0.78
Haemophilus influenzae	0.06	0.016	0.06	4.00	0.016
Escherichia coli	0.008	0.008	0.03	0.125	0.016
Klebsiella pneumoniae	0.13	0.13	0.13	0.50	0.06
Neisseria gonorrhoeae	0.016	0.016	0.016	0.06	0.008
Anerobic organisms					
Bacteroides fragilis	2.00	1.00	2.00	4.00	8.00
Propionibacterium acnes	0.25[b]	0.50	0.75	1.50	–

[a] MIC_{90} data are from Bauernfeind,[11] Osato et al.[12] and Ednie et al.[13]
[b] On file, Alcon Laboratories, Inc. Shaded = fourth-generation fluoroquinolones.
–Data not available
MSSA, methicillin-sensitive *S. aureus*.

in the treatment of localized filtering bleb infection in six consecutive patients with blebitis. These six patients were treated with oral gatifloxacin 400 mg tablets for 1 week (b.i.d. loading dose for 1 day followed by q.d. thereafter) in conjunction with a topically administered antibiotic q.i.d. (ofloxacin, ciprofloxacin, fortified ceftazidime, or fortified tobramicin). Excluded were those patients with frank bleb-associated endophthalmitis. Cultures of the superior conjunctiva were obtained in two patients revealing *S. pneumoniae* in one and *S. aureus* in the other. All patients had prompt resolution of bleb purulence, none developed clinical features of endophthalmitis, and all patients tolerated the treatment regimen well.[19]

The ideal oral anti-infective agent has several characteristics: It offers a broad spectrum of coverage for the organisms of concern, is bactericidal, is well tolerated, has excellent bioavailability with oral administration, and has rapid kill curves. We believe that these properties are intrinsic to the fourth-generation fluoroquinolones. Experience with these agents over time and further investigations will help elucidate the precise role of oral antibiotics in the management of endophthalmitis.

Oral and Intravitreal Antifungal Agents

Although fungal endophthalmitis is rare in the grand scheme of intraocular infection, it remains an important clinical problem in ophthalmology because of the potentially devastating consequences resulting from these infections. Additionally, ocular fungal infections have traditionally been very difficult to treat because of limited therapeutic options both systemically and intravitreally.

In the past few years there have been major strides in the development of antifungal agents, and their potential use in the treatment of fungal endophthalmitis needs to be explored. The new-generation triazoles such as voriconazole, posaconazole, and ravuconazole represent advances in the evolution of the triazole antifungal class and have been developed to address the increasing incidence of fungal infections and the limitations of the currently available agents.[20,21]

Voriconazole (VFend by Pfizer Pharmaceuticals) is a second-generation synthetic derivative of fluconazole. It was developed by Pfizer Pharmaceuticals as part of a program designed to enhance the potency and spectrum of activity of fluconazole (i.e., *in vitro* potency of voriconazole against yeasts is 60-fold higher than that of fluconazole). Voriconazole differs from fluconazole because of the addition of a methyl group to the propyl backbone and the substitution of a triazole moiety with a fluoropyrimidine group resulting in a marked change in activity (see Fig. 10.4). Voriconazole has 96% oral bioavailability and reaches peak plasma concentrations 2 to 3 hours after oral dosing. Previous *in vitro* studies have shown voriconazole to have a broad spectrum of fungistatic action against *Aspergillus* species, *Blastomyces dermatitidis*, *Candida* species, *Paecilomyces lilacinus*, *Coccidioides immitis*, *Cryptococcus neoformans*, *Histoplasma capsulatum*, *Penicillium* species, *Scedosporium* species, *Curvularia* species, and others.[20,21]

We designed a prospective, nonrandomized clinical study of 14 patients scheduled for elective pars plana vitrectomy surgery to investigate the aqueous and vitreous concentration achieved after oral administration of two 400 mg doses of voriconazole taken 12 hours apart before surgery. The percentages of plasma voriconazole concentration achieved in the vitreous and aqueous were 38.1% and 53.0%,

respectively. Mean inhibitory vitreous and aqueous MIC_{90} levels were achieved against a wide spectrum of yeasts and molds (e.g., the vitreous concentration of voriconazole achieved with this dosing regimen exceeded the MIC_{90} for *Candida albicans* by over 13-fold).[22] To determine if voriconazole could be used safely for intravitreal injection, our group also performed a histopathologic and electroretinographic study using a rodent model. Our studies demonstrated that voriconazole did not cause retinal toxicity on either electroretinogram (ERG) or histology studies when intravitreal concentrations were 25 μg per mL or less. This represents a level of antibiotic that is 50-fold greater than commonly encountered MIC_{90} levels. When the concentration reached 50 μg per mL, focal retinal necrosis was occasionally noticed on histologic examination (see Fig. 10.5).[23] While further studies are obviously needed to delineate the appropriate level of voriconazole to use in humans, we have utilized this agent in select cases alone or with another novel intravenous antifungal (caspofungin), without evidence of apparent toxicity.[24]

Orally administered voriconazole achieves therapeutic aqueous and vitreous levels in the noninflamed human eye and the activity spectrum appears to appropriately encompass the most frequently encountered fungal species involved in the various causes of exogenous and endogenous fungal endophthalmitis. In addition, oral or intravitreal voriconazole may present an alternate management technique for fungal endophthalmitis by which the risk of retinal toxicity associated with intravitreal amphotericin-B injection can be avoided.[25] Because of its broad spectrum of coverage, low MIC_{90} levels for the organisms of concern, good tolerability, and excellent bioavailability with oral administration,

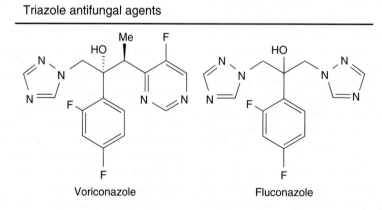

Triazole antifungal agents

Voriconazole   Fluconazole

FIGURE 10.4 ☐ Graphic structures of voriconazole and fluconazole.

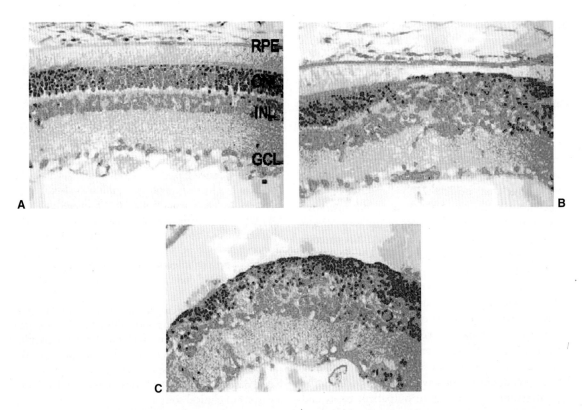

FIGURE 10.5 □ Intravitreal voriconazole toxicity in the rodent model. No retinal abnormalities were observed in group A (5 μg/mL, 10 μg/mL, 25 μg/mL) compared with control eyes injected with a balanced salt solution. Occasional small foci of retinal necrosis were observed in the outer retinal layers in group B (50 μg/mL). Occasional foci of more obvious photoreceptor degeneration and retinal disorganization were observed in group C (500 μg/mL).[23] RPE, retinal pigment epithelium; ONL, outer nerve fiber layer; INL, inner nerve fiber layer; GCL, ganglion cell layer.

voriconazole may be useful to the ophthalmologist in the primary treatment of intraocular fungal infections or as an adjunct in its current management.

Intraocular Corticosteroids

The precise role that intraocular or systemic corticosteroids play in managing the various settings and etiologies of endophthalmitis remains unclear at the present time. The use of intravitreal corticosteroids was excluded from the EVS, as it was controversial at that time, and still is. The results of a survey taken in 1998 at the American Academy of Ophthalmology revealed no consensus among ophthalmologists regarding the use of corticosteroids for endophthalmitis management. There are several theoretical benefits of corticosteroid use. Corticosteroids inhibit macrophage and neutrophil migration to the area of inflammation, reduce vascular permeability, and block the release of inflammatory mediators.

Shah et al. retrospectively investigated visual outcomes between patients with acute postoperative endophthalmitis that did or did not receive intravitreal corticosteroids and found that patients who received intravitreal corticosteroids had a significantly reduced likelihood of obtaining a three-line improvement in visual acuity. While the results are most likely predicated by case selection (corticosteroids may have been employed in cases where the surgeon felt the infection was more severe), their study does not provide support for the use of corticosteroids in the postoperative setting.[26] Das et al. evaluated the efficacy of intravitreal dexamethasone in the management of exogenous bacterial endophthalmitis. They reported that intravitreal dexamethasone aided in the early reduction of inflammation; however, its use had no independent influence on final visual outcome.[27]

At the present time the use of corticosteroids in the management of endophthalmitis remains unresolved and its use appears to be primarily based on clinical judgment and the surgeon's preference. It is not clear if this issue will ever be adequately studied in a controlled clinical trial.

Inpatient Versus Outpatient Management

As the ophthalmic community develops new treatment strategies for the management of endophthalmitis, we must all take cognizance of the cost-sensitive environment in which we work. The EVS found that hospitalization and the use of intravenous antibiotics for managing postoperative endophthalmitis alone cost tens of millions of dollars annually.[28] The EVS initially hoped that vitreous taps/biopsies would be performed outside of an operating room environment, thereby resulting in significant cost savings. As it turns out, many taps were performed in surgical operating rooms, therefore an analysis of true cost savings could not be ascertained.

Over the past several years, however, there has been a shift in the management of eye disease from the inpatient to the outpatient setting. When managing bacterial endophthalmitis, we routinely perform the tap/vitrectomy surgery on an outpatient basis, and send the patient home on oral moxifloxacin along with a topical fourth-generation fluoroquinolone. The literature does not support the use of any intravenous agent in the setting of endophthalmitis, even including antifungals such as amphotericin-B for fungal endophthalmitis, as therapeutic intravitreal levels are not achieved.[29] Therefore, hospitalization should be considered only in extenuating circumstances (i.e., noncompliance or very aggressive infection). From a socioeconomic standpoint, the shift of managing endophthalmitis from an inpatient to outpatient setting is a sensible one, which does not appear to compromise clinical outcome.

Conclusion

In the past 20 years, numerous significant advances have undoubtedly been made in the treatment of endophthalmitis, initially culminating with the employment of intravitreal antibiotics. The EVS provided us with excellent evidence-based data regarding visual and anatomic outcomes when comparing complete pars plana vitrectomy with vitreous tap. Both groups of patients received intravitreal antibiotics. Results were shown to be equal, if the presenting visual acuity was hand motions or better, otherwise vitrectomy was the favored procedure.

There have been significant advances in the development of new-generation antibiotics also. These agents, in particular the fourth-generation fluoroquinolones, are already playing a key role in the management of ocular infection, as well as in the prophylaxis against infection. However, there are numerous unresolved issues.

We need to rethink the applicability of the EVS data, given the availability of these "new weapons in the arsenal of ophthalmic antibiotics."[9] So while we do have evidence-based data from the EVS, with time the data has lost some of its significance, because of the new developments noted in the preceding text. Our next step is to develop new strategies for the management of intraocular infection utilizing these new fluoroquinolone agents, with a goal of limiting the impact of proven infection, or ideally eliminating the development of endophthalmitis in a cost-effective manner.

Even with the advancements over the past decade, unparalleled opportunities for the prevention and/or reduction of morbidity from intraocular infection continue to exist. While we would truly like to base all our therapeutic decisions on evidence-based data, we will still be forced to rely on data from a variety of clinical sources.

References

1. Endophthalmitis Vitrectomy Study Group. Results of the endophthalmitis vitrectomy Study: A randomized trial of immediate vitrectomy and of intravenous antibiotics for the treatment of postoperative bacterial endophthalmitis. *Arch Ophthalmol.* 1995;113:1479–1496.
2. el-Massry A, Meredith TA, Aguilar HE, et al. Aminoglycoside levels in the rabbit vitreous cavity after intravenous administration. *Am J Ophthalmol.* 1996;122:684–689.
3. Aguilar HE, Meredith TA, Shaarawy A, et al. Vitreous cavity penetration of ceftazidime after intravenous administration. *Retina.* 1995;15:154–159.
4. Doft BH. The endophthalmitis vitrectomy study. *Arch Ophthalmol.* 1991;109:487–489.
5. Han DP, Wisniewski SR, Wilson LA, Barza M, Vine AK, Doft BH, Kelsey SF, The EVS Group. Spectrum and susceptibilities of microbiologic isolates in the EVS. *Am J Ophthalmol.* 1996;122:1–17.
6. Endophthalmitis Vitrectomy Study Group. Microbiologic factors and visual outcomes in

The Endophthalmitis Vitrectomy Study. *Am J Ophthalmol.* 1996;122:830–846.

7. Johnson MW, Doft BH, Kelsey SF, et al. The Endophthalmitis Vitrectomy Study. Relationship between clinical presentation and microbiologic spectrum. *Ophthalmology.* 1997;104: 261–272.

8. Bannerman TL, Rhoden DL, McAllister SK, et al. The source of coagulase-negative staphylococci in the Endophthalmitis Vitrectomy Study: A comparison of eyelid and intraocular isolates using pulsed-field gel electrophoresis. *Arch Ophthalmol.* 1997;115:357–361.

9. Mather R, Karanchak LM, Romanowski EG, Fourth generation fluoroquinolones: New weapons in the arsenal of ophthalmic antibiotics. *Am J Ophthalmol.* 2002; 133:463–466.

10. Fiscella RG, Shapiro MJ, Solomon MJ, et al. Ofloxacin penetration into the eye after intravenous and topical administration. *Retina.* 1997;17:535–539.

11. Hariprasad SM, Blinder KJ, Shah GK, et al. Penetration pharmacokinetics of topically administered 0.5% moxifloxacin ophthalmic solution in human aqueous and vitreous. *Arch Ophthalmol.* 2005;123:39–44.

12. Hariprasad SM, Mieler WF, Holz ER. Vitreous and aqueous penetration of orally administered Gatifloxacin in humans. *Arch Ophthalmol.* 2003;121:345–350.

13. Hariprasad SM, Mieler WF, Holz ER. Vitreous penetration of orally administered Gatifloxacin in humans. *Tr Am Ophthalmol Soc.* 2002;100:153–160.

14. Fiscella RG, Nguyen TK, Cwik MJ, et al. Aqueous and vitreous penetration of levofloxacin after oral administration. *Ophthalmology.* 1999;106:2286–2290.

15. Hariprasad SM, Shah GK, Mieler WF, et al. Vitreous and aqueous penetration of orally administered moxifloxacin in humans. *Arch Ophthalmol.* 2006;124:178–182.

16. Keren G, Alhalel A, Bartov E, et al. The intravitreal penetration of orally administered ciprofloxacin in humans. *Invest Ophthalmol Vis Sci.* 1991;32:2388–2392.

17. Garcia-Saenz MC, Arias-Puente A, Fresnadillo-Martinez MJ, Human aqueous humor levels of oral ciprofloxacin, levofloxacin, and moxifloxacin. *J Cataract Refract Surg.* 2001;27: 1969–1974.

18. Aras C, Ozdamar A, Ozturk R, et al. Intravitreal penetration of Cefepime after systemic administration to humans. *Ophthalmologica.* 2002;216:261–264.

19. Hariprasad SM, Mieler WF, Orengo-Nania S, et al. The use of oral Gatifloxacin in the treatment of localized filtering bleb infections. In review.

20. Ghannoum MA, Kuhn DM. Voriconazole-better chances for patients with invasive mycoses. *Eur J Med Res.* 2002;7:242–256.

21. Sabo JA, Abdel-Rahman SM. Voriconazole: A new triazole antifungal. *Ann Pharmacother.* 2000;34:1032–1043.

22. Hariprasad SM, Mieler WF, Holz ER, et al. Determination of vitreous, aqueous, and plasma concentration of orally administered Voriconazole in humans. *Arch Ophthalmol.* 2004;122: 42–47.

23. Gao H, Pennesi M, Shah K, et al. Safety of intravitreal voriconazole- histopathologic and electroretinographic study. *Tr Am Ophthalmol Soc.* 2003;101:183–189.

24. Breit SM, Hariprasad SM, Mieler WF, et al. Management of endogenous fungal endophthalmitis with voriconazole and caspofungin. *Am J Ophthalmol.* 2005;139:135–140.

25. Axelrod AJ, Peyman GA, Apple DJ. Toxicity of intravitreal injection of amphotericin B. *Am J Ophthalmol.* 1973;76:578–583.

26. Shah GK, Stein JD, Sharma S, et al. Visual outcomes following the use of intravitreal steroids in the treatment of postoperative endophthalmitis. *Ophthalmology.* 2000;107:486–489.

27. Das T, Jalali S, Gothwal VK, et al. Intravitreal dexamethasone in exogenous bacterial endophthalmitis: Results of a prospective randomized study. *Br J Ophthalmol.* 1999;83:1050–1055.

28. Wisniewski SP, Hammer ME, Grizzard WS, et al. An investigation of the hospital charges related to the treatment of endophthalmitis in The Endophthalmitis Vitrectomy Study. *Ophthalmology.* 1997;104:739–745.

29. O'Day DM, Head WS, Robinson RD, et al. Intraocular penetration of systemically administered antifungal agents. *Curr Eye Res.* 1985;4: 131–134.

SECTION V

PEDIATRIC OPHTHALMOLOGY

CHAPTER 11

Retinopathy of Prematurity

Anna Ells, MD, FRCS (C)

Retinopathy of prematurity (ROP) is a vasoprolifera-tive retinopathy in infants who are born prematurely. It is the leading cause of preventable blindness in our pediatric population.[1,2] The degree of prematu-rity vulnerable to ROP varies between high human development countries (HHDC) and middle and low human development countries.[3] According to an electronic review of published studies in ROP, there have been 1,323 peer-reviewed articles published in the last 10 years and 795 published in the last 5 years. Both the basic and clinical sciences of ROP continue to have a great presence in ophthalmology and pedi-atrics. This chapter will review the landmark clinical trials in ROP in the last 20 years, which have provided much of the fundamental understanding and natural history of this disease.

Pathogenesis

ROP is multifactorial in origin, with prematurity of the retinal vasculature as a prerequisite. ROP does not occur in full-term infants. Normal vasculogenesis during early fetal development is determined by local "physiologic" hypoxia. This occurs as a consequence of increasing retinal thickness, which creates an increase in metabolic demand in advance of the development of intraretinal vessels. Astrocytes in this hypoxic vanguard respond by secreting vascular endothelial growth factor (VEGF) that promotes vascular development or angiogenesis, to meet this increasing metabolic demand.[4,5] Therefore, VEGF is secreted in response to physiologic hypoxia in the maturing avascular retina, just anterior to the

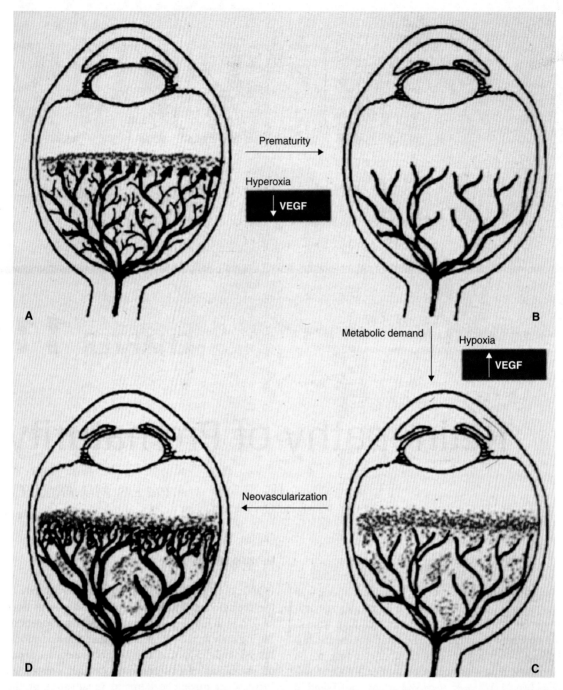

FIGURE 11.1 ☐ **A:** Neonatal resuscitation in the first few days of the premature infant's life results in a dramatic increase in the oxygen environment and subsequent hyperoxia. **B:** This hyperoxia causes vasospasm and shut down of sections of the retinal vasculature, resulting in retinal ischemia and capillary regression. **C:** The resultant retinal ischemia stimulates an overproduction of vascular endothelial growth factor (VEGF) causing, **D:** the neovascularization known as ROP. Pierce E, Foley E, Smith L. Regulation of vascular endothelial growth factor by oxygen in a model of retinopathy of prematurity. *Arch Ophthalmol.* 1996;114:1219-1228. Low IGF-I suppresses VEGF-survival signaling in retinal endothelial cells: Direct correlation with clinical retinopathy of prematurity. Hellstrom A, Perruzzi C, Ju M, et al. *Proc Natl Acad Sci U S A* 2001;98:5804–5808.

advancing retinal vessels, leading to normal retinal vessel vasculogenesis in a centripetal fashion from optic nerve to ora serrata. ROP, however, occurs as a result of an oxidative insult that impedes normal retinal vasculogenesis. Neonatal resuscitation in the first few days of the premature infant's life results in a dramatic increase in the oxygen environment and subsequent hyperoxia. This hyperoxia causes vasospasm and shut down of sections of the retinal vasculature, resulting in retinal ischemia and excessive capillary regression. The resultant retinal ischemia stimulates an overproduction of VEGF causing the neovascularization known as *ROP* (see Fig. 11.1).[5,6] Insulin-like growth factor-1 (IGF-1) has also been implicated in controlling VEGF activation, because when IGF-1 is low vessels do not grow. Thus, oxygen-independent IGF-1 and oxygen-dependent VEGF are complementary and synergistic.[7] Genetic factors, such as defects in Norrie's gene and Frizzled-4 gene, have also been implicated in the pathogenesis of ROP, and future studies in this area are in progress.[8,9] A recent study has provided evidence that some preterm babies may have a genetic predisposition toward greater production of VEGF,[10] which may have implications and opportunities for novel treatments such as the intravitreous injection of pegaptanib (Macugen, Eyetech Pharmaceuticals Inc) or other agents directed toward blocking the production-specific isoforms of VEGF within the premature eye.

International Classification for Retinopathy of Prematurity[11–13]

To understand and interpret information from clinical trials in ROP, the International Classification of ROP will first be reviewed.

1. *Location of retinopathy:* The retina is divided into three concentric circles or zones, centered on the optic disc (see Fig. 11.2). The lower the zone, the more severe the disease.

   a. Zone I—the posterior pole, consisting of a circle whose radius is twice the distance from the optic disc to the macula.

   b. Zone II—a doughnut shaped area of retina that extends from the edge of zone I to a position tangential to the nasal ora serrata and around an area near the temporal anatomic equator.

   c. Zone III—the outermost residual crescent of retina anterior to zone II.

2. *Severity of retinopathy:* The severity of the disease is attributed to the stage of the disease. The higher the stage, the more severe the disease.

   a. Stage 1: A demarcation line separating normal developing retina from avascular, peripheral retina

   b. Stage 2: Ridge of mesenchymal tissue with height and width in the region of the demarcation line

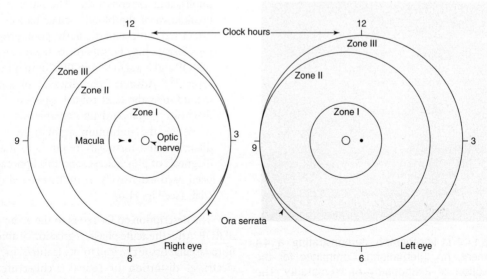

FIGURE 11.2 ■ Diagram illustrating zones and clock hours used in the classification of ROP. (The Committee for the Classification of Retinopathy of Prematurity. An International Classification of retinopathy of prematurity. *Arch Ophthalmol.* 1984;102:1130–1134.)

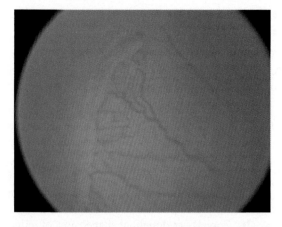

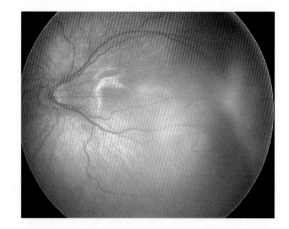

FIGURE 11.3 ◻ Photograph of the right eye highlighting stage 3 extra retinal fibrovascular proliferation and several "popcorn" lesions (stage 2). Note avascular retina anterior to the stage 3 retinopathy of prematurity.

FIGURE 11.5 ◻ Photograph demonstrating a 4B detachment. An International Committee for the Classification of Retinopathy of Prematurity. The international classification of retinopathy of prematurity revisited. *Arch Ophthalmol.* 2005;123: 991–999.

    c. Stage 3: The ridge develops extraretinal fibrovascular proliferation (EFP) or neovascularization (see Fig. 11.3)

    d. Stage 4: Partial retinal detachment

        i. Stage 4A—detachment that does not include the macula (see Fig. 11.4)

        ii. Stage 4B—detachment involves the macula (see Fig. 11.5)

    e. Stage 5: Complete retinal detachment

3. *Extent of retinopathy:* The extent of the disease is reported according to the circumferential accumulation of ROP, reported in clock hours in the appropriate zone.

4. *Plus disease:* Dilatation and/or tortuosity of posterior retinal vessels is present in at least two quadrants and may later increase in severity to include iris vascular engorgement, poor pupil dilation in response to medication (rigid pupil), and vitreous haze. The latter indicates breakdown of the blood–ocular barrier and is associated with a particularly poor prognosis. Plus disease may be superimposed on any stage of ROP and is a sign that ROP is, or may become, severe.[14,15] Advanced plus disease is obvious, but if mild, it is the least robust aspect of ROP to diagnose. A standard photograph can be used to define the minimum amount of vascular dilatation and tortuosity required to make the diagnosis of plus disease, and this approach has been used extensively in multicentered clinical trials (see Fig. 11.6)

The description so far refers to the acute phases of ROP. After the acute phase, regression of abnormal fibrovascular tissue can lead to late features, including cicatricial distortion of retinal architecture, with dragging of the retina usually toward the temporal retinal periphery and collapse of the temporal vessel arcade angle (see Fig. 11.7).[12]

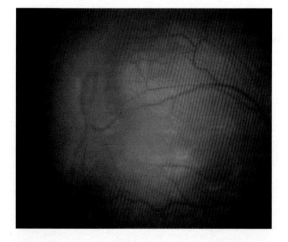

FIGURE 11.4 ◻ Photograph demonstrating a 4A detachment. An International Committee for the Classification of Retinopathy of Prematurity. The international classification of retinopathy of prematurity revisited. *Arch Ophthalmol.* 2005;123: 991–999.

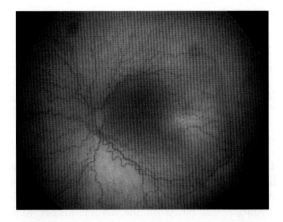

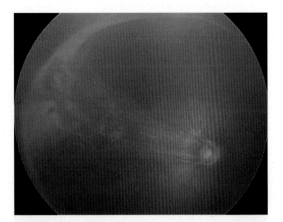

FIGURE 11.6 ☐ This photograph demonstrates vascular changes of the posterior pole vessels consistent with plus disease in all four quadrants. Note the zone I and temporal "flat" neovascularization and circumferential vessels, as seen in aggressive posterior retinopathy of prematurity (AP-ROP).

FIGURE 11.7 ☐ Wide-angle photograph of cicatricial ROP. Note the dragging of the retinal vessels and the significant collapse or narrowing of the temporal arcade angle. Also note the peripheral elevated fibrotic membrane, remnant of a stage-4B detachment, forming a macular fold. An International Committee for the Classification of Retinopathy of Prematurity. The international classification of retinopathy of prematurity revisited. *Arch Ophthalmol.* 2005;123:991–999

Revision of the International Classification of Retinopathy of Prematurity (2005)[13]

The 1984–1987 classification has recently been revisited and published for the first time, in its entirety. As a result of research and experiences gained over the past 20 years, the following amendments have been made:

1. Clarification of zone I. If the disc is seen at the edge of the retinal image when examining the retina with a 25 or 28 D lens, the approximate limit of zone I will be visualized at the opposite edge of the condensing lens.
2. Addition of pre-plus to the classification. Pre-plus is defined as increased dilation and/or tortuosity of retinal arteries and/or veins in at least two quadrants, which is not severe enough to meet the criteria of plus disease (see Fig. 11.8). Over time, the vessel abnormalities of pre-plus may progress to frank plus disease, or revert to normal.
3. Addition of "aggressive, posterior ROP" (AP-ROP). This is an uncommon form of ROP, which is severe and progresses rapidly to stages 4 and 5 if left untreated (see Figs. 11.9 and 11.10). AP-ROP has the following characteristics:
   a. Posterior location—usually zone I
   b. Plus disease without prominent ridge proliferation or classic stage 3
   c. Low-lying, tangled web of vessel (sometimes called "*flat neovascularization*")
   d. Typically extends circumferentially

Major Clinical Trials in Retinopathy of Prematurity

The Multicenter Trial of Cryotherapy for Retinopathy of Prematurity—1990

A multicenter randomized trial was conducted by the Cryotherapy for ROP Cooperative Group, which published its first outcome report in 1990.

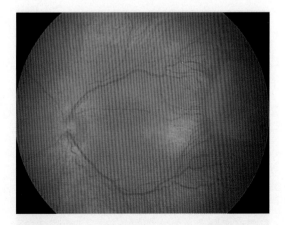

FIGURE 11.8 ☐ Photograph demonstrating pre-plus vascular changes in the temporal quadrants. Also note the "notch-type" configuration of stage 3 disease.

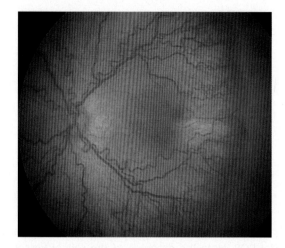

FIGURE 11.9 ◻ Photograph demonstrating AP-ROP (posterior, flat neovascularization, associated with plus disease in all four quadrants).

Study Questions

1. Does retinal ablation using cryotherapy of the peripheral avascular retina reduce the risk of significant visual loss (stage 4 or above; macular retinal fold; vision <20/200) in the treated eye?
2. Using natural history data from eyes, what are the factors associated with the development of severe ROP and unfavorable outcomes?

Inclusion Criteria

1. Birth weight <1,251 g
2. Survived at least 28 days

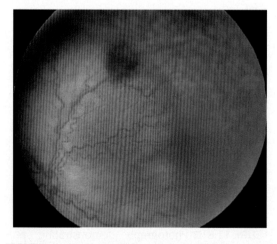

FIGURE 11.10 ◻ AP-ROP demonstrating near-confluent laser photocoagulation to the avascular retina.

Exclusion Criteria

1. The presence of lethal congenital abnormalities
2. Major ocular abnormalities
3. Progression beyond threshold disease in either eye, prior to randomization
4. Transfer of infant to a non-study hospital, or follow-up not feasible

Definition of Threshold Retinopathy of Prematurity

Threshold retinopathy of prematurity is defined as five continuous or 8 noncontinuous clock hours of stage-3 ROP, in the presence of plus disease. This definition was based on the natural history ROP data, indicating that there was a "threshold" amount of severe disease, which predictably resulted in significant cicatricial ROP and subsequent poor visual outcome.

Study Design

This is a multicenter randomized interventional study with a longitudinal natural history cohort. During serial biweekly or weekly ROP examinations, if both eyes developed "threshold ROP," one eye was randomized to receive treatment of the peripheral avascular retina for 360 degrees using cryotherapy and the fellow eye served as a control and did not receive treatment. If only one eye reached threshold ROP, then that eye was randomized to receive cryotherapy or to receive no treatment. Cryotherapy was performed within 72 hours of determination of threshold disease, to limit the risk of progression of disease to stage 4.

A detailed fundus examination was performed independently by two investigators at 3 and 12 months after cryotherapy and stereo photographs of the posterior pole and the anterior segment of the eye were then sent to a fundus photograph reading center where photographs were graded as depicting an "unfavorable outcome" or a "favorable outcome."

Unfavorable Outcome

An unfavorable **structural** outcome referred to a retinal fold involving the macula or retrolental tissue. An unfavorable **visual** outcome referred to the equivalent of Snellen visual acuity of <20/200. Visual acuity was measured using grating acuity and judged as poor compared to normal or blind.

Favorable Outcome

A favorable **structural** outcome referred to no retinal fold through the macula, with an attached retina. A favorable **visual** outcome referred to the equivalent of Snellen visual acuity of better than 20/200 using grating acuity and judged as normal or below normal for that particular age.

At later study examinations in verbal children, recognition visual acuity was used and unfavorable visual outcome was scored as <20/200.

Summary of Major Findings :

Major findings of the study are summarized (see Table 11.1)

1. Infants who reach "threshold ROP" should be treated because the risk of blindness is predicted to approach 50% at this level of disease severity. Of the control eyes, 50.6% were categorized as being blind or having low vision, whereas only 31.9% of the treated eyes showed acuity results in the blind or poor-vision category at the 1-year outcome.
2. Peripheral retinal ablation with cryotherapy reduced the incidence of retinal detachment by 50%, and reduced the incidence of an "unfavorable" visual outcome from 56.3% to 35.0% in treated eyes.
3. The average number of clock hours of stage 3, at the diagnosis of "threshold" was 9.6 in both treated and non-treated eyes.
4. Long-term follow-up of these children up to age 15 years confirms the continued benefits of treatment, but despite the best available treatment at that time, over 50% of children had a visual acuity of <20/200 in the treated eye at 10 years.[16] The proportion of eyes with visual acuity 20/200 or better was 25.9% in the control group and 48.9% in the treated group at the 15-year examination.

Implications for Clinical Practice

The question of whether ablation of the avascular retina with cryotherapy in the presence of a significant amount of EFP (threshold ROP) would prevent cicatricial ROP and the resultant loss of vision or blindness first led to the unification of the ROP classification and then the publication of the International Classification of ROP (ICROP). The Cryotherapy for ROP Cooperative Group was soon formed to study the question of treatment using cryotherapy for this potentially blinding disease. This clinical trial was not the first study addressing the treatment of ROP but it was the first multicenter randomized surgical clinical trial in the treatment of ROP.[20-23]

With the emerging technology of argon and diode lasers in treating other retinal diseases, publication of smaller studies demonstrating that ablation of the peripheral avascular retina reduced the likelihood of visual loss and blindness appeared in the literature in the early 1990s.[24-29] Soon laser photocoagulation for treatment of severe ROP quickly replaced cryotherapy in many centers throughout North America and the world. Transpupillary diode and argon retinal laser photocoagulation has subsequently been shown in small clinical studies to reduce the amount of myopia and improve visual outcomes from less pigment disruption in the macula, when compared to cryotherapy.[30,31]

An enormous amount of information about the natural history of ROP has been documented as the secondary objective of the CRYO-ROP study in the 1-, 5-, 10- and 15-year outcome reports. The salient points with clinical applications are summarized as follows:

1. *Age at onset of ROP:* ROP develops over a relatively narrow postmenstrual age (PMA) range

TABLE 11.1 ☐ Summary of the CRYO-ROP Outcomes Published to Date

CRYO-ROP Outcomes	1 year[17] Treated/Control	5.5 years[18] Treated/Control	10 years[16] Treated/Control	15 years[19] Treated/Control
Unfavorable structural outcome	25.1%/44.7%	26.9%/45.4%	27.2%/47.9%	30.0%/51.9%
Total retinal detachments	18.3%/33.0%	22.1%/38.6%	21.6%/41.4%	No data
Number of blind eyes	51%/80%	56%/85%	70%	69%
Unfavorable VA outcome	Recognition VA not measured at 1 y	47.1%/61.7%	44.4%/62.1%	44.7%/64.3%

VA, visual acuity.

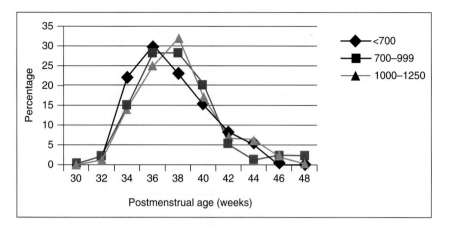

FIGURE 11.11 ◻ Graph showing the onset of threshold ROP by gestational age in the CRYO-ROP trial.[32]

and is related more to the stage of development of the infant, by PMA, than to the neonatal events (see Fig. 11.11).[32,33]

2. *Zone of involvement:* The propensity for severity is governed to a large extent by the state of retinal vascularization at birth so that zone is perhaps the most important predictor of outcome.[15,34] Therefore, incomplete vascularization in zone I carries a 54% risk of reaching the threshold but this falls to only 8% when vessels have reached zone II.

3. *Progression of disease* (see Fig. 11.12): The more premature the neonate, the more posterior the zone or location of the retinopathy and the

ROP status by gestational age

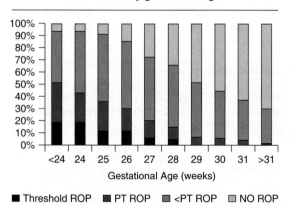

FIGURE 11.12 ◻ Graphic display of data from the natural history arm of the CRYO-ROP Study demonstrating progression of the disease. PT ROP, prethreshold ROP.

greater the potential for progression of disease. Therefore, zone I disease is very likely to progress to stage 3 needing treatment, but ROP confined entirely to zone III rarely requires treatment. As with the onset, the rate of progression is also governed predominantly by developmental age (i.e., PMA) rather than by postnatal age or neonatal events.[32] The median PMA at which the various stages develop is as follows: Stage 1, 34 weeks; stage 2, 35 weeks; stage 3, 36 weeks, and for threshold ROP, 37 weeks PMA. In the CRYO-ROP study, babies were randomized for treatment within 72 hours of diagnosis of threshold ROP, which was at a mean age of 37.7 weeks PMA (range 32 to 50 weeks).[17] This was confirmed by comparing the rate of progression in the CRYO-ROP and LIGHT-ROP trials.[35] It is important to note the extremes of this range. Subhani et al. (2001) reported threshold ROP at 31 weeks PMA, but almost all infants will develop severe ROP by 46.3 weeks PMA.[36] The no-treatment, natural history arm of the CRYO-ROP trial showed that once threshold develops there is progression to an unfavorable outcome in approximately 50% of eyes.

4. *Regression of ROP:* Most infants with stage 1 or 2 ROP will have spontaneous regression of the disease.[32,37] For infants born weighing <1,251 g, stage 1 ROP was the highest stage reached in 25.2% of infants, stage 2 ROP in 21.7%, and threshold in 6.0% of infants.[32]

Major Unanswered Questions or Limitations

1. Unfavorable outcome of visual acuity for the CRYO-ROP study was visual acuity <20/200 or structural outcome of macular fold, retrolental tissue or retinal detachment. Our management strategies in the new millennium aim for a favorable outcome of better than 20/40 visual acuity, preserved macular architecture, and minimal cicatricial peripheral retinal changes.[38,39]

2. Cryotherapy is no longer the primary modality of treatment for severe ROP.

3. "Threshold ROP" was the upper limit of severe disease beyond which blindness from retinal detachment and cicatricial ROP would occur. This was determined from a retrospective study and then used in the CRYO-ROP study.[40] According to the Early Treatment Trial for ROP (ET-ROP), it is not necessarily the amount of stage 3 disease that should determine the timing of treatment.[41]

Supplemental Therapeutic Oxygen for Prethreshold Retinopathy of Prematurity—A Randomized, Controlled Trial-2000[42]

Purpose of Study

To determine the efficacy and safety of supplemental therapeutic oxygen for infants with prethreshold ROP to reduce the probability of progression to threshold ROP.

Study Question

Does supplemental inspired oxygen therapy for premature infants at high risk for threshold disease, prevent the progression of disease? Are there any negative impacts from treating infants with higher oxygen levels?

Inclusion Criteria

Premature infants who reached prethreshold ROP in at least one eye and had a median pulse oximetry of <94% saturation (SaO_2) while breathing room air; no lethal anomalies; or congenital eye anomalies were included.

Study Definitions

1. *Threshold ROP:* Five continuous or eight non-continuous clock hours of stage 3 ROP in zone I or zone II, in the presence of plus disease.

2. *Prethreshold ROP:* Zone I ROP of any stage, less than threshold. Zone II, stage 3 ROP, less than threshold, or zone II, stage 2 ROP with plus disease.

Study Design

Multicenter, randomized, controlled clinical trial, comparing the effects of two oxygenation strategies on the progression of severe ROP. Infants with prethreshold disease ($n = 324$) were randomized to receive either supplemental or therapeutic inspired oxygen through nasal prongs titrated to an oxygen saturation of 96% to 99%, measured by pulse oximetry or conventional amounts of inspired oxygen ($n = 325$) to maintain target oxygen saturation levels of 89% to 94%.

Summary of Major Findings

1. There was a reduction in the rate of conversion from prethreshold ROP to threshold ROP from 48.5% for the conventional oxygen group down to 40.9% for the supplemental oxygen group. This was not a statistically significant result ($p = 0.032$).

2. There was a benefit for a subgroup of infants with prethreshold disease without plus disease. The conversion rate to threshold decreased from 46% in the conventional group to 32% in the supplemental oxygen group ($p = 0.004$).

3. Threshold disease took longer to develop in the supplemental oxygen group, suggesting an effect on the tempo of the disease, although this was not statistically significant.

4. Chronic lung disease was more common in infants randomized to supplemental oxygen (8.5% to 13.2%).

5. No adverse effect on ROP in the supplemental group was detected in the study.

Implications for Clinical Practice

1. The risks and benefits of supplemental oxygen for prethreshold ROP must be analyzed by the treating physicians for each infant. Infants without severe pulmonary disease with prethreshold ROP, without plus disease, may benefit from liberal use of inspired oxygen, without any additional risks to the infant.

2. If an infant requires supplemental oxygen for cardiac reasons, the increased levels can be given with the confidence that this will not have an adverse effect on the ROP.

Limitations

1. At most centers, two thirds of the prethreshold infants were excluded from the study for various

reasons. Infants were excluded if they had a pulse oximeter reading >94% at any time before enrollment. This establishes a potential study group with more severe prethreshold ROP (and lower birth weights and gestational ages) than the overall population of premature infants that reach prethreshold.[43]

2. Frequency of examinations in the STOP-ROP study was every 2 weeks before the development of prethreshold ROP. If weekly examinations had been performed, prethreshold ROP may have been detected at an earlier phase. Later detection of prethreshold ROP in the study may have had an impact on the outcomes.[43]

3. The majority of STOP-ROP infants in the supplemental oxygen group were maintained at a median pulse oximetry level of 96% or 97% (80% of infants). Only 1% of infants in the therapeutic group had a median pulse oximetry of 99%.[43]

Early Treatment for Retinopathy of Prematurity Study—2003[41]

Purpose of Study

To determine whether earlier treatment with retinal laser ablation in high-risk prethreshold ROP leads to improved visual function and improved retinal structure outcomes as compared with treatment at conventional threshold ROP.

Study Question

Does the treatment of ROP at an earlier stage than conventional threshold ROP improve structural and visual outcomes as compared to conventional timing of treatment?

Inclusion Criteria

1. Infants with birth weights <1,251 g
2. Development of prethreshold ROP

Definitions

1. *Prethreshold ROP:* Zone I, any stage ROP, less than threshold; zone II, stage 2, with plus disease or stage 3 without plus disease; zone II, stage 3 with plus disease, but less than the threshold
2. *Threshold ROP:* Zone I or zone II, with five continuous or 8 noncontinuous clock hours (30-degree sectors) of stage 3 ROP, in the presence of plus disease (see Fig. 11.13).

3. *Risk-Model for ROP Treatment-Risk-Model Retinopathy of Prematurity (RM-ROP):* Theoretical model based on infant risk factors used to assign risk of blindness without treatment. Risk factors observed about the infant and retina are correlated with the structural outcome. The model consists of five mathematical equations converted into a risk analysis computer program, on the basis of data from the CRYO-ROP study.[44,45]

4. Favorable visual outcome at a corrected age of 9 months was defined as vision better than 1.85 cycles per degree, using Teller Acuity testing. An unfavorable visual outcome was defined as vision worse than 1.85 cycles per degree, light perception or no light perception.

5. An unfavorable structural outcome at 6 and 9 months of corrected age was defined as: (i) Posterior retinal fold involving the macula (ii) Retinal detachment involving the macula (iii) Retrolental mass or tissue obscuring the view of the posterior pole.

Study Design

The Risk Management model for ROP (RM-ROP) was used to determine the theoretical risk of progression to an unfavorable outcome in the absence of treatment. This model is based on CRYO-ROP natural history data. RM-ROP "low-risk" prethreshold disease was defined as having a <15% risk of progression to unfavorable outcome if not treated and "high-risk" prethreshold disease was defined as having a >15% risk of progression to unfavorable outcome if not treated. Prethreshold eyes that were determined to have RM-ROP "high-risk" disease were therefore randomized to early treatment or conventional timing of treatment and RM-ROP "low-risk" infants continued to be screened for conventional timing of treatment (waiting until traditional threshold ROP occurred). Eight hundred and twenty-eight infants enrolled in the study reached prethreshold disease in one or both eyes and were analyzed using the RM-ROP-II model. Three hundred and twenty-nine infants were determined to have "low-risk" prethreshold disease and were not randomized, but continued to be screened. Four hundred and ninety-nine infants were determined to have "high-risk" prethreshold disease and were therefore eligible for randomization to early laser treatment or conventional treatment. If bilateral "high-risk" prethreshold disease was present, one eye was assigned to receive laser treatment within 48 hours and the fellow eye was followed up carefully and given treatment only if conventional "threshold" ROP developed. If unilateral "high-risk" prethreshold disease was present, that eye was randomized either to treatment within 48 hours or conventional management. If infants developed threshold ROP prior to randomization, they were excluded from the study.

Summary of Major Findings

1. At 9 months of postmenstrual age of follow-up, early treatment using Type I criteria reduced unfavorable visual outcomes from 19.5% to 14.5% (primary outcome) and reduced unfavorable structural outcome from 15.6% to 9.1% (secondary outcome); both were statistically significant.

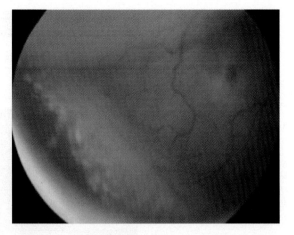

FIGURE 11.13 □ Photograph demonstrating confluent stage 3 ROP immediately following diode laser photocoagulation.

2. Using the RM-ROP 2 algorithm, 136 eyes with "high-risk" prethreshold ROP would have had favorable outcomes without treatment but would have been treated. In addition, 140/372 of "high-risk" eyes randomized to conventional treatment did not go on to the threshold. To address the concerns of "overtreatment," the study data were analyzed to identify "clinical" subgroups at high risk for progression to severe disease with unfavorable outcome that benefited from early treatment and another group that benefited from conventional treatment timing. These subgroups were termed Type I (early treatment) and Type II ROP (conventional ROP treatment timing). Because of the use of these clinical subtypes instead of the RM-ROP-II model, there would be a 35% reduction of eyes treated, while ensuring favorable outcomes.

Type I (Early treatment) Clinical Characteristics:

a. Zone I, any ROP with plus disease
b. Zone I, stage 3 with or without plus disease
c. Zone II, stage 2 or 3 with plus disease

Type II (Conventional treatment) Clinical Characteristics:

a. Zone I, stage 1 or 2 without plus disease
b. Zone II, stage 3 without plus disease

Implications for Clinical Practice

1. If one waits for CRYO-ROP threshold ROP definition, 6% of infants would require treatment;

if one were to add RM-ROP-II algorithm to the prethreshold definition, 9% of infants would require treatment and using ET-ROP Type 1 and 2 criteria (ICROP based), 8% of infants would likely require treatment.

2. Treat infants within 48 hours of observation of ET-ROP Type I clinical characteristics to maximize favorable anatomical outcomes.

3. Observe frequently for progression of ET-ROP Type II ROP. Surveillance or screening may be required as often as two times per week, in the presence of prethreshold criteria that do not meet Type I ET-ROP criteria for early treatment (see Fig. 11.14).[31]

4. Caveat: Use clinical judgment for the extent of stage 3, birth weight, and gestational age of the infant.

Major Unanswered Questions or Limitations

1. ET-ROP treatment decision is driven by the presence of plus disease; however, plus disease may be a relatively "soft" clinical sign.

   a. Clinical diagnosis of plus disease may vary from observer to observer and the inter-rater reliability has not been well studied.

   b. A standard photograph was used in the study to determine the presence of plus disease. This is not an objective measure and does not ensure accuracy or reproducibility.

   c. We are not able to objectively determine or quantify plus disease as yet, although

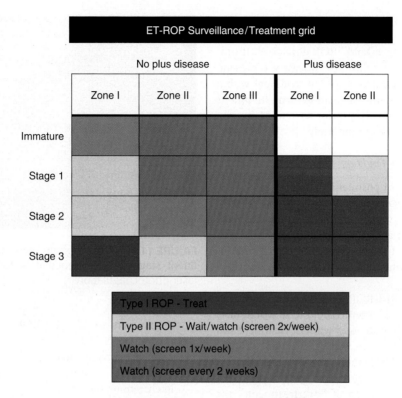

FIGURE 11.14 □ ET-ROP recommended surveillance and treatment grid.

recommendation of timing of intervention depends heavily on this clinical characteristic of severe disease.

d. No photographic documentation of plus disease was performed in the study although determination of prethreshold and threshold disease was confirmed by two study investigators.

2. ET-ROP type I and II criteria do not take into account the extent of stage 3 disease present; yet much of the clinical study and management decisions of the last 20 years have been based on the quantification of stage-3 disease. The ET-ROP study did not analyze the extent of stage-3 disease, as it related to the timing of the intervention. How then does the determination of "threshold ROP" for conventional timing of treatment relate to Type I criteria? There are some unanswered questions and relationships still to be studied.

3. A favorable visual outcome in both the CRYO-ROP and ET-ROP studies is defined as vision better than 20/200 or lack of macular fold. On the basis of other reports, a more reasonable favorable outcome for eyes treated for severe ROP should be a visual acuity of 20/50 or better with preservation of macular architecture.[30,46,47]

4. Timing of intervention may not be the only critical management factor in preventing visual loss from severe ROP. Data from longer follow-up periods may demonstrate factors other than the timing of the intervention, which may prevent visual loss.

Summary of Other Clinical Trials in Retinopathy of Prematurity that are Noteworthy

1. Lack of Efficacy of Light Reduction in Preventing Retinopathy of Prematurity (Light-ROP; 1998)[48] demonstrated that light reduction within the first 24 hours of birth until 31 weeks of postmenstrual age had no significant effect on the development of ROP or the conversion of prethreshold ROP to threshold ROP.

2. Vitamin E Meta-analysis of 6 controlled Clinical Trials[49] summarized data analysis from infants randomized to receiving vitamin E supplementation or not. No statistically significant difference

in the development of ROP was found between these two groups.

3. Evidence-Based Screening Criteria for Retinopathy of Prematurity—Natural History Data from the CRYO-ROP and Light-ROP Studies[35] is a report of compiled data from two prospective clinical trials in order to determine the approximate date for the initial ROP screening examination. The study recommended that the first examination should be at 31 weeks postmenstrual age or 4 weeks of chronological age, whichever is later.

4. Can Changes in Clinical Practice Decrease the Incidence of Severe Retinopathy of Prematurity in Very Low Birth Weight Infants:[50] This is a prospective study that reported a dramatic decrease (4.5% to 0%) in premature infants requiring laser photocoagulation for severe disease, after implementing early oxygen curtailment and enforcement of strict oxygen guidelines by the neonatal nursing staff. The findings from this report have led to the recent design of a multicenter randomized trial of early weaning of inspired oxygen in extremely premature infants.

5. Characteristics of Infants with Severe Retinopathy of Prematurity in Countries with Low, Moderate and High-Levels of Development: Implications for Screening Programs:[2] This observational study reports that infants from low and middle human development countries (MHDC) with severe ROP may have a different demographic profile from those of HHDC. Infants with severe ROP from low and moderate levels of human development are of greater gestational ages and of higher birth weights. ROP screening guidelines need to be tailored to the local population.

Important Note in Interpreting Clinical Trials

Epidemiology research published in the last 7 years has highlighted the demographic differences in the profile of infants at risk for severe disease requiring treatment.[2,3] Infants in HHDC treated for ROP are of lower gestational age and birth weight as compared to those in MHDC. Lower human development countries (LHDC), until recently, have had no blindness from ROP because of low survival rates of premature infants. Currently, with increasing technology and neonatal strategies in both MHDCs and LHDCs, combined with decreasing infant mortality rates,

ROP is emerging as the leading cause of preventable childhood blindness. The results and recommendations of the clinical trials that have been reviewed in this chapter apply to HHDCs and may have different implications in other parts of the world.

Acknowledgments

All digital ROP images were taken by either Anna Ells or Leslie MacKeen.

References

1. Gilbert C, Anderton L, Dandona L, et al. Prevalence of visual impairment in children: A review of available data. *Ophthalmic Epidemiol.* 1999;6:73–82.
2. Gilbert C, Fielder A, Gordillo L, et al. International NO-ROP Group. Characteristics of infants with severe retinopathy of prematurity in countries with low, moderate, and high levels of development: Implications for screening programs. *Pediatrics.* 2005;115:e518–e525.
3. Gilbert C, Rahi J, Eckstein M, et al. Retinopathy of prematurity in middle-income countries. *Lancet.* 1997;350:12–14.
4. Shih S, Ju M, Liu N, et al. Selective stimulation of VEGFR-1 prevents oxygen-induced retinal vascular degeneration in retinopathy of prematurity. *J Clin Invest.* 2003;112:50–57.
5. Pierce E, Foley E, Smith L. Regulation of vascular endothelial growth factor by oxygen in a model of retinopathy of prematurity. *Arch Ophthalmol.* 1996;114:1219–1228.
6. Alon T, Hemo I, Itin A, et al. Vascular endothelial growth factor acts as a survival factor for newly formed retinal vessels and has implications for retinopathy of prematurity. *Nat Med.* 1995;1:1024–1028.
7. Smith L. Pathogenesis of retinopathy of prematurity. *Growth Horm IGF Res.* 2004;14(Suppl A): S140–S144.
8. Shastry B, Pendergast S, Hartzer M, et al. Identification of missense mutations in the Norrie disease gene associated with advanced retinopathy of prematurity. *Arch Ophthalmol.* 1997;115:651–655.
9. Robitaille J, MacDonald M, Kaykas A, et al. Mutant frizzled-4 disrupts retinal angiogenesis in familial exudative vitreoretinopathy. *Nat Genet.* 2002;32:326–330.

10. Cooke R, Drury J, Mountford R, et al. Genetic polymorphisms and retinopathy of prematurity. *Invest Ophthalmol Vis Sci.* 2004;45:1712–1715.

11. The Committee for the Classification of Retinopathy of Prematurity. An international classification of retinopathy of prematurity. *Arch Ophthalmol.* 1984;102:1130–1134.

12. ICROP Committee for classification of late stages of ROP. An international classification of retinopathy of prematurity: II the classification of retinal detachment. *Arch Ophthalmol.* 1987;105:906–912.

13. An International Committee for the Classification of Retinopathy of Prematurity. The international classification of retinopathy of prematurity revisited. *Arch Ophthalmol.* 2005;123: 991–999.

14. Wallace D, Kylstra J, Chestnutt D. Prognostoc significance of vascular dilation and tortuosity insufficient for plus disease in retinopathy of prematurity. *J AAPOS.* 2000;4:224–229.

15. Schaffer D, Palmer E, Plotsky D, et al. The Cryotherapy for Retinopathy of Prematurity Cooperative Group. Prognostic factors in the natural course of retinopathy of prematurity. *Ophthalmology.* 1993;100:230–237.

16. Cryotherapy for Retinopathy of Prematurity Cooperative Group. Multicenter trial of cryotherapy for retinopathy of prematurity: Ophthalmological outcomes at 10 years. *Arch Ophthalmol.* 2001;119:1110–1118.

17. Cryotherapy for Retinopathy of Prematurity Group. Multicenter trial of cryotherapy for retinopathy of prematurity—one year outcome—structure and function. *Arch Ophthalmol.* 1990;108:1408–1413.

18. Cryotherapy for Retinopathy of Prematurity Cooperative Group. Multicenter trial of cryotherapy for retinopathy of prematurity. Snellen visual acuity and structural outcome at 5 1/2 years after randomization. *Arch Ophthalmol.* 1996;114:417–424.

19. Cryotherapy for Retinopathy of Prematurity Cooperative Group. 15-year outcomes following threshold retinopathy of prematurity: Final results from the multicenter trial of cryotherapy for retinopathy of prematurity. *Arch Ophthalmol.* 2005;123:311–318.

20. Hindle W. Cryotherapy for retinopathy of prematurity to prevent retrolental fibroplasia. *Can J Ophthalmol.* 1982;17:207–212.

21. Nagata M. Treatment of acute proliferative retrolental fibroplasia with xenon-arc photocoagulation: Its indication and limitations. *Jpn J Ophthalmol.* 1977;21:436–459.

22. Johnson L, Quinn GE, Abbasi S, et al. Effect of sustained pharmacologic vitamin E levels on incidence and severity of retinopathy of prematurity: A controlled clinical trial. *J Pediatr.* 1989;114:827–838.

23. Phleps DL, Rosenbaum AL, Isenberg SJ, et al. Tocopherol efficacy and safety for preventing retinopathy of prematurity: A randomized, controlled, double-masked trial. *Pediatrics.* 1987;79:489–500.

24. McNamara J, Tasman W, Brown G, et al. Laser photocoagulation for stage 3+ retinopathy of prematurity. *Ophthalmology.* 1991;98:576–580.

25. McNamara J, Tasman W, Vander J, et al. Diode laser photocoagulation for retinopathy of prematurity. Preliminary results. *Arch Ophthalmol.* 1992;110:1714–1716.

26. Iverson D, Trese M, Orgel I, et al. Laser photocoagulation for threshold retinopathy of prematurity. *Arch Ophthalmol..* 1991;109:1342–1343.

27. Landers M, Toth C, Semple H, et al. Treatment of retinopathy of prematurity with argon laser photocoagulation. *Arch Ophthalmol.* 1992; 110:44–47.

28. Goggin M, O'Keefe M. Diode laser for retinopathy of prematurity—early outcome. *Br J Ophthalmol.* 1993;77:559–562.

29. Seiberth V, Linderkamp O, Vardarli I, et al. Diode laser photocoagulation for stage 3+ retinopathy of prematurity. *Graefes Arch Clin Exp Ophthalmol.* 1995;233:489–493.

30. White J, Repka M. Randomized comparison of diode laser photocoagulation versus cryotherapy for threshold retinopathy of prematurity: 3-year outcome. *J Pediatr Ophthalmol Strabismus.* 1997; 34:83–87.

31. Phelps D. ETROP Cooperative Group. The early treatment for retinopathy of prematurity study: Better outcomes, changing strategy. *Pediatrics.* 2004;114:490–491.

32. Palmer E, Flynn J, Hardy R, et al. Incidence and early course of retinopathy of prematurity. *Ophthalmology.* 1991;98:1628–1638.

33. Quinn G, Johnson L, Abbasi S. Onset of retinopathy of prematurity as related to postnatal and postconceptional age. *Br J Ophthalmol.* 1992; 76:284–288.

34. Cryotherapy for Retinopathy of Prematurity Cooperative Group. The natural ocular outcome of premature birth and retinopathy. *Arch Ophthalmol.* 1994;112:903–912.

35. Reynolds J, Dobson V, Quinn G, et al. Evidence-based screening criteria for retinopathy of prematurity. *Arch Ophthalmol.* 2002;120:1470–1476.

36. Subhani M, Combs A, Weber P, et al. Screening guidelines for retinopathy of prematurity: The need for revision in extremely low birth weight infants. *Pediatrics.* 2001;107:656–659.

37. Repka M, Palmer E, Tung B, Group ftCfRoPC. Involution of retinopathy of prematurity. *Arch Ophthalmol.* 2000;118:645–649.

38. Ells A, Hicks M, Fielden M, et al. Severe retinopathy of prematurity: Longitudinal observation of disease and screening implications. *Eye.* 2004; 2004:1–7.

39. Hindle W. Is a 'favorable' outcome acceptable? *Arch Ophthalmol.* 1995;113:697–698.

40. Schaffer DB, Johnson L, Quinn GE, et al. Vitamin E and retinopathy of prematurity: Follow-up at one year. *Ophthalmology.* 1985;92: 1005–1011.

41. Early Treatment for Retinopathy of Prematurity Cooperative Group. Revised indications for the treatment of retinopathy of prematurity - results of the early treatment for retinopathy of prematurity randomized trial. *Arch Ophthalmol.* 2003;121:1684–1694.

42. The STOP-ROP Multicenter Study Group. Supplemental Therapeutic Oxygen for Prethreshold Retinopathy of Prematurity (STOP-ROP), A Randomized, Controlled Trial. I: Primary Outcomes. *Pediatrics.* 2000;105: 295–310.

43. Gaynon M, Stevenson D. What can we learn from STOP-ROP and earlier studies? *Pediatrics.* 2000;105:420–421.

44. Onofrey C, Feuer W, Flynn J. The outcome of retinopathy of prematurity: Screening for retinopathy of prematurity using an outcome predictive program. *Ophthalmology.* 2001; 108:27–34.

45. Hardy R, Palmer E, Dobson V, et al. Cryotherapy for Retinopathy of Prematurity Cooperative Group. Risk analysis of prethreshold retinopathy of prematurity. *Arch Ophthalmol.* 2003;121:1697–1701.

46. Connolly B, Ng E, McNamara J, et al. A comparison of laser photocoagulation with cryotherapy for threshold retinopathy of prematurity at 10 years: Part 2. Refractive outcome. *Ophthalmology.* 2002;109:936–941.

47. Ng E, Connolly B, McNamara J, et al. A Comparison of laser photocoagulation with cryotherapy for threshold retinopathy of prematurity at 10 years. *Ophthalmology.* 2002;109:928–935.

48. Reynolds J, Hardy R, Kennedy K, et al. Light Reduction in Retinopathy of Prematurity (LIGHT-ROP) Cooperative Group. Lack of efficacy of light reduction in preventing retinopathy of prematurity. *N Engl J Med.* 1998; 338:1572–1576.

49. Raju T, Langenberg P, Bhutani V, et al. Vitamin E prophylaxis to reduce retinopathy of prematurity: A reappraisal of published trials. *J Pediatr.* 1997;131:844–845.

50. Chow L, Wright K, Sola A. CSMC Oxygen Administration Study Group. Can changes in clinical practice decrease the incidence of severe retinopathy of prematurity in very low birth weight infants? *Pediatrics.* 2003;111:339–345.

CHAPTER 12

Amblyopia

Jonathan M. Holmes, BM, BCh , Michael X. Repka, MD , and Raymond T. Kraker, MSPH

A number of multicenter randomized controlled trials (RCTs) have been conducted by groups in North America and Europe addressing questions in the treatment of amblyopia. The Pediatric Eye Disease Investigator Group (PEDIG) in the United States[1] consists of approximately 200 pediatric ophthalmologists and pediatric optometrists across North America, both in academic and community-based private practice settings, who conduct large simple trials or simple data collection studies, each study mimicking clinical practice with the exception of randomization and standardized masked assessment of outcome measures. This chapter summarizes the major findings of completed PEDIG amblyopia studies,[2-9] and also describes several recent studies conducted by other investigator groups in Europe.[10-16]

To date, RCTs in amblyopia have exclusively addressed questions in the management of unilateral amblyopia caused by anisometropia, strabismus, or a combination of anisometropia and strabismus. No RCTs have been conducted in deprivation amblyopia, and therefore this chapter will not discuss the management of deprivation amblyopia or bilateral amblyopia.

Visual Acuity Testing in Amblyopia Studies

The standardization and masking of visual acuity (VA) measurement are critical for clinical trials in amblyopia. The use of age-appropriate clinical tests that incorporate a logMAR scale is important for the analysis and presentation of results. For children aged <7 years, PEDIG uses the amblyopia treatment study (ATS) VA protocol,[17] incorporating HOTV optotypes with surround bars. The test has been automated with a computer-based electronic visual acuity (EVA) tester.[18] Many children under 3 years are untestable with HOTV optotypes,[17] so PEDIG

studies of younger children with amblyopia have focused on 3- to <7-year olds. For children of aged 7 years or more, PEDIG uses an EVA version of the early treatment of diabetic retinopathy study (ETDRS) test (the e-ETDRS test),[19] presenting single optotypes with surround bars and yielding a letter score comparable to standard ETDRS testing. In the European studies, Clarke et al.[10] Stewart et al.[11,14,15] and Awan et al.[16] also used logMAR-based VA tests for outcome assessment.

Atropine versus Patching in Moderate Amblyopia

Background and Study Questions

Historically, advocates of atropine administered to the sound eye in the treatment of amblyopia have suggested that enhanced compliance and better binocular outcomes are advantages of atropine, while advocates of patching the sound eye have suggested that patching produces a more complete and more rapid response. In order to address this controversy, the first RCT conducted by PEDIG compared patching of the sound eye prescribed for at least 6 hours per day to atropine 1% one drop each morning to the sound eye.[2,3]

Patients Included in the Study

Children were <7 years old at the time of enrollment, and had to be able to complete optotype VA testing (HOTV matching), effectively limiting the study to 3- to <7-year olds. They had moderate amblyopia defined as 20/40 to 20/100 in the amblyopic eye, sound eye acuity of at least 20/40, and at least 3 logMAR lines of interocular difference to ensure that they had *bona fide* amblyopia. In addition, the presence or history of an amblyogenic (or more properly amblyopiogenic) factor that met criteria for strabismus, anisometropia, or both was required for enrollment. Patients could have had no more than 2 months of amblyopia therapy in the past 2 years and optimum spectacle correction (if needed) was required for at least 4 weeks.

Intervention and Outcome Measures

Randomization and follow-up schedule are shown in Figure 12.1. If the amblyopic eye had not improved by three lines or to at least 20/32 after 16 weeks of randomized treatment, the treatment was increased by either changing the spectacle lens over the sound eye to plano in the atropine group or increasing the patching to 12 or more hours per day in the patching group.

The primary outcome was amblyopic eye VA measured 6 months from enrollment and randomization. After 6 months of treatment according to randomization, investigators were allowed to treat each patient at their discretion. A long-term follow-up examination was then conducted at 2 years from enrollment.

Major Findings

At the 6-month primary outcome both groups showed similar improvement in the amblyopic eye VA (a mean improvement of 3.16 lines in the patching group and 2.84 lines in the atropine group). The difference in VA between treatment groups was small—equivalent to approximately 1.5 letters—and not clinically meaningful (mean difference 0.034 logMAR units 95% CI, 0.005 to 0.064). Improvement was initially faster in the patching group, with a mean improvement from baseline to five weeks of 2.22 lines in the patching group and 1.37 lines in the atropine group. Defining the 6-month outcome dichotomously as success or failure, with success defined as "20/32 or better in the amblyopic eye and/or improved from baseline by three or more lines," success was achieved in 79% of the patching group and 74% of the atropine group, which was not statistically different. The relative treatment effect did not vary according to age, depth of amblyopia, or cause of amblyopia.

Atropine had a slightly higher degree of acceptability when rated on a parental questionnaire[20,21]

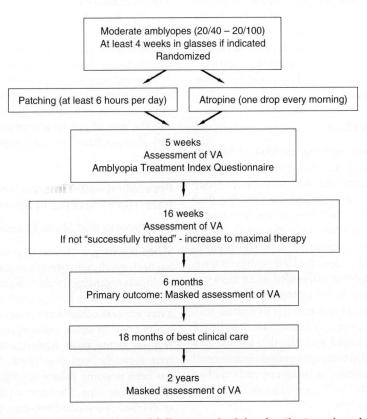

FIGURE 12.1 ☐ PEDIG RCT randomization and follow-up schedule of patients assigned to atropine versus patching in moderate amblyopia.

administered at the 5-week visit, before knowledge of any VA improvement.

Between 6 months and 2 years following randomization,[3] treatment was at the discretion of the investigator, but only about a quarter of the children underwent treatment using the other modality. At the 2-year outcome, the mean improvement in amblyopic eye VA was again similar in the patching and atropine groups (3.7 lines in the patching group and 3.6 lines in the atropine group). The difference in mean VA between the groups was very small (0.01 logMAR units 95% CI, −0.02 and 0.04). In both groups the mean amblyopic eye acuity at 2 years was approximately 20/32, 1.8 lines poorer than the mean sound eye acuity, which was approximately 20/20. It is noteworthy that only about half of the patients in each group reached 20/25 or better in the amblyopic eye. There was no difference in stereoacuity between patients in the patching and atropine groups when assessed at the 2-year outcome.

Implications for Clinical Practice

Both patching and daily atropine drops administered to the sound eye are excellent initial treatments for moderate anisometropic and strabismic amblyopia. It is reasonable to involve the parents and the child in deciding which treatment to start. If that treatment modality is unsuccessful, the child could be put on the alternative therapy.

Unanswered Questions

The optimum dose of patching and dose of atropine were not addressed in this study. The doses were selected as a consensus of the investigator group prior to initiating the RCT, and the patching dose was prescribed at the discretion of the investigator (starting with at least 6 hours per day in this study). Questions regarding optimum dose would begin to be addressed by studies described later in this chapter.

If a patient had not responded at 16 weeks to atropine therapy, the hypermetropic glasses correction over the sound eye was reduced to a plano lens. This would have the effect of further blurring the VA of the cyclopleged sound eye. Whether the use of a plano lens in addition to atropine results in increased effectiveness of treatment is being currently studied in an ongoing PEDIG RCT comparing atropine with and without a plano lens.

Analysis of fixation data and near VA data in patients randomized to atropine surprisingly revealed that fixation switch to the amblyopic eye was not necessary for VA improvement, and that patients who had better near VA in the sound eye while being cyclopleged with atropine could also show improvement in the amblyopic eye.[22] For practical reasons, this assessment was limited by performing these tests at the 5-week visit. The issues of fixation switch and near VA predicting success with atropine were also explored in the PEDIG RCT of atropine regimes, described later in the chapter.

At the 2-year outcome, only about half the children improved to 20/25 or better. This indicates that amblyopia is difficult to "cure." Future studies need to address the best treatment strategy for residual amblyopia. It is probable that a proportion of amblyopes have physical or functional deficits that cannot be completely reversed.

The role of "refractive adaptation," [12,13,23] that is, the optical treatment of amblyopia with spectacles alone was not addressed in this trial. The choice of "at least 4 weeks in glasses, if needed" was made as a compromise between those who wanted to start patching or atropine immediately and those who wanted to wait for maximal improvement. Subsequent work of Moseley, Stewart, Fielder et al.[12,13,23] has provided evidence that a great deal of improvement can be obtained with glasses alone in both strabismic and anisometropic amblyopia. In some cases patching or atropine may not be necessary. A further PEDIG study of optical treatment of amblyopia, to be published in 2006, will address the role of glasses alone and the role of patching over continued treatment with glasses when maximum improvement has been reached.

Prescribed Full-Time versus Prescribed Part-Time Patching in Severe Amblyopia

Background and Study Questions

When patching is chosen to treat amblyopia, there has been much controversy among pediatric ophthalmologists regarding the dose of patching to prescribe. Some practitioners have prescribed as little as 1 hour a day whereas others have prescribed as much as 24 hours a day. In severe amblyopia (20/100 to 20/400), regimes at the more intense end of the spectrum have typically been prescribed. Nevertheless, there has been ongoing debate regarding the necessity of full-time patching. Therefore an RCT was conducted to compare prescribed full-time patching (all or all but 1 waking hour a day) with prescribed 6 hours of daily patching.[6]

Patients Included in the Study

One hundred and seventy five children 3 to <7 years old with severe amblyopia (best corrected VA 20/100 to 20/400) secondary to strabismus, anisometropia, or both were enrolled. The VA in the sound eye was at least 20/40 or better. Patients could have had no patching treatment within 6 months and no other amblyopia treatment of any type other than spectacles within 1 month. Any significant refractive error had to be corrected for at least 4 weeks before enrollment.

Intervention and Outcome Measures

Randomization and follow-up schedule are shown in Figure 12.2. Due to debate regarding the need for near visual activities during patching, both groups were also prescribed at least 1 hour of near visual activities during patching. This study was not designed to test the maximum VA improvement, but rather to assess the initial response in the first 17 weeks.

Major Findings

At the 17-week primary outcome exam, VA in the amblyopic eye improved by a similar extent in both groups. The improvement in the amblyopic eye acuity from baseline to 17 weeks averaged 4.8 lines in the 6-hour group and 4.7 lines in the full-time group, with $p = 0.45$. The study concluded that 6 hours of prescribed daily patching produces an improvement in VA that is of similar magnitude to the improvement by prescribing full-time patching

in treating severe amblyopia in children 3 to <7 years of age. There was no difference in the rate of improvement.

Parental acceptance of both treatments was good, on the basis of the Amblyopia Treatment Index questionnaire.[20,21] The mean questionnaire scores and subscale scores (adverse effects, treatment compliance, and social stigma) were similar between part-time and full-time patching.

Implications for Clinical Practice

Since prescribing fewer hours per day of daily patching reduces the treatment burden for both the parents and the child, it would be reasonable to initially prescribe 6 hours of the daily patching in severe amblyopia caused by anisometropia and strabismus. The study did not support prescribing full-time patching as an initial treatment for amblyopia.

Unanswered Questions

This RCT did not address actual patch-wearing times, and it was acknowledged[6] that some of the children who were prescribed full-time patching might have worn the patch far less than full-time. Nevertheless, the RCT was designed as a real-world study of effectiveness and it is noteworthy that prescribing 6 hours of patching resulted in marked improvement in VA in these severe amblyopes. Stewart et al.[15] have conducted an RCT comparing 12 hours per day to 6 hours per day of patching. Although complete results are

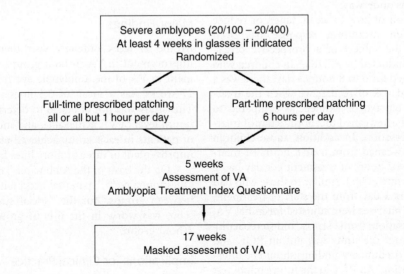

FIGURE 12.2 ◼ PEDIG RCT randomization and follow-up schedule of patients prescribed part-time versus full-time patching in severe amblyopia.

not available at this time, preliminary results[15] indicate that the actual patching time, measured using an occlusion dose monitor, was similar between groups (4.2 ± 1.7 hours vs. 6.2 ± 3.9 hours, $p = 0.06$).[15] These results indicate that the lack of superiority of more intense regimes might be due to reduced compliance with intense patching. Alternatively, there may be a ceiling effect on the rate of improvement of the amblyopic eye, which fewer hours can achieve, so that increased patching hours do not result in faster improvement.[6] These issues are worthy of further study.

The possibility of enhancing compliance is being addressed by Loudon and Simonsz[24] in another RCT comparing patching with compliance aids to standard patching. The results of this study will be forthcoming.

This PEDIG RCT[6] did not address whether the final VA of these children, after long-term treatment, might be different between treatment groups, but on applying these results to clinical practice it would seem reasonable to start treatment with 6 hours a day, since the initial response to treatment appears similar between prescribed part-time and prescribed full-time patching. It is possible that some children may require a more intense treatment later in the course, and further studies will need to address the issue of managing residual amblyopia.

Although the study prescribed 1 hour of "near visual activities" while being patched, the role of such near visual acuities remains controversial. The feasibility of conducting an RCT comparing patching with and without near activities was demonstrated in a recent pilot RCT conducted by PEDIG,[25] and a full-scale RCT is underway.

The question of how to wean, taper, or reduce treatment, when maximum response has been achieved, was the subject of a prospective observation study conducted by PEDIG.[8] In children who had been patched for 6 to 8 hours a day, there was a 4-fold increased risk of recurrence when the treatment was not tapered or weaned, as compared to those who had been weaned to 2 hours a day of treatment before cessation. In addition, those children who had been weaned from 6 or 8 hours of treatment per day to 2 hours of treatment per day had a low recurrence rate (14%), similar to those who had been on 2 hours a day from the start of treatment. Although these analyses were adjusted for initial VA, VA prior to cessation, tropia status, and stereoacuity prior to cessation, the study was not an RCT, and therefore these preliminary findings should be interpreted with caution. An RCT in the future might test the hypothesis that weaning or tapering of treatment is associated with a decreased recurrence rate.

Prescribed Six Hours A Day versus Prescribed Two Hours A Day Patching for Moderate Amblyopia

Background and Study Questions

The rationale for this RCT of patching regimens in moderate amblyopia was similar to that described above for comparing patching regimens in severe amblyopia. The optimum intensity of patching, that is, number of hours per day, has not been rigorously studied previously.

Patients Included in the Study

One hundred and eighty-nine children between 3 and 7 years of age with moderate amblyopia (20/40 to 20/80) due to strabismus and anisometropia or both were enrolled.[5] The VA in the sound eye had to be at least 20/40 or better, with an intraocular acuity difference of 3 logMAR lines or more. No patching treatment within the last 6 months and no other treatment except spectacles within the prior month were allowed. Any significant refractive error had to be corrected for at least 4 weeks before enrollment.

Intervention and Outcome Measures

Patients were randomized to either 2 hours per day of prescribed patching of the sound eye or 6 hours per day of prescribed patching. The follow-up schedule is shown in Figure 12.3. Due to the controversy of whether near activities during patching enhances the effect of patching, 1 hour per day of near activities during occlusion was also prescribed in each group.

Major Findings

At the 17-week outcome visit there was similar improvement in VA in both groups. The improvement in VA of the amblyopic eye from baseline to 17 weeks was a mean of 2.4 lines in each group. This study was not designed to determine the maximum level of VA achievable, and indeed only 62% of patients in each group achieved at least 20/32 or improvement of three or more lines from baseline.

On the basis of the Amblyopia Treatment Index Questionnaire,[20,21] parental acceptance was similar between groups, but the "social stigma" subscale score was worse in the 6-hour group than in the 2-hour group.

Implications for Clinical Practice

In moderate amblyopia (20/40 to 20/80), due to strabismus, anisometropia or both, it is reasonable to

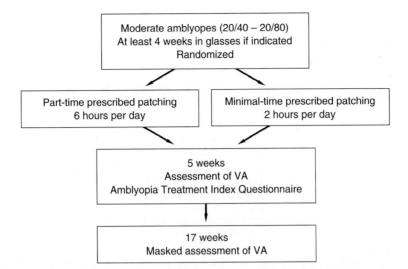

FIGURE 12.3 ☐ PEDIG RCT randomization and follow-up schedule of patients prescribed 6 hours per day of patching versus 2 hours per day patching in moderate amblyopia.

start patching by prescribing 2 hours a day combined with 1 hour of near visual acuities. This decreased burden of patching may be more acceptable to both the child and the parent.

Unanswered Questions

The possible role of refractive correction alone, before starting patching or atropine, has been discussed in the preceding text and has recently been studied by Moseley, Stewart, Fielder et al.[11–15,23] and by PEDIG (2006). As described above, the role of near activities during patching[25] is the subject on an ongoing PEDIG RCT.

It is also possible that <2 hours per day is effective in treating amblyopia. Recent data from Stewart et al.[14] suggests that only 1 hour per day of patching is effective in some children with amblyopia. There also appears to be a great deal of individual variability of response to treatment with a given dose of patching.[12,14] These issues will be the subject of future studies.

Daily versus Weekend Atropine for Moderate Amblyopia

Background and Study Questions

In the same way that, until recently, there have been few rigorous studies addressing patching regimes for amblyopia, there are even fewer studies addressing different dosing regimens of atropine. Once or twice a week atropine to the sound eye has been reported to be successful in some children with amblyopia[26] and therefore an RCT was conducted to compare weekend atropine (2 days a week) to daily atropine.

Patients Included in the Study

One hundred and sixty-eight children aged 3 to <7 years with moderate amblyopia (20/40 to 20/80), associated with strabismus, anisometropia, or both, were enrolled. VA in the sound eye was 20/40 or better with an intraocular acuity difference of at least 3 LogMAR lines. Children with myopia of −6.00 D in the amblyopic eye or more than −0.50 of myopia in the sound eye or with Down syndrome were excluded. It was felt that some degree of uncorrected hypermetropic refractive error at near in the sound eye would be needed for atropine to be effective, although this had not been rigorously studied.

Intervention and Outcome Measures

Patients were randomized to 1% atropine drops to the sound eye either daily or on the weekend (Saturday and Sunday). The randomization and follow-up schedule are summarized in Figure 12.4.

Major Findings

Both groups improved by an average of 2.3 lines from baseline to 17 weeks. The VA of the amblyopic eye at study completion, in follow-up extended until the

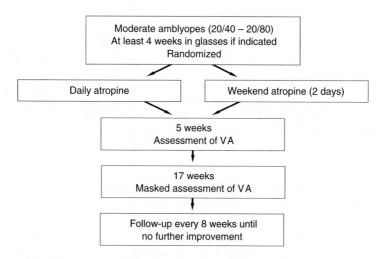

FIGURE 12.4 ☐ PEDIG RCT randomization and follow-up schedule of patients prescribed daily versus weekend atropine in moderate amblyopia.

child stopped improving, was at least 20/25 or better than or equal to the sound eye in 47% of the daily group and 53% of the weekend group. The VA of the sound eye at the end of long-term follow-up was reduced by two lines in one patient in each group at final follow-up. Stereoacuity was similar in both groups.

The impact of the treatment on the child and the family was similar between groups when assessed by the Amblyopia Treatment Questionnaire,[20,21] in all but the compliance subscale, which was slightly worse in the weekend group. It is possible that the children who were receiving daily atropine became accustomed to the routine, whereas the children who received atropine only on the weekend were less compliant.

The improvement in the amblyopic eye was similar in subgroups based on gender, age, cause of amblyopia, iris color, prior amblyopia treatment, and refractive error of the sound eye.

Implications for Clinical Practice

Since the first PEDIG RCT[2] provided evidence that both patching and atropine are effective in treating moderate amblyopia, the choice of initial treatment may be left to the parent and the child. If atropine is chosen, a reasonable approach would be to start with a twice-weekly dose of the 1% drop.

Unanswered Questions

It is possible that even less frequent administration of atropine might be effective in treating moderate amblyopia, and this should be studied further. It is also possible that atropine might be effective in treating more severe amblyopia, since in both this study and the previous atropine study,[2] improvement in the amblyopic eye was seen in children whose near VA of the cyclopleged sound eye on atropine was not reduced below the level of the amblyopic eye. We speculate that, in these conditions, the amblyopic eye might be used in conditions other than those evaluated with near VA testing. It is also possible that atropine selectively degrades higher spatial frequencies, which might be critical in the treatment of amblyopia, and that measurement of VA alone does not detect such an effect of atropine.

Ongoing PEDIG studies are comparing atropine with and without a plano lens and are also investigating the effectiveness of atropine in severe amblyopia. Recruitment is also ongoing for an additional atropine versus patching study for older amblyopic children (age 7 to 12 years).

Optical Treatment versus Optical Treatment Plus Patching and Atropine in 7- to 17-Year Olds

Background and Study Questions

Some eye care professionals have believed that the sensitive period for the treatment of amblyopia ends at the age of 6 or 7 years, and therefore have not offered treatment to older children. Other providers treat patients aged 9 years or even older and there are case reports and small cases series reporting successful treatment of amblyopia in still older children. In a pilot study[7] of children 10 to 17 years old with amblyopia treated with part-time patching, VA improved by two or more lines in 27% of patients. Therefore a formal RCT was designed to test the hypothesis that patching (with or without atropine) would be superior to optical correction alone.

Patients Included in the Study

Five hundred and seven patients aged 7 to 17 years with unilateral amblyopia secondary to strabismus, anisometropia, or both were enrolled (404 children aged 7 to 12 years and 103 aged 13 to 17 years). No amblyopia treatment other than spectacles in the prior month and no more than 1 month of amblyopia treatment in the last 6 months was allowed. Best corrected VA was 20/40 to 20/400, with sound eye acuity of 20/25 or better. No more than 6 D of myopia was allowed to exclude patients with possible organic retinal disease. For patients younger than 13 years, an additional eligibility criterion was no more than 0.5 D of myopia in the sound eye, since this group could be randomized to atropine in addition to patching.

Intervention and Outcome Measures

Patients were randomized to treatment with either optical correction alone or optical correction augmented with patching of the sound eye 2 to 6 hours a day, with 1 hour of near visual activities (see Fig. 12.5). A Game Boy (Nintendo, Redmond, Washington) was provided to be used for the near visual activities. Younger patients in the augmented treatment group (age 7 to 12 years) were also prescribed one drop of 1% atropine daily. In these children, glasses were provided for near work if they were unable to read grade-appropriate print. Patients aged 13 to 17 years were not prescribed atropine, due to the increased demands of their activities. The use of simultaneous atropine and patching in the younger children was based on the rationale that a first RCT of treatment in children over 7 years should be designed to maximize the probability of finding a treatment effect, beyond glasses, if one did in fact exist.

The primary outcome was defined as the proportion of patients in each group classified as a responder. The patient was classified as a responder if the amblyopic eye acuity was 10 or more letters (two

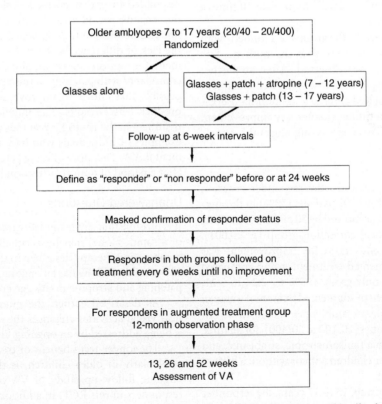

FIGURE 12.5 ◻ PEDIG RCT randomization and follow-up schedule of patients prescribed optical treatment versus optical treatment plus patching and atropine in 7- to 17-year olds.

lines) better than the baseline acuity. VA testing was performed at 6 weeks, 12 weeks, 18 weeks, and 24 weeks. The responder status was confirmed by a masked examiner. By the 24-week visit if the amblyopic eye had not improved by 10 or more letters, the patient was classified as a nonresponder. The patient could also be classified as a nonresponder at an earlier visit if there was no improvement from the prior visit or only minimal improvement from baseline, defined at the 6-week visit as a zero-letter improvement, <3-letter improvement from the baseline at the 12-week visit and <5-letter improvement from the baseline at the 18-week visit. Patients who did not complete the randomized trial and patients in the optical correction group who received additional amblyopia treatment were considered to be nonresponders in the primary analysis.

Due to concerns about inducing diplopia in these older children with patching, the patients (and parents) were asked at each visit if they ever saw two of the same thing and if so, the frequency. For both the patient and the parent, any diplopia was recorded as: "Less than once a week," "once a week," "once a day," "up to 10 times a day," "more than 10 times a day," and "all the time."

Responders in both groups continued with follow-up with visits every 6 weeks until no further improvement was observed. After no further improvement, responders to augmented treatment stopped treatment and entered a 12-month observation phase to determine whether any improvement was long lasting. This phase is ongoing at this time.

Major Findings

In the 7- to 12-year olds, the responder criterion was met by 106 of the 201 patients (53%) in the augmented treatment group and by 50 of the 203 patients (25%) in the optical correction group (p <0.001). The unadjusted odds ratio for improvement was 3.41 for the augmented treatment group compared to the spectacles-only group (95% CI 2.24 to 5.21, p <0.001). A benefit of augmented treatment was seen for both the moderate amblyopes (20/40 to 20/80) and severe amblyopes (20/100 to 20/400), for all three causes of amblyopia (anisometropic, strabismic, and combined) and for children with or without a history of prior treatment.

In the older group, 13 to 17 years, the responder criteria was met by 14 (25%) of the 55 patients in the treatment group, and by 11 (23%) of the 48

patients in the optical correction group (p = 0.47). The unadjusted odds ratio for improvement was 1.15 (95% CI 0.46 to 2.84, p = 0.38) Nevertheless, among patients who had not been previously treated for amblyopia, those in the augmented treatment group did show a greater improvement than those in the optical correction group, 47% versus 20%, adjusted p = 0.03.

No patient developed constant diplopia during the randomized trial phase.

Implications for Clinical Practice

In patients with amblyopia secondary to anisometropia and/or strabismus aged 7 to 12 years, augmenting optical correction with patching, near activities, and atropine should be offered. The 25% responder rate in the pure optical correction group was surprising and therefore it might be reasonable to start spectacle correction first to determine maximum acuity improvement prior to starting patching. This might be described as refractive adaptation,[13,23] or optical treatment of amblyopia, as described earlier in studies for children <7 years of age.

The fact that 23% of the 13- to 17-year olds responded to optical correction alone suggests that the sensitive period for treatment of amblyopia does not end before the teenage years. It is possible that the lack of difference between the augmented treatment and optical correction alone was due to poor compliance with patching in this age group. It is also possible that efforts to improve compliance might produce better results. The individual response to treatment in the 13- to 17-year olds was variable, with examples of individuals who had marked improvement in VA. Therefore offering patching to teenagers after a period of optical correction is reasonable.

Unanswered Questions

It is possible that single modality treatment (patching or atropine alone) may be as equally effective as the combination therapy described in this study for 7- to 12-year olds. PEDIG has an ongoing RCT comparing patching and atropine in this age group.

As described earlier, the question of whether near visual activities enhances the effect of patching is being addressed by an ongoing PEDIG RCT.

The longer-term benefit of treating amblyopia, particularly in older children, is the subject of an ongoing follow-up study of VA outcome, for the responders in this RCT. In addition, work is underway by several groups, investigating the "functional deficits in amblyopia."

Patching Dose Regimes Using Occlusion Dose Monitors to Record Compliance

Background and Study Questions

As described above, previous RCTs of patching regimes have not addressed actual patch-wearing times. Awan et al.[16] used occlusion dose monitors to record the actual wearing time during a RCT comparing 0, 3, and 6 hours of daily patching for moderate strabismic and mixed anisometropic/strabismic amblyopia. The occlusion dose monitors were flat discs placed on the patch, logging temperature differences between the front and back of the disc at 5-minute intervals.

Patients Included in the Study

Sixty newly diagnosed children, 37 with strabismic amblyopia and 23 with combined strabismic and anisometropic amblyopia were enrolled. Children wore glasses (if needed) for 6 weeks before the study started. VA ranged from 20/40 to 20/160. The mean age was approximately 4 ½ years.

Intervention and Outcome Measures

Children were randomized to one of three groups, no patching, 3 hours of daily patching, and 6 hours of daily patching (see Fig. 12.6). The primary outcome measure for this study was actual patch-wearing time. VA was also measured at a 12-week outcome exam.

Major Findings

The mean daily patching durations were 1 hour 43 minutes in the 3-hour group and 2 hours 33 minutes in the 6-hour group. The compliance represented as a proportion of patching hours prescribed was also similar (58% vs. 41%).

The mean improvement in VA over the 12-week study was similar between all 3 groups (0.24 logMAR with no patching, 0.29 logMAR with 3 hours per day, 0.34 logMAR with 6 hours per day). Although there was a positive correlation between hours of patching completed and the proportion of VA deficit corrected, there was marked individual variability. A post hoc analysis revealed that confirmed patching of 3 to 6 hours per day was significantly better than no patching.

Implications for Clinical Practice

In this small study there is controversial evidence that "on average" no patching is as good as prescribing 3 or 6 hours per day. Nevertheless, these children did not have a prolonged period of refractive adaptation[13] (optical treatment of amblyopia) until no further improvement was observed, so the true effect of patching will have been somewhat masked by the simultaneous optical treatment. In addition, poor compliance in a proportion of children assigned to patching likely masks the potential real effect of patching. The post hoc analysis suggests a real effect of patching, so treatment of amblyopia with patching should not be abandoned.

Improving compliance is clearly important in maximizing the chance of a successful outcome. Educating the families and the child on the importance of treatment and consequences of nontreatment may be a first step in improving compliance.[27,28] Other compliance aids are the topic of ongoing studies.[24]

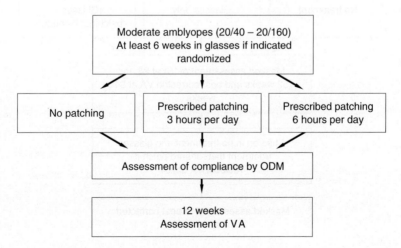

FIGURE 12.6 ☐ Randomization and follow-up schedule of patients prescribed patching for 6, 3, and 0 hours per day using occlusion dose monitors to measure compliance.

Unanswered Questions

The individual variability in response to a particular dose of patching is a noteworthy finding of this study[16] and the study of Stewart et al.[12] who also used occlusion dose monitors of a different design. Further studies are needed to establish why some children are resistant to treatment whereas others seem to respond quickly and completely.

As discussed above, further work is needed on techniques to improve compliance with patching. Whether educational programs or behavioral intervention will impact the proportion of children who respond to patching remains to be seen.

Unilateral Visual Impairment Detected at Preschool Vision Screening

Background and Study Questions

In the late 1990s, public health policy makers were questioning whether screening for amblyopia in the United Kingdom should be abandoned.[29] They argued that the benefits of patching had not been demonstrated in an RCT, that patching placed a severe psychological burden on the child and the family, and that it was unclear whether unilateral amblyopia actually created any true disability. In

that context Clarke et al.[10] designed an RCT with a completely untreated control group. They studied a population of children who had failed VA screening and were referred for possible amblyopia.

Patients Included in the Study

One hundred and seventy-seven children with a mean age of 4 years and with unilateral moderately decreased VA (20/30 to 20/120) with 20/20 VA in the fellow eye, were enrolled.

Intervention and Outcome Measures

Children were randomized to either no treatment, treatment with glasses alone, or treatment with glasses plus patching if indicated (see Fig. 12.7). The primary outcome was corrected VA at 54 weeks. Children in the no-treatment or glasses-only groups were then offered patching if needed, and best corrected VA was measured in all groups 6 months later, at 18 months from study enrollment.

Major Findings

Children who were treated with glasses alone or glasses plus patching had a better mean best corrected VA at 54 weeks than those who received no

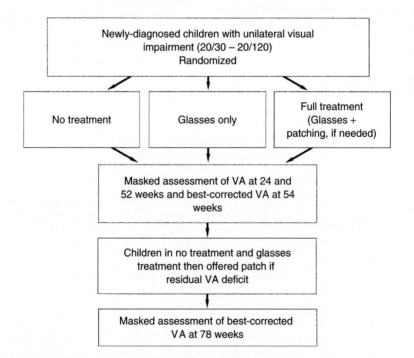

FIGURE 12.7 ◻ Randomization and follow-up schedule of patients assigned to no treatment versus glasses-only versus glasses plus patching in unilateral visual impairment.

treatment (mean differences of about a logMAR line). In a planned subgroup analysis, children with more severe VA deficit (20/60 to 20/120) showed additional improvement with patching (of approximately another logMAR line) over and above that with glasses alone. Children with a mild uncorrected VA deficit (20/30 to 20/40) had no significant improvement over no treatment, with glasses alone or glasses plus patching.

After subsequent full treatment (patching if needed) for 6 months the no-treatment group and glasses-only group improved to have corrected visual acuities indistinguishable from the originally fully treated group (glasses plus patching).

Implications for Clinical Practice

From a public health perspective, the results of Clarke's study are very important. Treating unilateral VA deficit with glasses and patching (if indicated) results in improvement of best corrected VA. Much of the VA deficit in this study may have been due to amblyopia, though an unknown proportion would have been purely refractive error. Children should continue to be screened for VA deficits and referred for treatment. Despite the dilution of the amblyopic cohort in this study, this RCT provided excellent evidence that patching works.

The improvement of children whose treatment was delayed for a year indicates that the sensitive period for treating amblyopia is not over by the age of 4 years. This lack of age effect is consistent with the findings of the several PEDIG studies,[2,5,9] in the 3- to 7-year age range, and has also been confirmed by others.[14,16]

Unanswered Questions

The failure of children with mild unilateral VA deficit in Clarke's study to improve with glasses and patching compared to no treatment raises the issue of pass/fail acuity criteria that should be used for screening. This topic is beyond the scope of this chapter, but it should be noted that "normal" VA for a 3- to 5-year old is not 20/20 and that there is some test–retest variability in VA testing. These factors should be taken into consideration when setting referral criteria.

In order that public health officials can make rationale decisions in allocating health care resources (e.g., preschool vision screening), the true lifetime disability of amblyopia needs to be better defined. Although there are data on the effect of losing the

better eye later in life,[30,31] there is little quality data on the effect of amblyopia on the day-to-day life of individuals who have residual or untreated amblyopia that lasts for the remaining decades of their lives. Extended follow-up is continuing in a subset of children who participated in the first ATS RCT of patching versus atropine.[2,3] Reading speed is being assessed at ages 10 and 15 years, which may yield further information regarding potential long-term sequelae of both successfully treated and residual amblyopia.

Conclusions

The evidence for the rational treatment of amblyopia is rapidly evolving. At the time of writing this chapter, there is excellent evidence for initially prescribing the best refractive correction for anisometropic and strabismic amblyopic children, and monitoring VA until it stabilizes. This may take several months and a proportion of patients will achieve equal VA with glasses alone. For residual anisometropic and strabismic amblyopia, the choice of patching or atropine should involve the parent and the child. The dose of prescribed patching or atropine may initially be quite modest, such as 2 hours of patching a day or twice weekly atropine. Treatment should be offered to children at least until the age of 12 years and even to teenagers.

Ongoing studies will define the role of near activities and the role of atropine in severe amblyopia. Future studies are needed to investigate the best treatment strategies for residual amblyopia, whether weaning treatment is needed at the end of a course, and how compliance can be enhanced. On the basis of the progress we have made in clinical amblyopia research over the last 5 years and the plethora of unanswered questions, it is likely that 5 years from now we will have new evidence that will again change how we manage this common condition.

References

1. Beck RW. The pediatric eye disease investigator group. *J AAPOS*. 1998;2:255–256.
2. Pediatric Eye Disease Investigator Group. A randomized trial of atropine versus patching for treatment of moderate amblyopia in children. *Arch Ophthalmol.*2002;120:268–278.
3. Pediatric Eye Disease Investigator Group. Two-year follow-up of a 6-month randomized trial of

atropine versus patching for treatment of moderate amblyopia in children. *Arch Ophthalmol.* 2005;123:149–157.

4. Pediatric Eye Disease Investigator Group. A randomized trial of atropine regimens for treatment of moderate amblyopia in children. *Ophthalmology.* 2004;111:2076–2085.

5. Pediatric Eye Disease Investigator Group. A randomized trial of patching regimens for treatment of moderate amblyopia in children. *Arch Ophthalmol.* 2003;121:603–611.

6. Pediatric Eye Disease Investigator Group. A randomized trial of prescribed patching regimens for treatment of severe amblyopia in children. *Ophthalmology.* 2003;110:2075–2087.

7. Pediatric Eye Disease Investigator Group. A prospective, pilot study of treatment of amblyopia in children 10 to <18 years old. *Am J Ophthalmol.* 2004;137:581–583.

8. Pediatric Eye Disease Investigator Group. Risk of amblyopia recurrence after cessation of treatment. *J AAPOS.* 2004;8:420–428.

9. Pediatric Eye Disease Investigator Group. Randomized trial of treatment of amblyopia in children aged 7 to 17 years. *Arch Ophthalmol.* 2005;123:437–447.

10. Clarke MP, Wright CM, Hrisos S, et al. Randomised controlled trial of treatment of unilateral visual impairment detected at preschool vision screening. *Br Med J.* 2003;327:1251–1256.

11. Stewart CE, Fielder AR, Stephens DA, et al. Design of the Monitored Occlusion Treatment of Amblyopia Study (MOTAS). *Br J Ophthalmol.* 2002;86:915–919.

12. Stewart CE, Moseley MJ, Stephens DA, et al. Treatment dose-response in amblyopia therapy: The Monitored Occlusion Treatment of Amblyopia Study (MOTAS). *Invest Ophthalmol Vis Sci.* 2004;45:3048–3054.

13. Stewart CE, Moseley MJ, Fielder AR, et al. Refractive adaptation in amblyopia: Quantification of effect and implications for practice. *Br J Ophthalmol.* 2004;88:1552–1556.

14. Stewart CE, Fielder AR, Stephens DA, et al. Treatment of unilateral amblyopia: Factors influencing visual outcome. *Invest Ophthalmol Vis Sci.* 2005;46:3152–3160.

15. Stewart CE, Moseley MJ, Stephens DA, et al. Modelling of treatment dose-response in amblyopia. *Invest Ophthalmol Vis Sci.* 2005;46: E-abstract 3595.

16. Awan M, Proudlock FA, Gottlob I. A randomized controlled trial of unilateral strabismic and mixed amblyopia using occlusion dose monitors to record compliance. *Invest Ophthalmol Vis Sci.* 2005;46:1435–1439.

17. Holmes JM, Beck RW, Repka MX, et al. The amblyopia treatment study visual acuity testing protocol. *Arch Ophthalmol.* 2001;119:1345–1353.

18. Moke PS, Turpin AH, Beck RW, et al. Computerized method of visual acuity testing: Adaptation of the amblyopia treatment study visual acuity testing protocol. *Am J Ophthalmol.* 2001;132:903–909.

19. Beck RW, Moke PS, Turpin AH, et al. A computerized method of visual acuity testing: Adaptation of the early treatment of diabetic retinopathy study testing protocol. *Am J Ophthalmol.* 2003;135:194–205.

20. Cole SR, Beck RW, Moke PS, et al. The Amblyopia treatment index. *J AAPOS.* 2001;5: 250–254.

21. Pediatric Eye Disease Investigator Group. Impact of patching and atropine treatment on the child and family in the amblyopia treatment study. *Arch Ophthalmol.* 2003;121:1625–1632.

22. Pediatric Eye Disease Investigator Group. The course of moderate amblyopia treated with atropine in children: Experience of the amblyopia treatment study. *Am J Ophthalmol.* 2003; 136:630–639.

23. Moseley MJ, Neufeld M, Fielder AR. Treatment of amblyopia by spectacles. *Ophthalmic Physiol Opt.* 2002;22:296–299.

24. Loudon SE, Polling JR, Simonsz HJ. Electronically measured compliance with occlusion therapy for amblyopia is related to visual acuity increase. *Graefes Arch Clin Exp Ophthalmol.* 2003;241:176–180.

25. Pediatric Eye Disease Investigator Group. A randomized pilot study of near activities versus non-near activities during patching therapy for amblyopia. *J AAPOS.* 2005;9:129–136.

26. Simons K, Stein L, Sener EC, et al. Full-time atropine, intermittent atropine and optical penalization and binocular outcome in treatment of strabismic amblyopia. *Ophthalmology.* 1997;104:2143–2155.

27. Newsham D. Parental non-concordance with occlusion therapy. *Br J Ophthalmol.* 2000;84: 957–962.

28. Newsham D. A randomised controlled trial of written information: The effect on parental non-concordance with occlusion therapy. *Br J Ophthalmol*. 2002;86:787–791.

29. Snowdon SK, Stewart-Brown SL. Preschool vision screening. *Health Technol Assess*. 1997;1:1–83.

30. Tomilla V, Tarkkanen A. Incidence of loss of vision in the healthy eye in amblyopia. *Br J Ophthalmol*. 1981;65:575–577.

31. Rahi J, Logan S, Timms C, et al. Risk, causes, and outcomes of visual impairment after loss of vision in the non-amblyopic eye: A population-based study. *Lancet*. 2002;360:597–602.

SECTION VI

OCULAR ONCOLOGY

CHAPTER 13

Uveal Melanoma: Approaches to Management

Ernest Rand Simpson, MD, FRCS (C)

Background

Choroidal melanoma is the most common primary intraocular malignancy in humans. The estimated incidence throughout North America is six to seven cases per million per year. Mortality from melanoma typically results from metastatic spread to the liver. Metastases are often delayed in presentation by many years. Historically, the primary therapy for choroidal melanoma was enucleation. The failure of enucleation to prevent metastatic disease has led to the exploration of adjunct therapies. In addition, therapeutic alternatives to enucleation emerged because of a desire to develop globe-sparing and potentially vision-sparing procedures. Evaluation of therapy for choroidal melanoma has proven difficult because of the relative rarity of the malignancy and the long time horizon for metastatic spread.

Collaborative Ocular Melanoma Study

Nearly 20 years ago, the Collaborative Ocular Melanoma Study (COMS) was launched to address the survival benefit of competing treatment options which, at the time, included enucleation and radiotherapy. The study addressed three clinical questions:

1. Does subtherapeutic external beam radiation before enucleation of large choroidal melanomas reduce metastases and mortality?

2. Is there a survival benefit to enucleation compared to radioactive iodine 125 (^{125}I) plaque application in patients with medium-sized choroidal melanoma?

3. What is the natural history of small choroidal melanomas?

For reasons of consistency in clinical comparison, size characteristics of choroidal melanoma were defined as small (1.0 to 3.0 mm in apical height and at least 5.0 mm in basal diameter), medium (2.5 to 10 mm in height and 16 mm or less in the largest basal diameter) and large (>10 mm in height or >16 mm in the largest basal diameter and at least 2 mm or more in height).

Methodology for Collaborative Ocular Melanoma Study Trials

A process of certification to establish clinical center uniformity required repeated certification of each investigator, clinical coordinator, plaquing surgeon, enucleating surgeon, examining ophthalmologist, radiation oncologist, radiation physicist, echographer, photographer, ophthalmic pathologist, and visual acuity examiner.

Patient eligibility and enrollment were determined by a rigid protocol, which included:

1. A complete ophthalmic and systemic evaluation
2. Color photographs and fluorescein angiography to document tumor size and characteristics
3. Standardized echography, including A and B scan evaluation

4. Eligibility confirmed and randomization provided by the Central Study Coordinating Center after full ophthalmologic, radiation, and medical oncology review

COMS Protocol Compliance

Overall protocol compliance in the COMS patients requiring radiation therapy for large tumors was >98%, and nearly 95% for medium tumors. Data was collected on standardized forms and submitted within a specific time frame to the COMS Central Coordinating Center and to specific resource centers.

COMS Small Choroidal Melanoma Observational Study

The Small Choroidal Melanoma Observational Study was an observation series of otherwise healthy adults with small choroidal melanomas. The primary end points were 5-year mortality and tumor growth. The overall 5-year mortality was low. Five-year all-cause mortality was 6.0% (95% confidence interval, 2.7% to 9.3%) and 8-year all-cause mortality was 14.9% (95% confidence interval, 9.6% to 20.2%.[1]

Of the small choroidal melanomas initially observed, 21% demonstrated growth by 2 years and 31% by 5 years.[2] Factors associated with time to growth were greater initial tumor thickness and diameter, presence of orange pigment, absence of drusen, and absence of retinal pigment epithelial alteration adjacent to the tumor. These observations have also been noted in other large case series of small choroidal

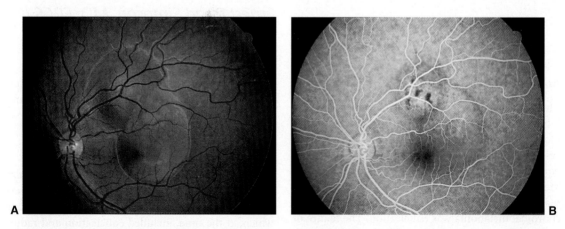

FIGURE 13.1 ☐ Small melanocytic choroidal mass with associated serous subretinal fluid. **A:** Clinical appearance showing surface lipofuscin and macular involvement with serous fluid. **B:** Fluorescein angiogram demonstrating abnormal hyperfluorescence at the level of the choroid with blocked fluorescence due to lipofuscin over the mass. Note the reduced fluorescence underlying the serous detachment extending into the foveal region.

melanoma and atypical choroidal nevi. In a separate study, Shields et al. found increased tumor thickness (>1 mm), proximity to the optic nerve, visual symptoms, presence of orange pigment, and presence of subretinal fluid to be predictive of future growth.[3] (see Fig. 13.1)

COMS Medium Choroidal Melanoma Trial

The medium tumor trial compared enucleation to radioactive ^{125}I plaque application. Patients included in the study met the following criteria (see Fig. 13.2):

1. Apical height between 2.5 and 10 mm and basal diameter of 16 mm or less
2. Visual acuity of at least 20/200 in fellow eye
3. No neovascular glaucoma
4. No iris involvement with tumor
5. No angle involvement with tumor
6. Clear ocular media
7. Tumor not contiguous with the optic disc
8. Tumor within 2 mm of the optic disc to fit within a 90-degree angle, with the apex at the center of the optic disc
9. The tumor "plaquable" in the opinion of the ophthalmologist

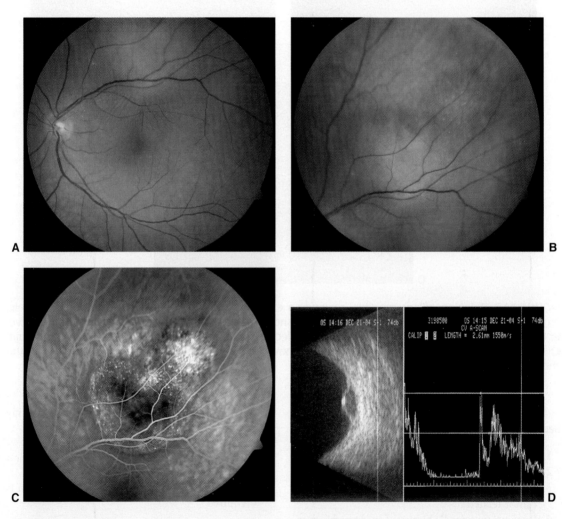

FIGURE 13.2 ☐ Medium choroidal melanoma with orange pigment, beginning to affect macular function. **A:** Clinical appearance of choroidal mass with overlying lipofuscin beginning to exert traction on paramacular retina. **B:** Margins of tumor are ill defined with an irregular contour. **C:** Fluorescein angiogram showing more specific contour of the mass, abnormal hyperfluorescence with partial blocking effect from orange pigment and dot-like fluorescence indicating Bruch membrane alteration. **D:** Ultrasonogram in B-mode showing dome-shaped low reflective mass with an A-mode height measurement of 2.61 mm.

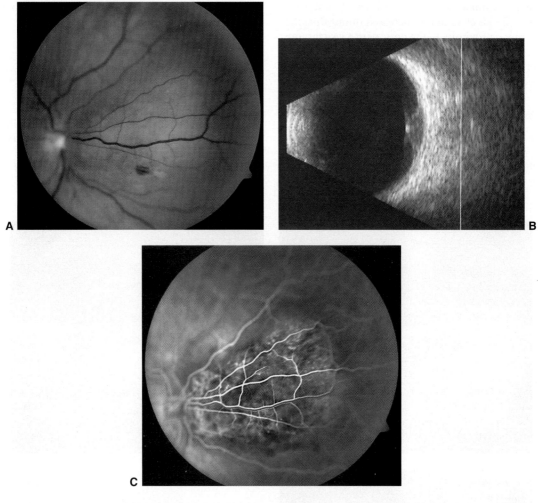

FIGURE 13.3 □ Juxtapapillary choroidal melanoma excluded from enrollment in the COMS owing to its proximity to the optic nerve. **A:** Clinical appearance showing the tumor involving 180 degrees of the nerve. **B:** Ultrasonogram in B-mode demonstrating low reflective dome-shaped mass with overlying serous fluid. **C:** Fluorescein angiogram of juxtapapillary mass showing mottled hyperfluorescence at the level of the choroid.

Patients evaluated in the COMS were excluded because of the following indications (see Fig. 13.3):

1. Use of immunosuppressive therapy
2. Previous treatment for choroidal melanoma
3. Previous intervention in the eye, which was tumor related
4. Previous fine needle biopsy of suspected tumor
5. Extrascleral extension of >2 mm
6. Diffuse "ring" or multiple melanoma
7. Other known primary tumors except cervical carcinoma *in situ* or nonmelanotic skin cancers
8. Any disease compromising survival
9. Involvement of 50% or more of the ciliary body with tumor
10. Tumor contiguous with the optic nerve
11. Contraindications to surgery or radiation therapy
12. Contraindication to anesthesia if enucleation is required

Twenty-two percent of patients evaluated for the study were deemed to be ineligible for enrollment. The most common reasons for exclusion were proximity of the tumor to the optic disc (40%), one or more primary cancers (20%), and melanoma that was present primarily in the ciliary body (11%).

Brachytherapy

Plaque radiotherapy is the most widespread method of delivering therapeutic doses of radiation to intraocular tumors, including choroidal melanoma. High-energy sources such as cobalt have been replaced by lower energy radioisotopes including iridium 192, ruthenium 106, palladium 103, and ^{125}I. There were a number of reasons why ^{125}I was the radioisotope chosen for the COMS. Eleven millimeters of lead are needed to block 50% of the photons emitted from a plaque employing cobalt, whereas only 1 mm of gold can arrest all radioactive emission from an ^{125}I-containing plaque. Although some investigators use different radioisotopes for various tumor shapes and volumes, the most commonly employed radioactive isotope is ^{125}I. With a half-life of 60 days, this isotope is relatively safe for both the patient and the operating surgeon to use and can be incorporated into the plaque structure on site with a high degree of accuracy and reproducibility. Iodine 125 can provide sufficient dose rates to the tumor without exposing the sclera to excessive radiation.

Plaque dosimetry for individual tumors is provided by the ocular oncologist and radiation oncologist in conjunction with the radiation physicist and according to precise clinical measurements obtained through ophthalmoscopy, ocular imaging, and echography; plaques are constructed to cover the tumor base with a 2.0-mm margin greater than the largest tumor base dimension (see Fig. 13.4). At the time of surgery, plaque placement is facilitated by either transillumination of the tumor margins or standard indirect ophthalmoscopic localization techniques with or without ultrasound assistance. The plaque is then secured to the sclera and the final position verified by either intraoperative echography or an indirect ophthalmoscopic-fiberoptic system (see Fig. 13.5).

Brachytherapy is usually applied to medium category tumors with the aim of treating the tumor apex with approximately 8,500 cGy, delivered over 3 to 7 days (see Fig. 13.6). Brachytherapy in the COMS employed ^{125}I plaques.

Complications of plaque therapy include treatment failure due to tumor recurrence, radiation vasculopathy, cataract formation, vitreous hemorrhage, optic neuropathy, and diplopia resulting from ocular muscle manipulation during plaque placement and removal.

COMS Medium Tumor Results

Of the 1,317 patients enrolled in the study of medium-sized choroidal melanomas, 660 were assigned to

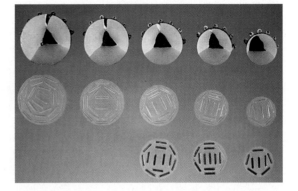

FIGURE 13.4 ☐ Structure of iodine 125 radioactive plaques employed in brachytherapy for choroidal melanoma. Seeds, silastic inserts, and gold backing disassembled. Plaque sizes range from 12 to 20 mm in diameter.

enuculation and 657 to ^{125}I brachytherapy. The primary outcome was mortality at 5 and 10 years (see Table 13.1). Eighty-one percent of patients had been followed up for 5 years and 32% for 10 years at the end of the 11.5-year accrual period. The unadjusted estimated 5-year survival rates were 81% and 82% respectively with no clinical or statistical difference in survival rates overall (see Table 13.2). Five-year rates of death with histopathologically proven melanoma metastasis were 11% and 9% following enucleation and brachytherapy, respectively (see Table 13.3).[4] The power of the study was sufficient to indicate that neither treatment was likely to increase or decrease mortality rates by as much as 25% relative to the other.

Although there was no significant survival advantage conferred by removal of the eye, the visual results

TABLE 13.1 ☐ **All-Cause Mortality Data for COMS Medium Tumors (COMS Report No. 18)**

| Interval (y) | Life Table Rates % (95% CI) | |
	Enucleation	^{125}I (%)
3	9 (7–11)	9 (7–12)
5	19 (16–23)	18 (15–21)
8	32 (28–36)	28 (24–32)
10	37 (33–42)	34 (30–39)

COMS, Collaborative Ocular Melanoma Study; CI, confidence interval.

of patients receiving treatment with radioactive ^{125}I plaque did show significant visual impairment due to radiation-related complications, particularly radiation retinopathy. At 3 years 50% of patients had a loss of six or more lines of visual acuity and 43% had a visual acuity <20/200.[5] The risk factors for visual loss at 3 years included:

1. Apical tumor height >5.0 mm
2. Distance to foveal avascular zone (FAZ) <2.0 mm
3. History of diabetes
4. Presence of tumor associated retinal detachment (RD)
5. Tumor not dome shaped

By 5 years following brachytherapy for choroidal melanoma, treatment failure resulting in enucleation occurred in 12.5% of patients. Treatment failure was the most common reason for enucleation within 3 years, and beyond 3 years, ocular pain was most common. The risk factors for treatment failure included older age at enrollment, larger tumors, and increasing proximity of the tumor to the fovea. Treatment failure was weakly associated with poorer survival. Almost all surviving patients retained good visual acuity in the fellow eyes throughout 5 years following treatment for choroidal melanoma.[6]

COMS Large Choroidal Melanoma Trial

Enucleation of eyes containing choroidal melanoma does not necessarily prevent metastatic disease from

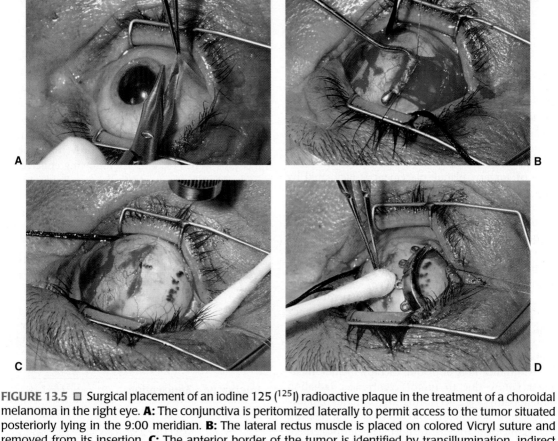

FIGURE 13.5 ◻ Surgical placement of an iodine 125 (^{125}I) radioactive plaque in the treatment of a choroidal melanoma in the right eye. **A:** The conjunctiva is peritomized laterally to permit access to the tumor situated posteriorly lying in the 9:00 meridian. **B:** The lateral rectus muscle is placed on colored Vicryl suture and removed from its insertion. **C:** The anterior border of the tumor is identified by transillumination, indirect ophthalmoscopy, or intraoperative ultrasound and marked on the scleral surface. **D:** A plaque without radioactivity identical to the proposed ^{125}I-containing plaque is placed to cover the marked sclera, and suture points are noted. **E:** The "dummy" plaque is removed and replaced with the radioactive plaque that is secured with Mersilene suture. **F:** The lateral rectus muscle is temporarily tied into the inferior fornix to be later resutured to the original insertion at the time of plaque removal. **G:** The conjunctiva is closed.

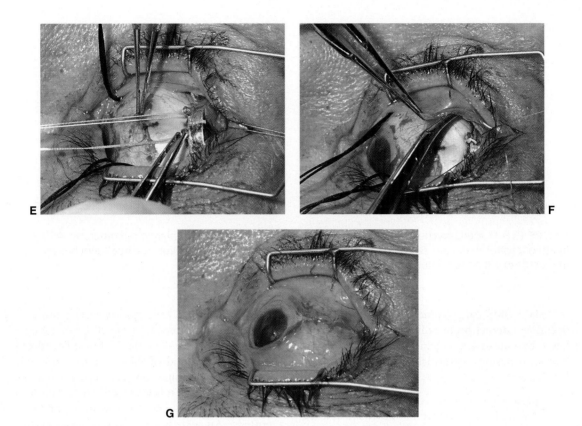

FIGURE 13.5 ☐ *(continued)*

presenting years later. The observations of Zimmerman et al.[7] and McLean et al.[8] raised the question of whether globe manipulation during enucleation disseminated viable tumor cells to produce metastases. This premise is often referred to as *The Zimmerman Hypothesis.* Adjunctive treatments have been proposed for large choroidal melanoma to reduce the possibility of tumor dissemination during enucleation. These have included pre- and postenucleation

irradiation of the globe and orbit as well as cryotherapy, chemotherapy, immunotherapy, and combinations thereof. The COMS was the first prospective randomized management strategy to assess preoperative radiation preceding enucleation. The primary outcome measure was mortality at 5 and 10 years.

TABLE 13.2 ☐ **Five-Year Mortality by Treatment and Age for COMS Medium Tumor Patients**

Age (y)	Enucleation (%)	^{125}I (%)	Log Rank *p* Value
<60	11	8	0.20
60–69	22	25	0.95
>69	29	28	0.57

COMS, Collaborative Ocular Melanoma Study.

TABLE 13.3 ☐ **Death with Confirmed Melanoma Metastasis for COMS Medium Tumor Patients**

Interval (y)	Life Table Rates, % (CI)	
	Enucleation (*n* = 660)	^{125}I (*n* = 657)
3	3.6 (2.4–5.3)	2.5 (1.5–4.0)
5	10.6 (8.3–13.4)	8.8 (6.7–11.4)
8	15.9 (12.8–19.5)	13.5 (10.7–17.0)

COMS, Collaborative Ocular Melanoma Study; CI, confidence interval.

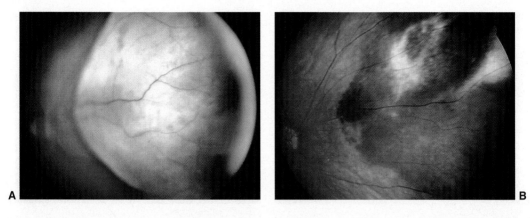

FIGURE 13.6 ◻ Medium choroidal melanoma treated by iodine 125 (^{125}I) plaque radiotherapy. **A:** Before treatment with ^{125}I plaque. **B:** The same tumor 2 years following treatment. Note the treatment has reduced the tumor to a flat pigmented remnant over this time.

The COMS Large Tumor Trial compared preoperative external beam radiation (2,000 cGy) followed by enucleation, to enucleation alone for large tumors. Inclusion criteria included the following (see Fig. 13.7):

1. Apical height >10 mm (or >8 mm whenever the proximal border of the tumor was too close to the optic nerve to qualify for the trial of enucleation vs. ^{125}I brachytherapy) or
2. Basal diameter >16 mm and apical height at least 2 mm

Five- and 10-year survival of patients with large choroidal melanoma randomized to either 2,000 cGy of preoperative external beam radiation followed by enucleation or enucleation alone was shown to be neither clinically nor statistically different between the treatment arms regardless of whether all-cause or disease-specific death was considered. At 5 years, the all-cause mortality and disease-specific death rates were 43% and 38% respectively. Ten-year all-cause mortality was 61% for patients in both treatment arms. The 10-year rate of disease-specific death was 45% in the pre-enucleation radiation arm and 40% in the enucleation only arm (see Table 13.4). Older age and larger basal tumor diameters were the most significant predictors of both all-cause and disease-specific mortality.[9]

Histopathologic Findings in COMS

The COMS yielded additional important clinical information. In particular, it confirmed the improved diagnostic accuracy for choroidal melanoma. Since first reported over 35 years ago, the misdiagnosis rate for choroidal melanoma fell from 20% to 1.4% over a 11-year period. In 1990, the COMS reviewed 413 specimens. Four hundred and eleven were correctly diagnosed as melanoma. One hemangioma and one melanocytoma were misdiagnosed. This established a misdiagnosis rate of 0.48%, the lowest rate ever reported.[10] An analysis based on 1,527 cases of enucleated eyes with uveal melanoma demonstrated a diagnostic accuracy for COMS centers of 99.7%.

The COMS also provided a large series of globes for evaluation to further characterize the pathology of choroidal melanoma. Histology showed the tumor cell type distribution to be spindle cell tumors in 9% of cases, mixed tumors in 86% of cases and epithelioid tumors in 5% of cases. Extensive local invasion of tumor was reported with rupture of Bruch membrane (87.7%), invasion of the retina (25.2%), vortex vein invasion (8.9%), and invasion into emissary canals (55.0%). Scleral invasion was noted in 55.7% of eyes with extension outside the sclera in 8.2%.

TABLE 13.4 ◻ **COMS Large Tumor Trial Melanoma-Specific Mortality (COMS Reports Nos 10 and 24)**

Interval (y)	Enucleation Alone (%)	Enucleation with Preop Radiation (%)
5	28	26
10	40	45

COMS, Collaborative Ocular Melanoma Study.

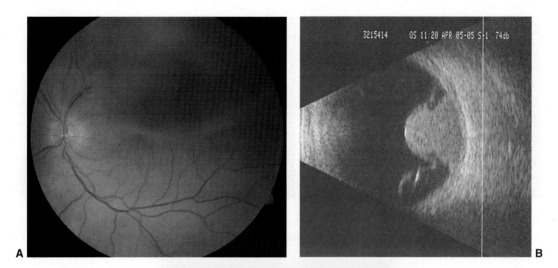

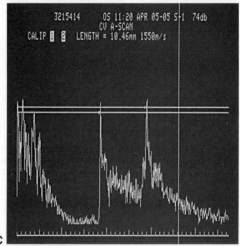

FIGURE 13.7 ▢ Large choroidal melanoma. **A:** Clinical appearance of a pigmented mass occupying the posterior pole with an associated serous retinal detachment. **B:** Ultrasonogram in B-mode demonstrating a collar-button shaped solid choroidal mass with associated serous retinal detachment. **C:** A-mode of the same tumor showing a vertical height of 10.46 mm.

This pathologic review reported 81.1% of eyes with involvement of the sclera by tumor in one form or another; these observations would suggest caution in accepting eye-wall resection as a treatment option for choroidal melanoma.[11]

Beyond COMS

Despite the success of the COMS many questions regarding the management of ocular melanoma remain. New therapies designed to avoid enucleation, preserve vision, and reduce metastatic deaths have emerged. Combination treatments incorporating radiation and laser have been suggested to reduce the secondary retinal complications of radiation. Specially designed plaques have allowed brachytherapy to tumors not considered treatable in the COMS protocol. The relative rarity of the tumor makes it difficult to evaluate all new therapeutic approaches with large clinical trials making clinicians reliant on the evaluation of multiple case series for treatment decisions.

Observation

Although the natural history of choroidal melanoma remains unclear with regard to its potential for malignancy, some small melanocytic tumors nevertheless

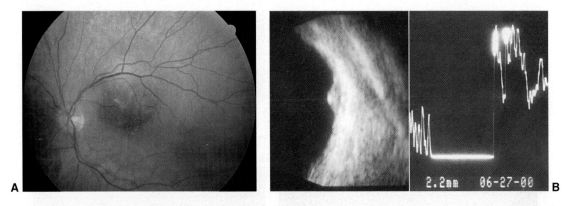

FIGURE 13.8 ◻ Small untreated choroidal melanoma observed over 2 years without change in clinical appearance. **A:** clinical appearance. **B:** Ultrasonogram demonstrating dome-shaped choroidal mass measuring 2.2 mm in vertical height.

appear clinically inactive and remain stable throughout long periods of observation (see Fig. 13.8). Shields et al. documented growth in 18% of 1,329 small melanocytic lesions and the COMS reported 31% growth in 204 patients with small choroidal lesions presumed to be melanomas over 5 years. Observation may therefore be appropriate for some slow-growing lesions, especially in visually critical situations, elderly or ill patients, or for cases in which the consequences of intervention might outweigh any perceived treatment benefit.

Transpupillary Thermotherapy

Infrared diode laser energy has been employed in the management of some small choroidal melanomas both as a primary treatment modality and as a secondary adjuvant therapy in patients receiving brachytherapy. Tumor death occurs through cellular necrosis as opposed to coagulative necrosis, a consequence of thermal laser energy, and has the theoretical advantage of providing tumor control with minimal collateral damage to normal tissue. The limited penetration of 810-nm light to a depth of approximately 4.0 mm permits the treatment of relatively flat primary tumors and small recurrences. Secondary adjuvant therapy has been proposed as a method to achieve complete tumor control while limiting the radiation dose at the tumor apex and the possibility of radiation retinopathy (see Fig. 13.9).

The evidence for transpupillary thermotherapy (TTT) to date is confined to a number of case series with variable duration of follow-up. Oosterhuis et al. published the first study on TTT as a treatment for choroidal melanoma in 1995.[12] Shields et al. reported reduced tumor thickness (27% in heavily pigmented tumors and 15% in amelanotic tumors) over 1.7 months.[13]

Several questions have been raised regarding the efficacy and long-term safety of TTT. Specifically, questions exist about the ability of TTT as a primary therapy to achieve tumor control given its limited penetration depth and the high incidence of cellular scleral invasion observed in medium-sized tumors. In addition, its role in amelanotic and variably pigmented tumors has been questioned. In one series, Stoffelns showed that despite apparent tumor regression, the choriocapillaris was incompletely destroyed in 90% of cases.[14] Harbour et al. reported retinal complications in 76% and treatment failure in 29% with primary TTT. Treatment failure occurred primarily at tumor margins.[15]

Brachytherapy for Peripapillary Melanoma

Plaques can be configured with indentations to treat juxtapapillary tumors with some success; however, the mechanical effect of this peripapillary plaque placement itself can restrict circulation to the optic nerve inducing significant early visual loss.

Charged Particle Radiotherapy

An alternative radiotherapeutic approach to treating choroidal melanoma employs charged particles in the form of protons or helium ions. This form of radiotherapy requires the surgical placement of tantalum markers sutured to the sclera for tumor localization, followed by the delivery of charged particle radiation

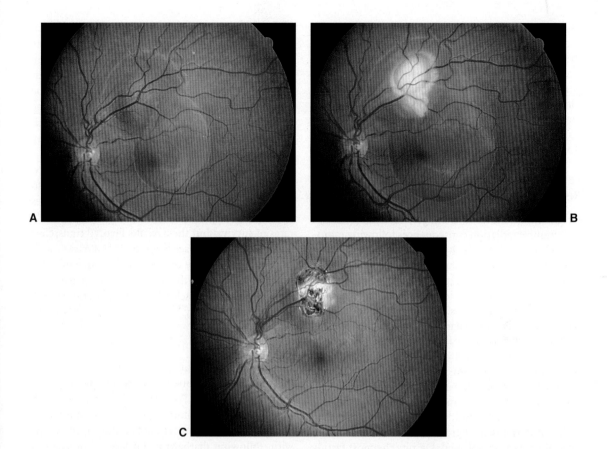

FIGURE 13.9 ☐ Transpupillary thermotherapy (TTT) treatment of a small choroidal melanoma (seen in Fig. 13.1). **A:** Clinical appearance of small melanoma with high-risk characteristics and associated serous detachment extending into the macula. **B:** Initial response immediately following TTT. **C:** One month following initial treatment with TTT. Note the absence of serous fluid with return of macular function.

in a highly focused system to the tumor. During treatment sessions, which last several minutes, 10- to 16-Gy fractions are delivered to achieve the desired total dose. Positively charged particles pass through tissue in a highly collimated beam path, ionizing surrounding atoms to a given ionization density known as the *Bragg Peak*. Collateral tissue damage is thereby minimized and tumor irradiation is more uniform, with the lateral irradiation dose dropping from 100% to 10% in <2.5 mm of the radiation field. A treatment margin of 2 to 3 mm is usually employed to account for a safety factor, an allowance for patient movement, and a factor to account for lateral spread of radiation. Although tumor control rates compare favorably with those reported for brachytherapy the use of charged particles results in a higher rate of neovascular glaucoma, cataract formation, keratoconjunctivitis, and lash loss.

A similar spectrum of tumors is treated with charged particle radiotherapy as with brachytherapy but because a significant amount of energy is delivered to the anterior aspect of the eye during treatment with charged particles, anterior complications are more prevalent than with radiation delivered posteriorly through the sclera. Gragoudas et al. reported that following proton beam radiation, radiation maculopathy occurred in approximately 75% of eyes with tumors within 1 disc diameter of the fovea and in 40% of eyes with tumors >1 disc diameter of the fovea.[16]

Other Teletherapy Approaches

More recently, other methods of radiotherapy employing either gamma knife or stereotactic hypofractionated radiation therapy have been evaluated in the treatment of choroidal melanoma. Gamma knife techniques have been associated with a higher incidence of neovascular glaucoma and there remains uncertainty in optimal dose delivery. Linac-based stereotactic radiotherapy has provided satisfactory control of juxtapapillary choroidal melanomas when plaque radiotherapy was not considered appropriate, and has the advantage of delivering radiation (usually 70 Gy in five fractions) without the need for surgical intervention (see Fig. 13.10).[17]

Lamellar and Full Thickness Eye-wall Resection

Originally intended to manage iridociliary tumors to minimize radiation consequences following radiotherapy, this technically challenging surgery is accomplished now with less frequency, owing to observed complications over time. In 1986, Foulds and Damato recommended resection for tumors 10 to 15 mm in diameter.[18] In lamellar sclerouvectomy, the tumor base is defined and a free margin around the tumor is outlined. After a scleral flap is fashioned, the deep scleral lamella is incised down to the choroid. The tumor is dissected from the retina, delivered with the scleral wall and the scleral flap is replaced. A full thickness resection includes removal of all layers of the eye wall beneath the tumor, including the retina. A corneoscleral graft repairs the defect and a vitrectomy is accomplished. Despite the most fastidious surgical technique, often employing hypotensive anesthesia, frequent complications including

vitreous and choroidal hemorrhage, retinal detachment, cataract formation, and residual tumor are frequently observed. The most compelling argument against eye-wall resection for treating ciliochoroidal melanoma, however, is the COMS enucleation experience, which reported local invasion of the sclera in 81.1% of eyes, suggesting a significant potential for viable melanoma cells to remain within the eye following treatment.

One matched case–control study compared transscleral resection to iodine brachytherapy for choroidal melanomas 6 mm or greater in thickness in 49 pairs of patients. The authors found similar rates of survival but their results favored transscleral resection for the preservation of 20/200 vision while avoiding some of the major complications of iodine brachytherapy, but the risk of local recurrence is increased with transscleral resection as compared to iodine brachytherapy.[19]

Internal Resection

Internal resection or endoresection of choroidal melanomas is a globe-saving technique first performed by Gholam Peyman in 1984 and described in 1986.[20] The technique involves the creation of an arcuate retinotomy or retinal flap during vitrectomy with, following diathermy and laser photocoagulation, resection of all visible tumor down to bare sclera under hypotensive anesthesia. The retina is

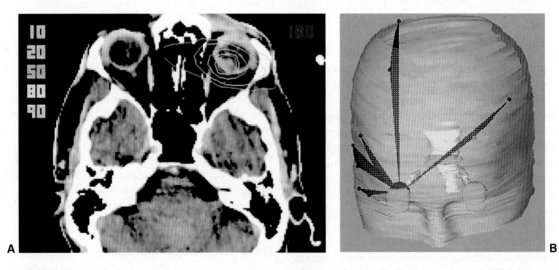

FIGURE 13.10 ☐ Linac-based stereotactic radiotherapy. **A:** Computed tomograph showing the isodose distribution in the treatment plan for a choroidal melanoma. **B:** 3D graphic demonstrating a non-coplanar arc plan for stereotactic hypofractionated radiation therapy to achieve a total dose of 70 Gy. This form of radiotherapy is administered as five fractions on alternate days.

then reposited during an air–fluid exchange and laser applied to the edges of the retinotomy and liberally to the resection bed in an effort to destroy any remaining viable melanoma cells. A scleral buckle is placed and the eye filled with silicone oil.[21] In one series of 32 patients followed for a mean of 40.1 months, 3 developed distant metastases and succumbed to their disease, only one of which was associated with a local recurrence, and 10 eyes (31.2%) had visual acuities ≥20/200.[21] This modality seems best suited to highly elevated posterior tumors, although the COMS findings of relatively common local invasion into the retina and sclera would suggest caution in the use of this technique.

Enucleation

For large tumors with extensive ocular involvement with intractable glaucoma, which are unresponsive to radiotherapy or demonstrate significant extrascleral extension or orbital invasion, enucleation is appropriate and remains the standard management option for some choroidal melanomas (see Fig. 13.11).[22] The COMS evaluated the use of adjunctive preoperative external beam radiation prior to enucleation

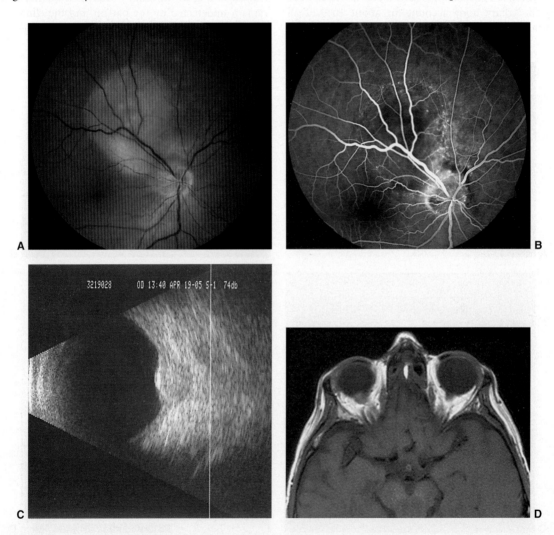

FIGURE 13.11 ▢ Juxtapapillary choroidal melanoma with extrascleral extension. **A:** Clinical appearance of a juxtapapillary choroidal melanoma with retained foveal vision. **B:** Fluorescein angiogram of the same tumor showing mottled fluorescence at the level of the choroid. **C:** Ultrasonogram in B-mode revealing a solid mass involving the choroid and extending through sclera posteriorly. **D:** Magnetic resonance imaging, T1 weighted, demonstrating the tumor occupying the choroid with extension through the sclera. This patient required enucleation with an extensive tenonectomy.

for patients with large choroidal melanoma and determined that there was no survival benefit following administration of 20 Gy before surgery. Nevertheless, surgical techniques to minimize globe manipulation seem valid. Wrapped implants and scleral shell/implant connections can result in highly effective cosmetic results.

Ciliary Body Melanoma

Ocular melanoma accounts for <0.5% of all human malignant neoplasms, and uveal melanoma is 1/10 as common as mucocutaneous melanoma. Melanomas of the ciliary body account for about 10% of all uveal melanomas. Since the human eye is devoid of lymphatics, the tumor spreads hematogenously or by local invasion.

Certain characteristics of the ciliary body in the human eye complicate the evaluation of this intraocular structure during routine ocular assessments. Since the ciliary body is situated posterior to the iris base, the anterior location of ciliary body melanomas permit substantial growth to proceed hidden from both the patient and the clinician.[23]

Clinical Evaluation

Although a growing ciliary body melanoma can remain undetected by the patient and the clinician for years, certain features suggest their presence.

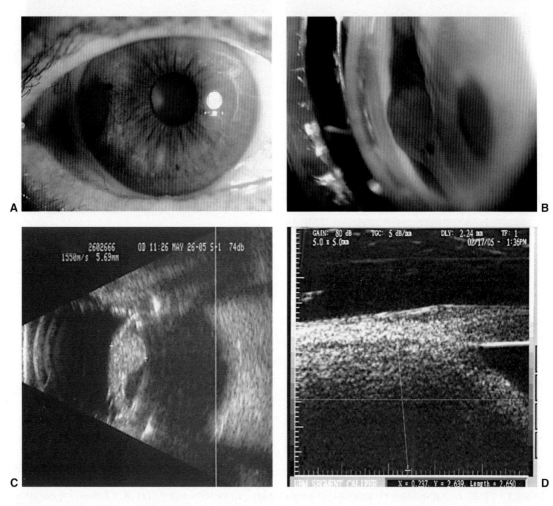

FIGURE 13.12 ◻ Ciliary body melanoma with extension into the anterior chamber. **A:** Clinical appearance of anterior extension of ciliary body melanoma into the iris base. **B:** Appearance of tumor involvement of angle structures. **C:** Ultrasonogram in the B-mode (standoff) to show the main body of the tumor occupying the ciliary body. **D:** Ultrasound biomicroscopy showing the anterior aspect of the ciliary body melanoma involving chamber angle.

Large tumors can be associated with dilated episcleral vasculature, bulging of the iris, sector cataract, lens deformation, and focal episcleral pigmentation. Such tumors can invade the anterior chamber or progress posteriorly to involve the peripheral choroid (ciliochoroidal). Transillumination may provide assistance in localization but the presence of retinal detachment and ciliary band shadows can confuse interpretation. Medium-sized ciliary body tumors can be defined by B scan (standoff) echography and are frequently dome shaped with low internal reflectivity. Tumor characteristics, including anterior and posterior margins, are more easily defined with ultrasound biomicroscopy (UBM), which can provide valuable information when considering biopsy, resection, or radiotherapeutic intervention (see Fig. 13.12).[24] Small ciliary body melanomas are usually discovered incidentally following peripheral retinal examination for other disease. Tumors under 3.0 mm in thickness change very little over time and can be followed carefully with UBM (see Fig. 13.13). The clock hour extent of these tumors should be noted with care to avoid overlooking early diffuse or ring tumor configuration which, although rare, presents a more grave management issue and ultimate prognosis. The "ring" variety of ciliary body melanoma occurs with a frequency of about 3 cases per 1,000 uveal melanomas and is commonly overlooked if it is not considered as the underlying cause for unilateral glaucoma, refractory to treatment. Owing to the generally large size of ring melanomas at the time of diagnosis, the prognosis is poor and management is limited to enucleation.

Management of Ciliary Body Melanoma

Tumor size, extent of intraocular involvement, systemic health, and patient preference must be considered when managing patients with ciliary body melanoma. Fine needle aspiration biopsy (FNAB) has been helpful in difficult diagnostic situations[25] but care in the interpretation of findings is essential. Although the majority of small tumors of the ciliary body demonstrate little or no growth over time, if growth should occur or if other ocular structures should become compromised, treatment is usually considered. Brachytherapy has been shown to achieve effective tumor control for medium-sized tumors with relatively well preserved vision. Cataract formation, radiation vasculopathy, vitreous hemorrhage, and chronic keratitis are notable complications. Charged particle radiotherapy employing protons has demonstrated a similar treatment benefit in managing ciliary body melanoma although neovascular glaucoma and lash loss are somewhat more prevalent as complicating factors. Large tumors of the ciliary body including ring melanomas usually require enucleation, and in some cases, exenteration if significant extrascleral or intraorbital invasion has developed.

Although local ciliary body tumor resection is achievable with small- and medium-sized tumors and has the advantage of providing histopathologic diagnosis, complications including cataract formation, vitreous hemorrhage, retinal detachment, and visual distortion can be hazardous. More compelling, however, is the concern that the resection margins may be incompletely excised despite the most fastidious surgical technique. The application of a radioactive plaque over the resection site may add an element of security in some cases but a significant survival benefit has yet to be demonstrated following this adjunctive measure.

Iris Melanoma

Considered the most common primary iris malignancy, malignant melanoma involving the iris nevertheless comprises only 5% to 10% of all uveal melanomas. The disease is usually noted in later life, shows no sex predilection, and if confined to the iris,

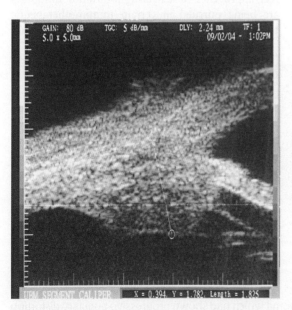

FIGURE 13.13 ▫ Small ciliary body melanoma. Ultrasound biomicrocopy through the ciliary body showing a small melanoma or nevus occupying the ciliary body and involving the iris base.

is associated with a low disease-specific mortality, in the range of 4% to 8%. Metastasis is rare.

Iris melanomas have a variable pattern of presentation including solitary nodular, plaque-like and diffuse varieties with different degrees of pigmentation and vascularity. Most iris pigment proliferations do not require intervention but if accurate follow-up discloses a changing pattern of growth, increasing iris distortion, related intraocular pressure elevation or involvement of intraocular structures, more definitive management is usually considered. Pigment dispersion or direct tumor invasion into the anterior chamber angle is thought to induce secondary glaucoma and cataract formation usually develops in close association to the tumor. Other findings associated with iris melanomas including heterochromia, spontaneous hyphema, and uveitis have been reported with less frequency. UBM not only provides detailed imaging of iris tumor dimensions and characteristics but can also define anterior and posterior tumor margins in relation to other ocular structures. Such information is essential to assess growth patterns and to provide information if intervention is to be considered (see Fig. 13.14).

Management of Iris Melanoma

Although features such as tumor size, iris margin distortion, intrinsic tumor vascularity and sector cataract formation may support a diagnosis of malignancy, documented growth with or without

associated ocular morbidity usually determines the need for intervention. Sector iridectomy, occasionally combined with cataract removal, is an appropriate approach to therapy for tumors with no more than 2 to 3 clock hours of involvement. Also, brachytherapy, in most instances, using ^{125}I, has been employed in the treatment of certain iris melanomas and has provided satisfactory local tumor control with acceptable anterior segment preservation. The application of plaque radiotherapy employing a safety margin around the tumor would seem to gain a theoretic advantage in this form of intervention. Lesions extending into the ciliary body can be managed by iridocyclectomy or plaque radiotherapy.[26] Large or diffuse tumors of the iris with intractable glaucoma are often best managed with enucleation.[27]

Conclusion

Over the last two decades, intraocular melanoma, with its variable presentation, has become easier to diagnose and is being defined with greater accuracy. Local tumor control is generally successful and can be achieved with various interventions. To increase long-term survival and improve the quality of life, however, there is a need to combine local management of this malignancy with measures to detect and treat micrometastatic disease. Direct and indirect approaches to activating antitumor immunity are being pursued in certain immunotherapeutic treatment models. Continuing genetic description

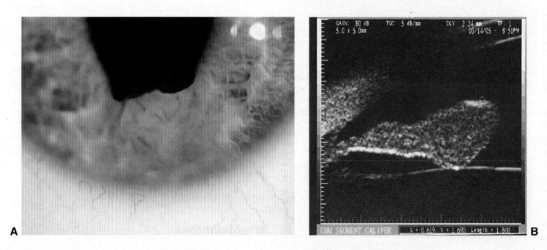

FIGURE 13.14 ☐ Clinical appearance of an iris melanoma which had shown progressive pupillary distortion over 2 years. **A:** Pigmented vascularized mass involving the iris in the 6:00 position. **B:** Ultrasound biomicrocopy of the same tumor occupying full thickness iris with early angle involvement measuring 1.8 mm at its thickest point. This tumor underwent iodine 125 plaque radiotherapy that achieved good local control.

relating to the normal and aberrant control of cellular growth and replication will improve our understanding of oncogenesis and will bear directly on our understanding of choroidal tumor production. Angiomanipulatory research aimed at inhibiting or modifying tumor-related angiogenesis coupled with the discovery of novel drug delivery systems continues to hold promise as a mechanism to modify both local and metastatic disease processes. Our continuing investment in the field of ocular oncology must be to encourage the appropriate scientific application of such novel approaches to the control of this and other malignancies.

Acknowledgments

The author wishes to acknowledge the contribution and support of Dr Charles Pavlin, the many physicians, and allied professionals of the Ocular Oncology Clinic of Princess Margaret Hospital with special thanks to Allan Connor and Keith Oxley of PhotoGraphics, University Health Network and Lee Penney, Manager of the Ocular Oncology Clinic, Princess Margaret Hospital.

References

1. Collaborative Ocular Melanoma Study Group. Factors predictive of growth and treatment of small Choroidal melanoma. COMS Report No. 5. *Arch Ophthalmol.* 1997;115:1537–1544.

2. Collaborative Ocular Melanoma Study Group. Mortality in patients with small choroidal melanoma. COMS Report No. 4. *Arch Ophthalmol.* 1997;115:886–893.

3. Shields CL, Shields JA, Kiratli H, et al. Risk factors for growth and metastasis of small choroidal melanocytic lesions. *Ophthalmology.* 1995;102:1351–1361.

4. Collaborative Ocular Melanoma Study Group. The Collaborative Ocular Melanoma Study (COMS) randomized trial of iodine 125 brachytherapy for choroidal melanoma.III. Initial mortality findings. COMS Report No. 18. *Arch Ophthalmol.* 2001;119:969–982.

5. Collaborative Ocular Melanoma Study Group. The Collaborative Ocular Melanoma Study (COMS) randomized trial of I-125 brachytherapy for medium choroidal melanoma. Visual acuity after 3 years. COMS Report No. 16. *Ophthalmology.* 2001;108:348–366.

6. Collaborative Ocular Melanoma Study Group. The COMS randomized trial of iodine 125 brachytherapy for choroidal melanoma. Local treatment failure and enucleation in the first 5 years after brachytherapy. COMS Report No. 19. *Ophthalmology.* 2004;111:1514.

7. Zimmerman LE, Mclean IW. An evaluation of enucleation in the management of uveal melanomas. *Am J Ophthalmol.* 1979;87:741–760.

8. Mclean IW, Zimmerman LE, Foster WD. Survival rates after enucleation of eyes with malignant melanoma. *Am J Ophthalmol.* 1979;88: 794–797.

9. Collaborative Ocular Melanoma Study Group. The Collaborative Ocular Melanoma Study (COMS) randomized trial of pre-enucleation radiation of large choroidal melanoma. IV. Ten- year mortality findings and prognostic factors. COMS Report No. 24. *Am J Ophthalmol.* 2004;138:936–951.

10. Collaborative Ocular Melanoma Study Group. Accuracy of diagnosis of choroidal melanomas in the Collaborative Ocular Melanoma Study. COMS Report No. 1. *Arch Ophthalmol.* 1990; 108:1268–1273.

11. Collaborative Ocular Melanoma Study Group. Histopathologic characteristics of uveal melanomas in eyes enucleated from the Collaborative Ocular Melanoma Study. COMS Report No. 6. *Am J Ophthalmol.* 1998;125:745–766.

12. Journee-de Korver JG, Oosterhuis JA, Van Best JA, et al. Xenon arc photocoagulator used for transpupillary hyperthermia. *Doc Ophthalmol.* 1991;78:183–187.

13. Shields CL, Shields JA, De Potter P, et al. Transpupillary thermotherapy in the management of choroidal melanoma. *Ophthalmology.* 1996;103:1642–1650.

14. Stoffelns BM. Primary transpupillary thermotherapy (TTT) for malignant choroidal melanoma. *Acta Ophthalmol Scand.* 2002;80: 25–31.

15. Harbour JW, Meredith TA, Thompson PA, et al. Transpupillary thermotherapy versus plaque radiotherapy for suspected choroidal melanomas. *Ophthalmology.* 2003;110:2207–2215.

16. Gragoudas ES, Lane AM, Regan S, et al. A randomized controlled trial of varying radiation doses in the treatment of choroidal melanoma. *Arch Ophthalmol.* 2000;118:773–778.

17. Emara K, Weisbrod DJ, Sahgal A, et al. Stereotactic radiotherapy in the treatment of juxtapapillary choroidal melanoma: Preliminary results.
Int J Radiat Oncol Biol Phys. 2004;59:94–100 .

18. Foulds WS, Damato BE. Alternatives to enucleation in the management of choroidal melanoma.
Aust N Z J Ophthalmol. 1986;14:19–27.

19. Kivela T, Puusaari I, Damato B. Transscleral resection versus iodine brachytherapy
for choroidal malignant melanomas 6 millimeters or more in thickness: A matched
case-control study. *Ophthalmology*. 2003;110:
2235–2244.

20. Peyman GA, Cohen SB. Ab interno resection of
uveal melanoma. *Int Ophthalmol*. 1986;9:29–36.

21. Kertes PJ, Johnson JC, Peyman GA. Internal
resection of posterior uveal melanomas. *Br J
Ophthalmol*. 1998;82:1147–1153.

22. Shields JA, Shields CL, Donoso LA. Management
of posterior uveal melanoma. *Surv Ophthalmol*.
1991;36:161–195.

23. Simpson ER. Ciliary body melanoma: A special
challenge. *Can J Ophthalmol*. 2004;39:365–371.

24. Maberley DAL, Pavlin CJ, McGowan HD, et al.
Ultrasound biomicroscopic imaging of the ante-
rior aspect of peripheral choroidal melanomas.
Am J Ophthalmol. 1997;123:506–514.

25. Grossniklaus HE. Fine-needle aspiration biopsy
of the iris. *Arch Ophthalmol*. 1992;110:969–976.

26. Finger PT. Plaque radiation therapy for malignant melanoma of the iris and ciliary body. *Am
J Ophthalmol*. 2001;132:328–335.

27. Shields CL, Shields JA, Materin M, et al.
Iris melanoma: risk factors for metastasis in
169 consecutive patients. *Ophthalmology*. 2001;
108:172–178.

SECTION **VII**

NEURO-OPHTHALMOLOGY

CHAPTER **14**

Optic Neuritis

Jonathan D. Trobe, MD

Overview

The treatment of optic neuritis has been explored in several randomized controlled trials (RCTs).[1–13] In the Optic Neuritis Treatment Trial (ONTT),[1–6] the largest trial to date, high-dose intravenous methylprednisolone (IVMP) treatment accelerated visual recovery but had no impact on final visual outcome. Three smaller RCTs on optic neuritis[9–11] found similar results. Two RCTs of intravenous immunoglobulin, one in acute optic neuritis[12] and the other in chronic residual optic neuropathy following optic neuritis,[13] failed to demonstrate any treatment benefit. The ONTT also found that high-dose IVMP treatment temporarily retarded the development of clinically definite multiple sclerosis (CDMS).[2,3] Two RCTs[7,8] of interferon β-1a in the treatment of acute optic neuritis and other "clinically isolated" neurologic syndromes that predict multiple sclerosis (MS) found that this treatment significantly reduced the development of CDMS and the accumulation of magnetic resonance imaging (MRI) abnormalities typical of MS.

The major findings of these trials are: (i) Neither corticosteroid (CS) nor intravenous immunoglobulin (IVIG) treatment appears to have a meaningful effect on visual outcome; CS treatment has no long-term impact on neurologic outcome; (ii) continuous treatment of acute optic neuritis with interferon β-1a reduces the development of new MS-like neurologic manifestations and accumulation of MS-like MRI abnormalities, but there is still no evidence that it reduces long-term neurologic disability; and (iii) acute optic neuritis, even if untreated, has a relatively benign neurologic course as compared to other

283

clinically isolated neurologic syndromes (weakness, ataxia, diplopia).

We will examine each of these findings separately.

Impact of Corticosteroid or Intravenous Immunoglobulin Treatment on Visual Outcome in Optic Neuritis

The treatment of acute optic neuritis with oral, intravenous, and retrobulbar CS was common before the first publication of the ONTT in 1992,[1] based largely on anecdotal and small-trial evidence.[1]

The ONTT was the first large RCT to study the effect of IVMP and low-dose oral prednisone (OP) on acute optic neuritis. In the ONTT, 457 patients with acute optic neuritis were randomized to three groups: (i) IVMP 250 mg four times per day for three days, followed by OP 1 mg per kg for 11 days; (ii) OP 1 mg per kg for 14 days; or (iii) placebo. Acute optic neuritis was defined as a monocular visual deficit of no more than 8 days' duration with an ipsilateral afferent pupillary defect in patients aged between 18 and 46 years. Patients were entered into the trial only if they had no previous episodes of optic neuritis in that eye, no previous CS treatment for MS, and no other systemic condition associated with optic neuritis apart from MS.

The ONTT end points were visual acuity, visual fields (Humphrey and Goldmann), color vision (Farnsworth-Munsell 100-hue), contrast sensitivity (Pelli-Robson chart), and other neurologic deficits as assessed by a neurologist. All patients underwent brain MRI and blood tests for antinuclear antibody and treponemal antigen, and a chest X-ray directed at sarcoidosis. Lumbar puncture was optional and less than half the cohort underwent the same. The examining neurologists were masked as to the treatment but the patients who received IVMP knew that they had received it.

Neither CS regimen produced any benefit on the visual outcome. Visual function improved more rapidly in the IVMP group but the difference was relatively trivial. These findings held in the follow-up evaluations up to 10 years after study entry. Patients who had been treated with OP without a preceding regimen of IVMP had a doubling of the recurrence rate of optic neuritis in the affected and the contralateral eyes. The IVMP group had a reduction in the development of CDMS after 2 years, but that effect had evaporated by 3 years after study entry.

The upshot of the treatment aspects of the ONTT is that this IVMP regimen, chosen because it was common in the treatment of organ transplant rejection, had no impact on visual recovery, and only a temporary effect on conversion to MS. OP had no impact on visual recovery and doubled the recurrence rate of optic neuritis.

Similarly defined cohorts of 66 optic neuritis patients in an English RCT[9] and a Japanese RCT[10] also found no benefit on visual recovery of an IVMP regimen similar to that of the ONTT. A Danish RCT[11] of 60 patients found that oral MP of 500 mg per day for 3 days with a 10-day taper had exactly the same impact on visual recovery as did the ONTT IVMP regimen.

Like IVMP, IVIG appears to have no meaningful impact on visual recovery in optic neuritis. In a Danish RCT of 68 patients with acute optic neuritis, five infusions of IVIG of 0.4 g per kg body weight administered on days 0, 1, 2, 30, and 60 after symptom onset produced no benefit in standard measures of visual function at 6 months.[12] An IVIG RCT from the Mayo Clinic, using a similar regimen, showed that there was no meaningful impact on visual function in 55 patients with persistent visual dysfunction from optic neuritis in MS.[13]

Impact of Interferon β on the Conversion of Optic Neuritis to Multiple Sclerosis

Multiple trials of patients with relapsing-remitting multiple sclerosis (RRMS) have established that chronic interferon β or glatiramer acetate treatment reduces the clinical relapse rate by 30% to 35% and reduces the accumulation of MRI signal abnormalities over a 2- to 3-year period.[14] Because these agents also attenuate the immune process involved in MS, they have been called *immune-modulating agents* (IMAs).

It was logical, then, to explore whether chronic treatment with any of the IMAs, begun shortly after the onset of acute optic neuritis or brain stem or spinal cord manifestations typical of MS (called *clinically isolated syndromes*), would reduce the conversion to CDMS and the accumulation of MRI abnormalities.

Two interferon β-1a trials, one conducted in the United States with Avonex (the controlled high risk subjects Avonex multiple sclerosis prevention study [CHAMPS] trial)[7] and the other conducted in Europe with Rebif (the early treatment of multiple sclerosis [ETOMS] trial),[8] included patients who had at least two MRI signal abnormalities typical of MS (see Fig. 14.1). (Earlier trials had shown that such abnormalities would predict a high likelihood of later development of CDMS.)

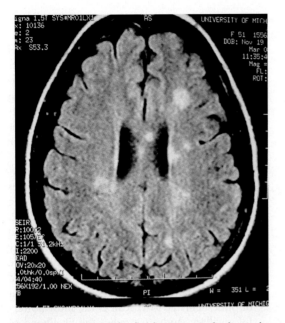

FIGURE 14.1 ☐ Axial fluid-attenuated inversion recovery (FLAIR) magnetic resonance imaging (MRI) shows multiple focal high-signal abnormalities characteristic of multiple sclerosis (MS). Such abnormalities, which are found in approximately 50% of patients with typical acute optic neuritis even if they have no history or physical evidence of other neurologic deficits, markedly increase the likelihood that a patient with optic neuritis will later develop clinically definite MS ("high-risk MRI").

The CHAMPS trial[7] of 393 patients found that Avonex reduced the 3-year conversion to MS from 50% to 35% and the accumulation of MRI signal abnormalities. The ETOMS trial[8] of 309 patients found a 2-year reduction in the conversion to MS from 45% to 34%.

Although the RRMS trials and the CHAMPS and ETOMS trials have clearly shown a reduction in neurologic relapses and MRI accumulation, the effect is not striking. More importantly, no RCT has been carried out long enough to determine whether any of the IMAs has a beneficial effect on long-term neurologic disability.[14] Many investigators are predicting that there will be such a benefit because a rapid early relapse rate[15] and an early accumulation of MRI signal abnormalities[16] have been associated with a higher long-term disability rate. Another basis for this prediction is that axonal loss, which occurs within inflammatory MS plaques,[17] is believed to be associated with long-term disability.[18] If IMAs can suppress inflammation, the argument goes, they could reduce axonal loss.[18]

The implications of these facts for the management of acute optic neuritis are still unclear.[19] Some commentators have stated that therapy with interferon β-1a should be recommended to all patients with acute optic neuritis who have an MRI scan showing signal abnormalities typical of MS, even when there are no history or current physical findings suggestive of MS. Extrapolating from the equivalently beneficial effects of interferon β-1b and glatiramer acetate on RRMS, other observers have suggested that physicians should not limit the recommendation to interferon β-1a, but consider treating with *any of the IMAs*. A less aggressive position is to wait to see if the disease is active, as determined by a brief interlude to relapse or rapid accumulation of MRI signal abnormalities.[19] This latter position is based on the robust evidence that the natural history of untreated optic neuritis is very good—much better than that of clinically isolated acute brain stem or spinal cord manifestations (see The Natural History of Optic Neuritis).

The Natural History of Optic Neuritis

The greatest contribution of the ONTT has been to verify the relatively "benign" long-term visual and neurologic outcome in patients with acute optic neuritis. In the ONTT, visual function remained remarkably stable after the one-year measurement. At 10 years after study entry, 69% of patients had 20/20 or better acuity in both eyes. As many as 86% of patients had a visual acuity of 20/20 or better in at least one eye. More than 99% of patients would be eligible for a driving license.[5] Recurrent optic neuritis occurred in either eye (with equal frequency in initially affected and unaffected eyes) in 35% of patients, but visual loss was not greatly diminished by the recurrences. These results are comparable to other large series which had less rigorous monitoring than the ONTT.[20,21]

At 10 years, only 38% of ONTT patients had developed CDMS.[4] Even among those with abnormal MRIs at study entry, who were generally not treated with IMAs but were often considered candidates for such treatment, only slightly more than half (56%) had developed CDMS. And among the 38% of ONTT patients who developed CDMS, only 14% had severe disability (were nonambulatory).[6]

A large natural history study conducted in France[22] showed that lower long-term disability was associated with complete recovery from the initial episode, a long latency until a relapse occurred, and few relapses within the first five years.

MS initiated by optic neuritis appears to have a relatively favorable prognosis relative to MS initiated by other clinically isolated syndromes. A long-term Swedish study found that clinically isolated syndromes of brain stem or spinal cord dysfunction have a threefold greater rate of severe disability than does optic neuritis.[23] Thus, typical optic neuritis—even with MS-like lesions on MRI—does not always lead to CDMS; if it does, the disability is relatively mild. Previous observers had suspected this, and called optic neuritis–initiated MS *benign MS*.

The ONTT has also confirmed that brain MRI is the best predictor of whether CDMS is likely to follow optic neuritis.[4] A single >2-mm diameter high T2 MRI signal abnormality was enough to increase the 10-year risk of developing CDMS from 22% to 56%.[4] In the ONTT, the number of MRI signal abnormalities (MRI "lesion load") was not correlated with long-term neurologic disability.[6] But in other studies, long-term neurologic disability has been correlated with MRI lesion load,[16] infratentorial lesions,[24] early accumulation of MRI signal abnormalities,[16] and early development of brain stem and spinal cord manifestations.[23]

In the ONTT, blood tests directed at connective tissue disease and syphilis, and a chest X-ray directed at sarcoidosis were unrevealing.[1] MRI disclosed a pertinent abnormality other than MS (a pituitary tumor) in only 1 of 457 studies. Lumbar puncture disclosed signs of autoimmune inflammation in some cases, but these signs had relatively little predictive value compared to MRI in terms of whether the patient would later develop CDMS.

Conclusions

The major clinical trials in acute optic neuritis have provided the following information:

1. *Impact of corticosteroid treatment.* A single standard IVMP/CS regimen (MP 1 gm per day for 3 days, OP for 11 days) mildly accelerates visual recovery in acute optic neuritis but does not affect final visual outcome. Low-dose OP (1 mg per kg) without preceding IVMP is harmful in that it significantly increases the recurrence rate of optic neuritis. High-dose OP (oral MP 500 mg per day × 3 days with a 10-day taper) probably accelerates visual recovery to the same degree as the standard IVMP/CS regimen. One-time administration of CS has no long-term benefit on the rate of conversion to CDMS. Whether periodic retreatment with a CS regimen would be beneficial is yet unknown.

2. *Impact of immunomodulatory treatment.* Continuous interferon β-1a (Avonex, Rebif) treatment reduces the conversion to CDMS and the accumulation of MRI signal abnormalities in patients with optic neuritis and other clinically isolated syndromes accompanied by at least two typical MRI signal abnormalities at outset. However, there is no evidence yet that this prophylactic treatment has any effect on the long-term neurologic disability of MS.

3. *Visual and other neurologic outcomes in optic neuritis.* The 10-year visual and neurologic outcomes in patients with acute optic neuritis without a prior diagnosis of MS are relatively favorable. Even among those patients who are not treated with IMAs, fewer than 5% will become visually or neurologically disabled. Only slightly more than 1/3 of the patients will even be diagnosed as having CDMS 10 years after the initial bout of optic neuritis. MRI scan is the most powerful ancillary study to predict the likelihood of developing CDMS. IMA treatment can be most reasonably justified in patients with optic neuritis who develop brain stem or spinal cord manifestations within a short interval after developing optic neuritis, or perhaps in those with an initially high MRI "lesion load" or rapid accumulation of MRI signal abnormalities. These considerations have prompted the notion that patients with isolated optic neuritis and normal MRI scans undergo repeat MRI scanning within a 3- or 6-month interval to determine if pertinent signal abnormalities have appeared.

Current Practices

There is no broad consensus on the proper management of first-time optic neuritis. However, a large 1999 survey of ophthalmologists and neurologists practicing in the United States[25] indicated that most practitioners had accepted the findings of the ONTT and were at least offering a standard regimen of IVMP followed by OP to patients with typical acute optic neuritis. Whether this approach reflects current practices in the United States and other countries is unknown. It is also unknown how frequently practitioners are treating these patients with immunomodulatory agents. Outside the United States, where health care is usually underwritten by government agencies, CS treatment is often not covered, and immunomodulatory treatment is almost never covered in these circumstances.

Notwithstanding these facts, the following guidelines are generally accepted as reasonable:

1. Exclude "atypical" optic neuritis associated with underlying infectious or non-infectious inflammatory disorders (syphilis, herpes zoster, Wegener's granulomatosis, sarcoidosis, idiopathic pachymeningitis) that must be managed according to the underlying diagnosis. Use history, physical findings, and perhaps ancillary studies to determine this.

2. If the diagnosis is "typical optic neuritis" (no underlying disorder except perhaps MS), consider performing a brain MRI largely to determine whether there is ample imaging evidence of subclinical demyelinization ("high-risk MRI").

3. To patients with high-risk MRI, offer IVMP 1 gm/day for 3 days followed by OP 1 mg per kg for 11 days, explaining that there is only a short-term benefit. To patients without high-risk MRI, explain that there is no evidence for any benefit of this treatment.

4. In patients with high-risk MRI, discuss the option of starting immunomodulatory agents. The benefit of such treatment lies in slightly reducing the accumulation of MRI signal abnormalities and the development of MS-like relapses. There is yet no evidence that this treatment reduces long-term disability.

Principal ONTT Findings

1. CS treatment of typical acute optic neuritis had no long-term benefits. It slightly hastened visual recovery. In patients with high-risk MRI scans (multiple high-signal abnormalities typical of MS), the 2-year conversion to MS was reduced by 50%, but by 3 years after trial entry, the conversion to MS was equal in corticosteroid-treated and placebo-treated patients. Treatment with OP without a preceding regimen of IVMP was harmful in that it doubled the recurrence rate of optic neuritis.

2. Brain MRI was by far the best predictor of whether a patient with optic neuritis would develop clinically definite MS. That is, a single cerebral high-signal abnormality measuring at least 2 mm in diameter raised the 10-year risk of MS from 22% to 56%.

3. The long-term visual outcome after optic neuritis was favorable. At 10 years after study entry, 69% of patients had 20/20 or better visual acuity in affected eyes. As many as 86% of patients had 20/20 or better visual acuity in one eye. Over 10 years, optic neuritis recurred in 35% of patients but these recurrences did not substantially lower long-term visual function.

4. The long-term nonvisual neurologic outcome after optic neuritis was favorable compared to that of patients whose initial demyelinating event involves the brain stem or spinal cord. After 10 years, only 38% of patients had developed clinically definite MS. Even among patients whose entry MRIs were high-risk, only 56% had developed clinically definite MS. Among the patients who developed MS, only 14% had severe neurologic disability (nonambulatory status).

References

1. Beck RW, Cleary PA, Anderson MM, et al. A randomized, controlled trial of corticosteroids in the treatment of acute optic neuritis. *N Engl J Med*. 1992;326:581–588.

2. Beck RW, Cleary PA, Trobe JD, et al. The effect of corticosteroids for acute optic neuritis on the subsequent development of multiple sclerosis. *N Engl J Med*. 1993;329:1764–1769.

3. Optic Neuritis Study Group. The 5-year risk of MS after optic neuritis: Experience of the optic neuritis treatment trial. *Neurology*. 1997; 49:1404–1413.

4. Optic Neuritis Study Group. High and low risk profiles for the development of multiple sclerosis within ten years after optic neuritis. Experience of the optic neuritis treatment trial. *Arch Ophthalmol*. 2003;121;944–949.

5. Optic Neuritis Study Group. Visual function more than 10 years after optic neuritis: Experience of the optic neuritis treatment trial. *Am J Ophthalmol*. 2004;137:77–83.

6. Optic Neuritis Study Group. Neurologic impairment ten years after optic neuritis. *Arch Neurol*. 2004;61:1386–1389.

7. Jacobs LD, Beck RW, Simon JH, et al. Intramuscular interferon beta-1a therapy initiated during a first demyelinating event in multiple sclerosis. CHAMPS Study Group. *N Engl J Med*. 2000;343:898–904.

8. Comi G, Filippi M, Barkhof F, et al. Effect of early interferon treatment on conversion to definite multiple sclerosis: A randomised study. *Lancet*. 2001;357:1576–1582.

9. Kapoor R, Miller DH, Jones SJ, et al. Effects of intravenous methylprednisolone on outcome in MRI-based prognostic subgroups in acute optic neuritis. *Neurology*. 1998;50: 230–237.

10. Wakakura M, Mashimo K, Oono S, et al. Multicenter clinical trial for evaluating methyl-prednsiolone pulse treatment of idiopathic optic neuritis in Japan. *Jpn J Ophthalmol.* 1999;43: 133–138.

11. Sellebjerg F, Nielsen HS, Frederiksen JL, et al. A randomized, controlled trial of oral high-dose methylprednisolone in acute optic neuritis. *Neurology.* 1999;52:1479–1484.

12. Roed HG, Langkilde A, Sellebjerg F, et al. A double-blind, randomized trial of IV immuno-globulin treatment in acute optic neuritis. *Neurology.* 2005;64:804–810.

13. Noseworthy JH, O'Brien PC, Petterson TM, et al. A randomized trial of intravenous immunoglob-ulin in inflammatory demyelinating optic neuri-tis. *Neurology.* 2001;56:1514–1522.

14. Kieseier BC, Hartung H-P. Current disease-modifying therapies in multiple sclerosis. *Semin Neurol.* 2003;23:133–145.

15. Weinshenker BG, Bass B, Rice GP, et al. The natural history of multiple sclerosis: A geographically based study. 1. Clinical course and disability. *Brain.* 1989;112:133–146.

16. Brex PA, Ciccarelli O, O'Riordan JI, et al. A longitudinal study of abnormalities on MRI and disability from multiple sclerosis. *N Engl J Med.* 2002;346:158–164.

17. Trapp BD, Peterson J, Ransohoff RM, et al. Axonal transection in the lesions of multiple sclerosis. *N Engl J Med.* 1998;338:278–285.

18. Rudick RA. Evolving concepts in the patho-genesis of multiple sclerosis and their therapeutic implications. *J Neuroophthalmol.* 2001;21:279–283.

19. Miller D, Barkhof F, Montalban X, et al. Clin-ically isolated syndromes suggestive of multiple sclerosis, part 2: Non-conventional MRI, recov-ery processes, and management. *Lancet Neurol.* 2005;4:341–348.

20. Bradley WG, Whitty CWM. Acute optic neu-ritis: Prognosis for development of multiple sclerosis. *J Neurol Neurosurg Psychiatry.* 1968;31: 10–18.

21. Cohen M, Lessell S, Wolf P. A prospective study of the risk of developing multiple sclerosis in uncomplicated optic neuritis. *Neurology.* 1979;29:208–213.

22. Confavreux C, Vukusic S, Adeleine P. Early clinical predictors and progressive of irreversible disability in multiple sclerosis: An amnesic process. *Brasin.* 2003;126:770–782.

23. Eriksson M, Andersen O, Runmarker B. Long-term follow-up of patients with clinically isolated syndromes, relapsing remitting and secondary progressive multiple sclerosis. *Mult Scler.* 2003;9:260–274.

24. Minneboo A, Barkhof F, Polman CH, et al. Infratentorial lesions predict long term disabil-ity in patients with initial findings suggestive of multiple sclerosis. *Arch Neurol.* 2004;61: 217–221.

25. Trobe JD, Sieving PC, Fendrick AM, et al. The impact of the optic neuritis treatment trial on the practices of ophthalmologists and neurologists. *Ophthalmology.* 1999;106:2047–2053.

SECTION VIII
OCULOPLASTICS

CHAPTER **15**

Thyroid Eye Disease

Louise A. Mawn, MD

Thyroid eye disease (TED) is an immune-mediated inflammatory condition involving the soft tissues of the orbit. Although most commonly associated with hyperthyroidism, patients with low levels of thyroid hormone (hypothyroid) and even normal levels of thyroid hormone (euthyroid) can exhibit the clinical manifestations of TED. The overwhelming majority of patients with active Graves ophthalmopathy are hyperthyroid (>90%) and those who are euthyroid have thyroid autoantibodies on careful laboratory analysis.[1,2] The onset of the eye changes occur within ±18 months around the onset of hyperthyroidism.[1,3] Graves ophthalmopathy is most commonly diagnosed at or within a year after the diagnosis of hyperthyroidism.[4–6] Many similar terms such as thyrotoxic exophthalmos, endocrine exophthalmos, thyroid ophthalmopathy,

or Graves ophthalmopathy are used to describe the condition.[7]

The weighted mean incidence of thyroid disease in the United States is estimated to be 13.9 per 100,000 per year.[8] Up to 50% of patients with thyroid disease will develop overt eye changes, and a greater number will have subclinical ophthalmopathy and increased intraocular pressure.[9,10] Bartley et al. studied the incidence of Graves ophthalmopathy in Olmstead County, Minnesota.[2] One hundred and twenty patients with Graves Disease were identified and used as the basis for several studies examining the chronology, clinical features, treatment, and long-term follow-up of Graves ophthalmopathy.[2,4,11–13] The patients described by Bartley et al. were all white.[2] Few studies examine nonCaucasian cohorts.[14–17] Women are affected five times more frequently than men.[2,5] Although most patients are middle aged,

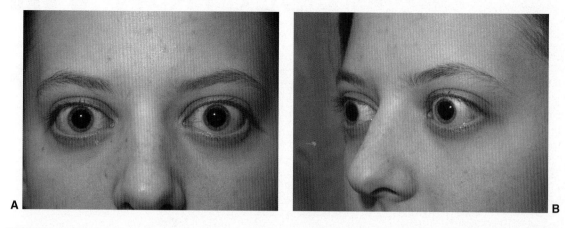

FIGURE 15.1 ☐ Seventeen-year-old girl with concurrent development of tachycardia, proptosis, and lid retraction who underwent elective total thyroidectomy for her hyperthyroidism.

children and elderly individuals can also develop TED.[1,2,18–20] Children make up <5% of patients with TED.[2] Thyroid disease in children occurs more commonly in the teenage years.[19,20] (see Fig. 15.1)

The clinical features seen in TED include lid retraction (Dalrymple sign), lateral flare of the upper lid, lid lag on downgaze (von Graefe sign), injection of the recti muscle insertions, proptosis, orbital congestion and inflammation, lid swelling, dry eyes, restriction of extraocular muscle movement and, in some cases, visual loss.[7,12] Patients commonly complain of an orbital ache or pressure behind the eye or in the eye socket, photophobia, dry gritty eyes, tearing, double vision, and blurred vision. The eyes

are not the only secondary organs involved in thyroid disease. Involvement of the skin can include inflammation over the tibia (pretibial myxedema or dermopathy) and thickening of the skin of the digits with digital clubbing (acropachy).[21,22] Dermopathy and acropachy are associated with severe ophthalmopathy and are thought to result from a similar autoimmune mechanism.[22] (see Fig. 15.2) The disease typically has an active phase in which the inflammatory component dominates and a late fibrotic component in which the late permanent effects of the previous orbital inflammation predominate. This curve of disease involvement was first described by Rundle in 1957 and is commonly referred to as Rundle's curve.[23]

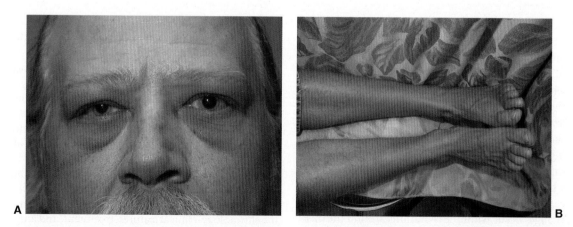

FIGURE 15.2 ☐ Fifty-one-year-old man who smokes 1.5 packs of cigarettes per day complained of two and a half months of periorbital edema, double and blurred vision, rash on his legs, insomnia, weight loss of 18 pounds, fatigue, heat intolerance, leg pain, and irritability. Laboratory results were remarkable for free T4 of 2.24 (0.6 to 1.8 ng/dL), a suppressed TSH of 0.005 (0.3 to 5 μU/mL) and markedly positive thyroid peroxidase antibodies at 3,928 (0 to 2 U/mL).

Graves ophthalmopathy has a measured profound negative impact on patients' quality of life.[24–26] The disease affects both physical and mental functioning, eroding self-confidence and socially isolating Graves ophthalmopathy patients.[25–27] Facial disfigurement resulting from the lid retraction, eyelid swelling, and retraction in Graves disease is reliably recognized by lay persons, endocrinologists, ophthalmologists, and Graves ophthalmopathy patients.[28] A Graves ophthalmopathy quality of life questionnaire, assessing both visual function and psychosocial function, developed in the Netherlands was first studied for validity and then used to assess improvement from treatment.[27,29] In a prospective cohort study, this instrument showed a 10 to 20 point change after radiotherapy or decompression and a 3 to 10 point change after strabismus and lid surgery.[30] The Dutch quality of life questionnaire was translated, slightly modified, and studied in Australian patients with Graves ophthalmopathy with similar findings.[24]

Both environmental and genetic features may influence the course of the disease. Cigarette smoking has been shown to be associated with a greater likelihood of developing TED in patients with thyroid disease.[31–34] A summary of nine studies found an average of 67% (range 44% to 95%) prevalence of smokers among patients with Graves ophthalmopathy.[35] Increased cigarette use has also been associated with more severe eye disease.[34,36–39] The risk relationship between tobacco and Graves ophthalmopathy is not seen in former smokers with comparable lifetime tobacco consumption.[34] In a European study of childhood Graves ophthalmopathy, prevalence of eye disease correlated with teenage smoking prevalence ($p = 0.0001$) in various countries.[20] The strong relationship reported between current tobacco use and risk for TED argues that patients should be counselled to stop smoking.[40,41] A prospective study of 155 newly diagnosed Graves disease patients showed a prevalence of Graves ophthalmopathy of 42% among Europeans and 7.7% for Asians ($p = 0.0002$). Twin studies have shown a higher incidence of thyroid disease.[42,43] However, no specific genetic loci have been found and environmental factors may have a greater influence on the development of TED than genetic factors.[44] Radioactive iodine may also exacerbate TED activity, particularly in patients who smoke.[45–47]

The immune disorder is thought to be caused by antibodies directed toward the thyroid-stimulating hormone (TSH) receptor.[48] This receptor is common to the organs affected by thyroid disease.[49] In thyroid disease, the antibodies to the TSH receptor lead to excess production of thyroid hormone.[49–52] Eye changes result from the intraorbital inflammation and enlargement of the orbital adipose tissue and muscles.[53] The orbit is invaded by CD4 + T cells.[54,55] Cytokines amplify the reaction and cause fibroblasts to synthesize and secrete glycosaminoglycans. The orbital soft tissue volume increases both because of cytokine-stimulated glycosaminoglycan accumulation within the extraocular muscles and adipogenesis.[52,56]

Systemic intervention is most likely to change the outcome in the early active phase of the TED; once the fibrotic phase has occurred, medical intervention is unlikely to improve the eye disease. Endocrine evaluation should be performed on all patients suspected of having TED. Laboratory studies should include TSH, tri-iodothyronine (T3), free thyroxine (FT4), and the thyroid antibodies including antithyroid peroxidase and antithyroglobulin. Imaging with computed tomography (CT) helps define the position of the globes in the bony orbit (particularly if the optic nerve is on stretch or if proptosis exists) and the size of the extraocular muscles and the relationship of the enlarged muscles to the optic nerve at the orbital apex (see Fig. 15.3). Considerable controversy exists regarding the treatment of TED.

Medical Treatment of Systemic Thyroid Abnormality

There are various methods for treating the systemic hyperthyroid disease. Most commonly the disease will first be treated with drugs that block thyroid hormone synthesis: Methimazole, carbimazole, and propylthiouracil through both a block and replace (higher dose antithyroid medication concurrent with thyroid hormone) method or a titration method (reduction based on thyroid hormone concentration).[57]

Two randomized prospective clinical trials showed progression of ophthalmopathy in some patients treated with radioactive iodine.[45,58] This progression can be managed with steroid administration.[45] A prospective, observational study of 72 patients examining radioiodine in minimally active Graves ophthalmopathy showed no change in TED when hypothyroidism was prevented.[59]

Because functional somatostatin receptors are expressed on activated lymphocytes and fibroblasts, somatostatin analogs have been considered as possible modulators of Graves ophthalmopathy. A double-blind placebo-controlled trial of octreotide

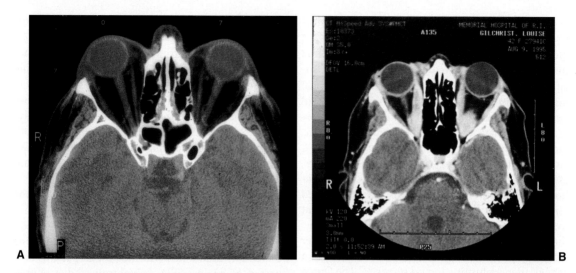

FIGURE 15.3 ☐ Axial computed tomography image at the midorbit level of two patients with Graves-related optic neuropathy. The image on the left shows stretching of the optic nerve from axial displacement by the increase in orbital fat. The image on the right shows enlarged recti muscles causing compression at the orbital apex.

long-acting repeatable (LAR) was studied in 50 euthyroid patients with active Graves ophthalmopathy. Patients received either 30 mg LAR every 4 weeks for 16 weeks or placebo. Both were followed by 30 mg for 16 to 32 weeks, and then no treatment for an additional 24 weeks. There was no significant difference in clinical outcomes between the groups.[60]

Medical Treatment of Orbitopathy

Rundle described the course of Graves ophthalmopathy as first having a Bell-shaped active phase in which inflammation occurred and later a severity curve which plateaus with permanent fibrotic involvement.[23] Studies examining treatment effects need to account for the natural tendency of Graves ophthalmopathy to improve with time. Only the active phase is expected to respond to immunosuppressive therapies.

Steroids are used to decrease the complications of the active phase of the disease. Several randomized controlled trials (RCTs) address whether steroids shorten the duration of the active phase and improve the outcome. A randomized, prospective, open comparison of intravenous methylprednisolone versus oral prednisone in 33 patients with mild or moderate TED showed an insignificant difference but a trend of less additional treatment needed after intravenous steroid.[61]

A later study evaluated 70 euthyroid patients with various stages of Graves ophthalmopathy randomized to either once weekly intravenous methylprednisolone 0.5 g for 6 weeks and then 0.25 g for 6 weeks or oral prednisolone 0.1 g per day, tapering the dose by 0.01 g per week. Clinical signs such as proptosis, lid width, and diplopia were used as outcome measures. The patients treated with intravenous steroid achieved better results than the oral steroid group ($p < 0.01$). Additional treatments were less frequently required in the intravenous group. Intravenous treatment was also associated with fewer adverse events than oral treatment ($p < 0.001$).[62] Smokers had worsening of ophthalmopathy in spite of steroids.[62] Oral steroids were associated with >3 kg weight gain in 26%.[62] A randomized trial comparing 19 patients treated with oral prednisone and 21 treated with immunoglobulin revealed side effects of steroids in 84% with severe hypertension and psychic disorders in two patients.[63] A study of radiation therapy treatment with either oral or intravenous steroid showed greater steroid-related side effect in the oral steroid group ($p < 0.01$).[64] One of the possible deleterious effects of intravenous steroids is liver failure; the recommended cumulative dose of intravenous methylprednisolone is 6 to 8 g.[65,66]

Direct injection of steroids into the orbit has also been studied. A randomized prospective study compared 25 patients treated with 4 doses of 20 mg of triamcinolone acetate 40 mg per mL injected into the inferolateral quadrant versus no treatment controls. Patients with compressive ophthalmopathy were excluded. Motility ($p = 0.0122$) and the superior rectus levator complex size ($p = 0.0060$) significantly improved with the injections.[67]

Other immunosuppressive agents have been evaluated for treatment of Graves ophthalmopathy. Cyclosporine was compared to prednisone in a prospective, randomized masked study of 36 patients. Prednisone was associated with a better response but was not tolerated as well ($p = 0.018$). Combination therapy was effective in the patients who did not respond to either of the drugs used singly.[68] A randomized study of 64 patients treated with antithyroid medication (28) or antithyroid medication and azathioprine (36) showed that only 1/36 patients treated with immunosuppression developed Graves ophthalmopathy as compared to the 7/28 treated with antithyroid medication alone. Four patients treated with azathioprine had gastrointestinal side effects or leucopenia[69] Azathioprine was also used as a steroid-sparing drug in a case series study of 40 patients treated with radiation and immunosuppression.[70]

Steroid immunosuppression, both intravenous and oral, has been compared with irradiation and irradiation with concurrent steroid treatment. These studies are summarized in Table 15.1. Steroids and irradiation were shown in one study to be equally effective, though the steroid group had more short-term side effects.[71] A combination of steroid and irradiation therapy was found to be more effective than either treatment modality alone.[72,73] Medical treatment has also been compared with surgical treatment. Fifteen patients with active Graves ophthalmopathy and optic neuropathy were randomized to treatment with either surgical decompression (6) or intravenous methylprednisolone (9) for 2 weeks followed by oral prednisone for 4 months. Patients were switched to the other treatment if they did not improve with one. Immediate surgery did not result in improved outcome. This study was limited by the small number of patients.[74]

Irradiation for Thyroid Eye Disease

Irradiation of the orbits in TED theoretically decreases the activity of the activated lymphocytes and fibroblasts.[75] Radiation to treat Graves ophthalmopathy was initially directed to the pituitary as it was thought to be the source of an exophthalmic inducing factor.[76] Potential side effects of radiation include cataracts, radiation retinopathy, and exacerbation of dry eye. Irradiation is contraindicated in patients at risk for retinal vascular disease such as patients with diabetes. Radiation has been considered as an alternative to immunosuppression with steroids.

Several randomized prospective, placebo-controlled studies have conflicting conclusions regarding the benefit of radiation for TED (see Table 15.1). Mourtis et al. randomized 60 moderate Graves ophthalmopathy patients in the Netherlands to sham radiation or irradiation in a prospective double-blind study. The only significant result was better motility in the treated group; in spite of the improved motility, a similar number in the irradiated and placebo groups underwent strabismus surgery.[77] Gorman et al. prospectively studied 42 patients at the Mayo Clinic, one orbit was irradiated, and then 6 months later the other control orbit was also irradiated. No benefit was found from irradiation.[78] In a second study by the Netherlands group, patients in the early stage of mild disease were irradiated and compared with patients treated with sham irradiation; this study found no significant effect of the irradiation.[79] All of these studies have limitations because of the difficulty in controlling for the disease phase.[80] The median duration of eye disease in the Mayo study was 16 months.[78] The Mayo study was most strongly criticized for treating patients who were in the nonactive phase of TED.[81] The median duration in the first Netherlands study was only slightly shorter at 13 and 14.5 months, for the treated, and the placebo groups, respectively.[77] The median duration in the second Dutch study was 17 and 15 months, for the treated and the placebo groups, respectively.

Subsequent to both the Mayo and the Dutch studies, a prospective study of 66 consecutive patients showed that disease activity could predict the response to treatment.[82] In the patients with moderately severe Graves ophthalmopathy, euthyroid for 2 months preceding treatment with radiation therapy for either restriction of extraocular motility or proptosis >25 mm, response could be predicted on the basis of several features. A model to predict both response and outcome was developed from this analysis. Duration of ophthalmopathy >16 months had a 10 times lower probability of response to radiotherapy.[82]

Several studies have compared radiation dose and have also had conflicting results. Kahaly et al. compared 3 doses (10 and 20 Gy over 2 weeks and 20 Gy over 20 weeks) and concluded that a low-dose regimen of 20 Gy in 20 weekly fractions was more

TABLE 15.1 ◻ Summary of Studies Comparing the Different Modalities of Treatment of Graves Ophthalmopathy

Radiotherapy

Author (Date)	Study Design/Purpose	Study Participants	Treatment Protocol	Outcome	Conclusion/Limitations
Mourtis (2000)[77]	Single-center, double-blind, randomized, placebo control trial	60 outpatients with moderately severe TED (30 assigned to irradiation; 30 assigned to sham irradiation)	Treatment group: 6 MV photon beam from Elekta SL 15 accelerator (20 Gy in 10 fractions over 12 d)	Qualitative treatment outcome: Observed in 18/30 irradiated patients and 9/29 sham patients (RR = 1.9; 95% CI 1.0−3.6, $p = 0.04$). Motility improvement: Observed in 14/17 irradiated patients, 4/15 sham patients (RR = 3.1; 95% CI 1.3−7.4, $p = 0.004$)	Study concludes that irradiation does not improve outcome in terms of reducing eyelid retraction, swelling, or proptosis; may be some indication that irradiation may improve motility
	To assess whether retrobulbar irradiation lessens severity of TED	Diagnosed by the following symptoms: Eyelid retraction, swelling, proptosis, impaired motility, including intraocular pressure in upward gaze, including intraocular fat	Placebo Group: Same protocol without irradiation; all patients examined 1 d before and 4, 12, 24 wk after treatment by the same clinician	Eyelid swelling: Observed in 4/11 irradiated patients, and 5/12 sham patients (RR = 0.9; 95% CI 0.3−2.4, $p > 099$)	
				Diplopia improvement: (in extremes of gaze) observed in 9/12 irradiated patients, and 1/4 sham patient; (no diplopia) 2/5 irradiated, 1/11 sham patient	
				Follow-up: No significant difference between groups in terms of number of additional therapies needed (3 irradiated, 4 sham—needed no additional therapy); Orbital decompression—9 irradiated patients, 14 sham patients	

Study	Study design	Objective / Population	Treatment	Results	Conclusions
Gorman (2001)[78]	Single-center, double-blind, randomized, placebo control trial	To evaluate efficacy of irradiation therapy in TED; 42 Graves patients with moderate TED (one eye from each patient randomly allocated to receive irradiation, other eye sham irradiation); Diagnosed with the following symptoms: +TSI level, euthyroid, eyelid edema, lid lag, lid retraction, bulging eyes, proptosis, restriction in major muscle motion	Treatment: 6 MV photons delivering 20 Gy of external beam irradiation at 10 fractions over 12 d, directed at one orbit (initial treatment at 3 mo and second eye treated at 6 mo); treated orbit compared to untreated orbit at 3, 6, and 12 mo	Treated orbit at 3 and 6mo: Muscle volume—11 mL (treated) and 10.4 mL (untreated); Proptosis—21.8 mm (treated) vs. 21.3 mm (untreated); These were statistically but not clinically significantly different; No other parameters were statistically significantly different; patients treated earlier in the course of the disease showed no difference in treatment outcome compared to patients with longer disease duration	Study unable to find a clinically or statistically significant difference between treated and nontreated orbit; therefore concludes that radiotherapy does not improve outcome in patients with moderate TED
Gorman (2002)[78a]	Noncomparative interventional case series (follow-up period following RCT)	42 patients with moderate TED (details described above)	Same as above	3-y outcome: Ancillary rehabilitation procedures—orbital decompression ($n = 8$), extraocular muscle surgery ($n = 11$), eyelid surgery ($n = 18$)	Uncontrolled study failed to identify any benefit to orbital irradiation, and suggests that orbital irradiation should no longer be considered a treatment option for mild to moderate TED

(continued)

TABLE 15.1 ▫ (Continued)

Author (Date)	Study Design/Purpose	Study Participants	Treatment Protocol	Outcome	Conclusion/Limitations
	To evaluate long-term improvement (3 y) following orbital irradiation in moderate TED patients			Orbital changes in patients who were not surgically decompressed ($n = 31$)—orbital fat increased from 12.1–14.0 cc ($p <0.001$) and muscle volume decreased from 10.7–8.4 cc ($p <0.001$); monocular range of motion showed no significant change, proptosis decreased 0.7 mm below the baseline and at 3 y ($p = 0.01$) Orbital changes in patients who were surgically decompressed ($n = 7$)—orbit volume increased from 27–34.6cc, proptosis decreased from 23.2–18.9 mm ($p = 0.01$)	
Gerling (2003)[78b]	Multicenter, blind, randomized study to compare results of irradiation with 2.4 Gy and 16 Gy	97 Graves patients with active TED (43 irradiated with 2.4 Gy; 43 irradiated with 16 Gy)	6-MeV linear accelerator; 8 fractions of 0.3 or 2.0 Gy over 16 d two opposing asymmetrical fields	Appearance: Graded from 0–100 $p = 0.42/0.09$ Hertel measurements for two eyes added: $p = 0.28$ Eye movements: Vertical ductions measured on Goldmann added for two eyes $p = 0.99$ Muscle thickness: Mean of three cross-sectional areas of eight muscles on MRI, $p = 0.26$	Symmetrical differences found with 2.4 and 16 Gy. Study concludes that irradiation should not exceed 2.4 Gy. Study did not examine effectiveness of irradiation

Study	Study type	Patients	Protocol/methods	Results	Conclusions
Prummel (2004)[79]	Single-center, blind, randomized study to compare irradiation to no treatment.	88 Graves patients euthyroid for 2 mo with untreated mild ophthalmopathy (44 irradiated and 44 sham-irradiated patients)	5 MeV linear accelerator; treated in 10 divided fractions over 2 wk. Patients examined at 3, 6, and 12 mo. All patients examined by same ophthalmologist for eyelid aperture, soft tissue involvement, proptosis, motility, diplopia, and visual acuity. Data from the most affected eye was studied	Complaints: 0–100 analog scale of five modalities, $p = 0.19$ Clinical measures: 23/44 responded in irradiated group, 12/44 sham group ($p = 0.02$). No further treatment was needed in 15/44 of irradiated group and 7/44 of sham group ($p = 0.049$) Quality of life assessment: No difference was found (visual function 8.2 in treatment group vs. 10.5 in placebo group) Cost assessment: No difference in costs—(5,007€ in treatment group and 4,465 € in placebo group)	The study concludes that orbital radiotherapy improves motility but had no beneficial effect on soft tissue involvement. The quality of life scores improved in a similar manner for both groups and observation was recommended as a good alternative strategy.

Corticosteroids and orbital irradiation

Study	Study type	Patients	Protocol/methods	Results	Conclusions
Marcocci (2001)[64]	Single blind, randomized study	82 Graves patients with moderate to severe cases of TED	IVGC protocol: Methylprednisolone acetate (15 mg/kg for 4 cycles, 7.5 mg/kg for 4 cycles) cycle = 2 infusions/2 wk	Proptosis: Significantly decreased in IVGC group from 23.3–21.6 mm ($p <0.0001$), and ORGC group from 23–21.7 mm ($p <0.0001$); final exophthalmometer readings did not differ between groups($p = 0.41$)	Study found that there is not much difference between IV and oral treatment of TED; however, IV administration seems to be better tolerated with less side effects than the oral method

(continued)

TABLE 15.1 ■ (Continued)

Author (Date)	Study Design/Purpose	Study Participants	Treatment Protocol	Outcome	Conclusion/Limitations
	To evaluate the effect of oral glucocorticoids (ORGC) vs. IVGC in association with orbital irradiation		ORGC protocol: Prednisone (100 mg/d for 7 d, with gradual weekly reduction until 25 mg dose is reached); then tapered to 5 mg/2 wk Duration of treatment = 22 wk Radiotherapy: 20 Gy delivered to each eye in 10 fractionated doses over 2 wk Ocular evaluation carried out by the same examiner	Diplopia: Disappeared in 10/27 and did not change in 12/27 IVGC patients, disappeared in 12/33 patients and did not change in 16/33 patients receiving ORGC; amelioration rate did not significantly differ between the 2 treatment groups (chi-squared = 0.06, p = 0.82) Overall clinical response: Statistical difference found in clinical response to therapy between IVGC and ORGC groups (p = 0.02) Adverse effects: IVGC better tolerated than ORGC	Lid width: Width did not differ between groups(p = 0.65)

Study	Design	Population/Objective	Treatment	Results	Conclusions
Bartalena (1983)[72]	Randomized control trial	48 patients with active Graves ophthalmopathy (24 patients with active TED randomly treated with radiation/methylprednisolone (12) or methylprednisolone alone (12), 24 additional patients with active TED submitted to combined therapy); patients were assessed in terms of ophthalmology index and clinical observations	Radiotherapy: 10 daily doses of 2 Gy for 2 wk	Significant improvement in both groups—patients receiving combination therapy or methylprednisolone alone.	Study concludes that patients receiving combined therapy showed a more significant improvement in clinical and ophthalmology indices. There was an inverse relationship between duration of ophthalmopathy and efficacy of treatment, more favorable results when symptoms were of <2 y duration.
		To evaluate the effect of radiation in combination with methylprednisone vs. methylprednisolone alone	Methylprednisolone: 70–80 mg/d for 3 wk, gradually tapered by 5 mg weekly until a daily dose of 20 mg is reached; subsequently reduced by 2.5–5 mg every 2–3 wks; discontinued after 5–6 mo	Ophthalmology index: Mean final index significantly reduced in combination group (decrease is 4.8 in combination group and 3.2 in methylprednisolone group, $p < 0.005$)	Major limitations to this study design may limit the applicability of results, including unbalanced treatment groups and differences in data collection
Marcocci (1991)[73]	Randomized control trial to evaluate the effect of radiation therapy combined with corticosteroids vs. radiation therapy alone	30 patients with active TED (26 patients completed the study) 13 patients in group 1 received combination therapy; 13 patients in group 2 received radiation alone	Radiotherapy: 4 MeV linear accelerator; 20 Gy delivered in 10 fractionated daily doses over 2 wk	Evaluation at 6–9 mo indicated that regression or substantial improvement occurred in all patients except one in group 1 and in only half in group 2	Study concludes that combined therapy produced more favorable results in terms of soft tissue changes and extraocular muscle involvement

(continued)

TABLE 15.1 ☐ (Continued)

Author (Date)	Study Design/Purpose	Study Participants	Treatment Protocol	Outcome	Conclusion/Limitations
			Prednisone: 100 mg/d for 7 days, weekly reduction to 25 mg was reached, then tapered by 5 mg/d for 2 wk; Duration of protocol 5–6 wk	Mean Ophthalmology Index was significantly different between the two groups (−3.39 in group 1 and −1.85 in group 2; $p = 0.043$); when evaluated clinically, the study did not find a statistical significance difference between groups ($p = 0.23$); adverse effects: Cushingoid features occurred in some cases during combined therapy because of corticosteroids	Limitations: Study size may limit the broad applicability of results
Prummel (1993)[71]	Randomized double-blind study to compare the efficacy of radiation with that of oral prednisone	56 patients with moderate to severe Graves ophthalmopathy (28 patients received oral prednisone and sham radiation; 28 received radiation and placebo capsules)	Radiation group: 5 MeV linear accelerator; ten 2 Gy doses over 2 wk Medication group: Prednisone 60 mg for 2 wk, 40 mg for 2 wk, 30 mg for 4 wk, 20 mg for 4 wk, tapered by 2–5 mg per wk. Patients examined 0, 4, 12, and 24 wk after treatment by the same ophthalmologist	No specs class: 13/28 radiation patients improved; 14/28 prednisone patients improved Monocular eye movements: 8/28 radiation improved, 7/28 prednisone patients improved	Study concludes there is a similar response rate to radiation and prednisone after 24 wks. Both treatments had minimal effect on proptosis. Seventy-one percent of prednisone group had moderate or severe side effects and study concluded that radiotherapy should replace prednisone treatment. The study was limited by inadequate follow-up time to detect the side effects of radiation

RCT, randomized controlled trial; TED, thyroid eye disease.

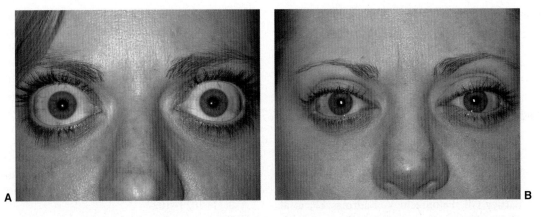

A B

FIGURE 15.4 ▣ Thirty-two-year-old woman with proptosis and lid retraction who underwent subcaruncular medial wall and swinging eyelid floor decompression followed by correction of upper lid retraction.

effective and better tolerated. The evaluation of response was completed 4 weeks after the last treatment in the 20 Gy over 20 week group and 22 weeks after the last treatment in the 10 Gy and 20 Gy over 2 weeks groups, so the conclusions of this study are limited. A Japanese study of 31 patients concluded that 24 Gy of radiation was more effective than 10 Gy when combined with systemic corticosteroids.[83]

Deleterious effects from radiation are often not realized until long after the treatment. Long-term follow-up of 250 patients irradiated for progressive Graves ophthalmopathy failed to show a difference in radiation-induced cancer death but did not have sufficient numbers to determine a difference.[84] A second long-term follow-up study also failed to show a difference in mortality in 245 patients but did show a significant risk of retinopathy ($p = 0.0002$).[85] Lifetime risk of radiation-induced cancer is dependent on the age and the dose of radiation.[86] The calculated risk of radiation-induced cancer after retrobulbar irradiation for Graves ophthalmopathy is 1.2%.[87]

Surgical Treatment

Orbital, strabismus, and lid surgery are most commonly performed as part of the rehabilitative phase of TED treatment (see Fig. 15.4). A randomized trial of 15 patients with very active Graves ophthalmopathy and optic neuropathy compared surgical decompression to steroid treatment. Immediate surgery did not result in a better outcome.[74] Most of the studies summarized in Table 15.1 show that radiation and immunosuppression do not change proptosis. Decompression surgery has been shown to reduce proptosis.[88,89] A quality of life survey showed a significant correlation between improvement in proptosis and quality of life ($p = 0.05$).[90]

Conclusions

Active phase thyroid disease improves naturally in many patients. The literature on the therapy for Graves ophthalmopathy consists largely of single-center RCTs, retrospective case series, and prospective cohort studies. Most randomized controlled studies indicate that radiation does not provide any clinically or statistically significant improvement in the outcomes over placebo or steroids. Radiation has been associated with retinopathy, particularly in diabetic patients. Radiation may also be associated with a higher lifetime risk of cancer. The dose of steroids needed for immunosuppression of active phase disease is associated with side effects in most patients. These side effects range from weight gain to liver failure. Neither steroids nor radiation reduce the need for decompression or rehabilitative surgery. Current cigarette smoking is strongly associated with prevalence of Graves ophthalmopathy and the level of cigarette use correlates with the severity of eye disease. Decompression surgery correlates with improvement in quality of life metrics.

The benefits of active phase treatment must be weighed against the risks. The disease duration has been shown to predict response to immunosuppressive therapy; the failure to show a benefit of radiation could be secondary to inclusion of patients in later phases of the disease process. An evidence-based benefit has not been shown with radiation, and given that there is a known risk of retinopathy and a theoretical risk of cancer, radiation should only be considered in older patients who are also at low risk for retinopathy. Concurrent steroid treatment may improve the outcome. High dose steroids should only be used when the pathology and treatment benefit outweigh the risks of the side effects. Liver function needs to be monitored during steroid treatment.

References

1. Marcocci C, Bartalena L, Bogazzi F, et al. Studies on the occurrence of ophthalmopathy in Graves' disease. *Acta Endocrinol (Copenh)*. 1989;120(4):473–478.

2. Bartley GB, Fatourechi V, Kadrmas EF, et al. The incidence of Graves' ophthalmopathy in Olmsted County, Minnesota. *Am J Ophthalmol*. 1995;120(4):511–517.

3. Gorman CA. Temporal relationship between onset of of Graves' ophthalmopathy and diagnosis of thyrotoxicosis. *Mayo Clin Proc*. 1983; 58:515–519.

4. Bartley GB, Fatourechi V, Kadrmas EF, et al. Chronology of Graves' ophthalmopathy in an incidence cohort. *Am J Ophthalmol*. 1996;121(4): 426–434.

5. Noth D, Gebauer M, Muller B, et al. Graves' ophthalmopathy:Natural history and treatment outcomes. *Swiss Med Wkly*. 2001;131(41–42): 603–609.

6. Burch HB, Wartofsky L. Graves' ophthalmopathy: Current concepts regarding pathogenesis and management. *Endocr Rev*. 1993;14(6): 747–793.

7. Bartley GB, Gorman CA. Diagnostic criteria for Graves' ophthalmopathy. *Am J Ophthalmol*. 1995;119(6):792–795.

8. Jacobson D, Gange S, Rose N, et al. Epidemiology and estimated population burden of selected autoimmune diseases in the United States. *Clin Immunol Immunopathol*. 1997;84:223–243.

9. Jacobson DH, Gorman CA. Diagnosis and management of endocrine ophthalmopathy. *Med Clin North Am*. 1984;69:973–988.

10. Gamblin GT, Harper DG, Galentine P, et al. Prevalence of increased intraocular pressure in Graves' disease—evidence of frequent subclinical ophthalmopathy. *N Engl J Med*. 1983; 308(8):420–424.

11. Bartley GB, Fatourechi V, Kadrmas EF, et al. Long-term follow-up of Graves ophthalmopathy in an incidence cohort. *Ophthalmology*. 1996; 103(6):958–962.

12. Bartley GB, Fatourechi V, Kadrmas EF, et al. Clinical features of Graves' ophthalmopathy in an incidence cohort. *Am J Ophthalmol*. 1996; 121(3):284–290.

13. Bartley GB, Fatourechi V, Kadrmas EF, et al. The treatment of Graves' ophthalmopathy in an incidence cohort. *Am J Ophthalmol*. 1996; 121:200–206.

14. Joffe B, Gunji K, Panz V, et al. Thyroid-associated ophthalmopathy in black South African patients with Graves' disease: Relationship to antiflavoprotein antibodies. *Thyroid*. 1998; 8(11):1023–1027.

15. Tellez M, Cooper J, Edmonds C. Graves' ophthalmopathy in relation to cigarette smoking and ethnic origin. *Clin Endocrinol (Oxf)*. 1992; 36(3):291–294.

16. Tsai CC, Kau HC, Kao SC, et al. Exophthalmos of patients with Graves' disease in Chinese of Taiwan. *Eye*. 2006;20(5):569–573.

17. Joffe BI, Panz VR, Yamada M, et al. Thyroid-associated ophthalmopathy in black South Africans with Graves' disease: Relationship to serum antibodies reactive against eye muscle and orbital connective tissue autoantigens. *Endocrine*. 2000;13(3):325–328.

18. Prummel MF, Bakker A, Wiersinga WM, et al. Multi-center study on the characteristics and treatment strategies of patients with Graves' orbitopathy: The first European Group on Graves' orbitopathy experience. *Eur J Endocrinol*. 2003;148(5):491–495.

19. Durairaj VD, Bartley GB, Garrity JA. Clinical features and treatment of graves ophthalmopathy in pediatric patients. *Ophthal Plast Reconstr Surg*. 2006;22(1):7–12.

20. Krassas GE, Segni M, Wiersinga WM. Childhood Graves' ophthalmopathy: Results of a European questionnaire study. *Eur J Endocrinol*. 2005;153(4):515–521.

21. Fatourechi V, Pajouhi M, Fransway AF. Dermopathy of Graves disease (pretibial myxedema). Review of 150 cases. *Medicine (Baltimore)*. 1994; 73(1):1–7.

22. Fatourechi V, Bartley GB, Eghbali-Fatourechi GZ, et al. Graves' dermopathy and acropathy are markers of severe Graves' ophthalmopathy. *Thyroid*. 2003;13(12):1141–1144.

23. Rundle FF. Management of exophthalmos and related ocular changes in Graves' disease. *Metabolism*. 1957;6:36–47.

24. Park JJ, Sullivan TJ, Mortimer RH, et al. Assessing quality of life in Australian patients with Graves' ophthalmopathy. *Br J Ophthalmol.* 2004;88:75–78.

25. Gerding MN, Terwee CB, Dekker FW, et al. Quality of life in patients with Graves' ophthalmopathy is markedly decreased: Measurement by the medical outcomes study instrument. *Thyroid.* 1997;7(6):885–889.

26. Terwee C, Wakelkamp I, Tan S, et al. Long-term effects of Graves' ophthalmopathy on health-related quality of life. *Eur J Endocrinol.* 2002;146(6):751–757.

27. Terwee CB, Gerding MN, Dekker FW, et al. Development of a disease specific quality of life questionnaire for patients with Graves' ophthalmopathy: The GO-QOL. *Br J Ophthalmol.* 1998;82(7):773–779.

28. Terwee CB, Dekker FW, Bonsel GJ, et al. Facial disfigurement: Is it in the eye of the beholder? A study in patients with Graves' ophthalmopathy. *Clin Endocrinol (Oxf).* 2003;58(2):192–198.

29. Terwee CB, Gerding MN, Dekker FW, et al. Test-retest reliability of the GO-QOL: A disease-specific quality of life questionnaire for patients with Graves' ophthalmopathy. *J Clin Epidemiol.* 1999;52(9):875–884.

30. Terwee CB, Dekker FW, Prummel MF, et al. Graves' ophthalmopathy through the eyes of the patient: A state of the art on health-related quality of life assessment. *Orbit.* 2001;20(4):281–290.

31. Bartalena L, Bogazzi F, Tanda ML, et al. Cigarette smoking and the thyroid. *Eur J Endocrinol.* 1995;133:507–512.

32. Bartalena L, Martino E, Marcocci C, et al. More on smoking habits and Graves' ophthalmopathy. *J Endocrinol Invest.* 1989;12(10):733–737.

33. Prummel MF, Wiersinga WM. Smoking and risk of Graves' disease. *JAMA.* 1993;269(4):479–482.

34. Pfeilschifter J, Ziegler R. Smoking and endocrine ophthalmopathy: Impact of smoking severity and current vs lifetime cigarette consumption. *Clin Endocrinol (Oxf).* 1996;45:477–481.

35. Bartalena L, Pinchera A, Marcocci C. Management of Graves' ophthalmopathy: Reality and perspectives. *Endocr Rev.* 2000;21(2):168–199.

36. Hagg E, Asplund K. Is endocrine ophthalmopathy related to smoking? *Br Med J.* 1987;295:634–635.

37. Shine B, Fells P, Edwards OM, et al. Association between Graves' ophthalmopathy and smoking. *Lancet.* 1990;1:1261–1263.

38. Winsa B, Mandahl A, Karlsson FA. Graves' disease, endocrine ophthalmopathy and smoking. *Acta Endocrinol (Copenh).* 1993;128(2):156–160.

39. Tallstedt L, Lundell G, Taube A. Graves' ophthalmopathy and tobacco smoking. *Acta Endocrinol (Copenh).* 1993;129(2):147–150.

40. Hegedius L, Brix TH, Vestergaard P. Relationship between cigarette smoking and Graves' ophthalmopathy. *J Endocrinol Invest.* 2004;27(3):265–271.

41. Keltner JL. Is Graves ophthalmopathy a preventable disease? *Arch Ophthalmol.* 1998;116:1106–1107.

42. Brix TH, Christensen K, Holm NV, et al. A population-based study of Graves disease in danish twins. *Clin Endocrinol.* 1998;48:397–400.

43. Brix TH, Kyvik KO, Christensen K, et al. Evidence for a major role of heredity in Graves' disease: A population-based study of two Danish twin cohorts. *J Clin Endocrinol Metab.* 2001;86:930–934.

44. Prabhakar BS, Bahn RS, Smith TJ. Current perspective on the pathogenesis of Graves' disease and ophthalmopathy. *Endocrine Reviews.* 2003;24(6):802–835.

45. Bartalena L, Marcocci C, Bogazzi F, et al. Relation between therapy for hyperthyroidism and the course of Graves' ophthalmopathy. *N Engl J Med.* 1998;338(2):73–78.

46. Wiersinga WM. Preventing Graves' ophthalmopathy. *N Engl J Med.* 1998;338:121–122.

47. Wiersinga WM, Bartalena L. Epidemiology and prevention of Graves' ophthalmopathy. *Thyroid.* 2002;12(10):855–860.

48. Bahn RS. A possible role for the thyrotropin receptor in thyroid-associated ophthalmopathy. *Orbit* 1996;15:119–128.

49. Feliciello A, Porcellini A, Ciullo I, et al. Expression of thyrotropin-receptor mRNA in healthy and Graves' disease retro-orbital tissue. *Lancet* 1993;342:337–338.

50. Heufelder AE, Dutton CM, Sarkar G, et al. Detection of TSH receptor RNA in cultured fibroblasts from patients with Graves' ophthalmopathy and pretibial dermopathy. *Thyroid.* 1993;3:297–300.

51. Hiromatsu Y, Sato M, Inoue Y, et al. Localization and clinical significance of thyrotropin receptor mRNA expression in orbital fat and eye muscle

tissues from patients with thyroid-associated ophthalmopathy. *Thyroid*. 1996;6(6):553–562.

52. Mengistu M, Lukes YG, Nagy EV, et al. TSH receptor gene expression in retroocular fibroblasts. *J Endocrinol Invest*. 1994;17:437–441.

53. Kumar S, Leontovich A, Coenen M, et al. Gene expression profiling of orbital adipose tissue from patients with Graves' ophthalmopathy: A potential role for secreted frizzled-related protein-1 in orbital adipogenesis. *J Endocrinol Invest*. 2005;90(8):4730–4735.

54. Otto EA, Ochs K, Hansen C, et al. Orbital tissue-derived T lymphocytes from patients with Graves' ophthalmopathy recognize autologous orbital antigens. *J Clin Endocrinol Metab*. 1996;81(8):3045–3050.

55. Pappa A, Calder V, Ajjan R, et al. Analysis of extraocular muscle-infiltrating T cells in Thyroid-Associated Ophthalmopathy (TAO). *Clin Exp Immunol*. 1997;109(2):362–369.

56. Kumar S, Coenen MJ, Scherer PE, et al. Evidence for enhanced adipogenesis in the orbits of patients with Graves' ophthalmopathy. *J Clin Endocrinol Metab*. 2004;89(2):930–935.

57. Abraham P, Avenell A, Park CM, et al. A systematic review of drug therapy for Graves' hyperthyroidism. *Eur J Endocrinol*. 2005;153:489–498.

58. Tallstedt L, Lundell G, Torring O, et al. Occurrence of ophthalmopathy after treatment for Graves' hyperthyroidism. *N Engl J Med*. 1992;326:1733–1738.

59. Perros P, Kendall-Taylor P, Neoh C, et al. A prospective study of the effects of radioiodine therapy for hyperthyroidism in patients with minimally active Graves' ophthalmopathy. *J Clin Endocrinol Metab*. 2005;90(9):5321–5323.

60. Dickinson AJ, Vaidya B, Miller M, et al. Double-blind, placebo-controlled trial of octreotide Long-Acting Repeatable (LAR) in thyroid-associated ophthalmopathy. *J Clin Endocrinol Metab*. 2004;89(12):5910–5915.

61. Kauppinen-Makelin R, Karma A, Leinonen E, et al. High dose intravenous methylprednisolone pulse therapy versus oral prednisone for thyroid-associated ophthalmopathy. *Acta Ophthalmol Scand*. 2002;80(3):316–321.

62. Kahaly GJ, Pitz S, Hommel G, et al. Randomized, single blind trial of intravenous versus oral steroid monotherapy in Graves' orbitopathy. *J Clin Endocrinol Metab*. 2005;90(9):5234–5240.

63. Kahaly G, Pitz S, Muller-Forell W, et al. Randomized trial of intravenous immunoglobulins versus prednisolone in Graves' ophthalmopathy. *Clin Exp Immunol*. 1996;106(2):197–202.

64. Marcocci C, Bartalena L, Tanda ML, et al. Comparison of the effectiveness and tolerability of intravenous or oral glucocorticoids associated with orbital radiotherapy in the management of severe Graves' ophthalmopathy: Results of a prospective, single-blind, randomized study. *J Clin Endocrinol Metab*. 2001;86(8):3562–3567.

65. Marino M, Morabito E, Brunetto MR, et al. Acute severe liver damage associated with intravenous glucocorticoid pulse therapy in a patient with Graves' ophthalmopathy. *Thyroid*. 2004;14:403–406.

66. Marcocci C, Marino M, Rocchi R, et al. Novel aspects of immunosuppressive and radiotherapy management of Graves' ophthalmopathy. *J Endocrinol Invest*. 2004;27:272–280.

67. Ebner R, Devoto MH, Weil D, et al. Treatment of thyroid associated ophthalmopathy with periocular injections of triamcinolone. *Br J Ophthalmol*. 2004;88(11):1380–1386.

68. Prummel MF, Mourits MP, Berghout A, et al. Prednisone and cyclosporine in the treatment of severe Graves' ophthalmopathy. *N Engl J Med*. 1989;321(20):1353–1359.

69. Huszno B, Trofimiuk M, Golkowski F, et al. Assessment of early immunosuppressive therapy in the prevention of complications of Graves' disease. *Przegl Lek*. 2004;61(8):868–871.

70. Claridge KG, Ghabrial R, Davis G, et al. Combined radiotherapy and medical immunosuppression in the management of thyroid eye disease. *Eye*. 1997;11(Pt 5):717–722.

71. Prummel MF, Mourits M, Blank L, et al. Randomized double blind trial of prednisone versus radiotherapy in Graves' ophthalmopathy. *Lancet*. 1993;342:949–954.

72. Bartalena L, Marcocci C, Chiovato L, et al. Orbital cobalt irradiation combined with systemic corticosteroids for Graves' ophthalmopathy: Comparison with systemic corticosteroids alone. *J Clin Endocrinol Metab*. 1983;56:1139–1144.

73. Marcocci C, Bartalena L, Bogazzi F, et al. Orbital radiotherapy combined with high dose systemic glucocorticoids for Graves' ophthalmopathy is more effective than radiotherapy alone: Results

of a prospective randomized study. *J Endocrinol Invest.* 1991;14:853–860.

74. Wakelkamp I, Baldeschi L, Saeed P, et al. Surgical or medical decompression as first-line treatment of optic neuropathy in Graves' ophthalmopathy? A randomized controlled trial. *Clin Endocrinol.* 2005;63(3):323–328.

75. Bartalena L, Marcocci C, Tanda ML, et al. Orbital radiotherapy for Graves' Ophthalmopathy. *Thyroid.* 2002;12(3):245–250.

76. Mandeville FB. Roentgen therapy of orbital-pituitary portals for progressive exophthalmos following subtotal thyroidectomy. *Radiology.* 1943;41:268.

77. Mourits MP, van Kempen-Harteveld ML, Garcia MB, et al. Radiotherapy for Graves' orbitopathy: Randomised placebo-controlled study. *Lancet.* 2000;355(9214):1505–1509.

78. Gorman CA, Garrity JA, Fatourechi V, et al. A prospective, randomized, double-blind, placebo-controlled study of orbital radiotherapy for Graves' ophthalmopathy. *Ophthalmology.* 2001;108:1523–1534.

78a. Gorman CA, Garrity JA, Fatourechi V, et al. The aftermath of orbital radiotherapy for graves' ophthalmopathy. *Ophthalmology.* 2002;109(11):2100–2107.

78b. Gerling J, Kommerell G, Henne K, et al. Retrobulbar irradiation for thyroid-associated orbitopathy: Double-blind comparison between 2.4 and 16 Gy. *Int J Radiat Oncol Biol Phys.* 2003;55(1):182–189.

79. Prummel MF, Terwee CB, Gerding MN, et al. A randomized controlled trial of orbital radiotherapy versus sham irradiation in patients with mild Graves' ophthalmopathy. *J Clin Endocrinol Metab.* 2004;89(1):15–20.

80. Perros P, Krassas GE. Orbital irradiation for thyroid-associated orbitopathy: Conventional dose, low dose or no dose? *Clin Endocrinol (Oxf).* 2002;56(6):689–691.

81. Kazim M. Perspectives - Part II Radiotherapy for Graves orbitopathy: The Columbia Experience. *Ophthal Plast Reconstr Surg.* 2002;18(3):173–174.

82. Terwee CB, Prummel MF, Gerding MN, et al. Measuring disease activity to predict therapeutic outcome in Graves' ophthalmopathy. *Clin Endocrinol (Oxf).* 2005;62(2):145–155.

83. Nakahara H, Noguchi S, Murakami N, et al. Graves' ophthalmopathy: MR evaluation of 10-Gy versus 24-Gy irradiation combined with systemic corticosteroids. *Radiology.* 1995;196(3):857–862.

84. Schaefer U, Hesselmann S, Mickie O, et al. A long-term follow-up study after retro-orbital irradiation for Graves' ophthalmopathy. *Int J Radiat Oncol Biol Phys.* 2002;52(1):192–197.

85. Wakelkamp IMMJ, Tan H, Saeed P, et al. Orbital irradiation for Graves' ophthalmopathy: Is it safe? A long-term follow-up study. *Ophthalmology.* 2004;111:1557–1562.

86. Broerse JJ, Snijders-Keilholz A, Jansen JTM, et al. Assessment of a carcinogenic risk for treatment of Graves' ophthalmopathy in dependence on age and irradiation geometry. *Radiother Oncol.* 1999;53:205–208.

87. Snijders-Keilholz A, Keizer RJW, Goslings BM, et al. Probable risk of tumour induction after retro-orbital irradiation for Graves' ophthalmopathy. *Radiother Oncol.* 1996;38:69–71.

88. Ben Simon GJ, Schwarcz RM, Mansury AM, et al. Minimally invasive orbital decompression: Local anesthesia and hand-carved bone. *Arch Ophthalmol.* 2005;123(12):1671–1675.

89. Goh MS, McNab AA. Orbital decompression in Graves' orbitopathy: Efficacy and safety. *Intern Med J.* 2005;35(10):586–591.

90. Tehrani M, Krummenauer F, Mann WJ, et al. Disease specific assessment of quality of life after decompression surgery for Graves' ophthalmopathy. *Eur J Ophthalmol.* 2004;14(3):193–199.

CHAPTER 16

Traumatic Optic Neuropathy

Louise A. Mawn, MD

Trauma is the leading cause of blindness in subjects <40 years old.[1] One cause of traumatic vision loss is injury to the optic nerve. Traumatic optic neuropathy (TON) is defined as traumatic loss of vision that occurs without obvious evidence of external or internal injury to the eye or its nerve.[2] TON is most commonly seen in the setting of cranial facial trauma.[3] The prevalence of TON after facial trauma is between 1.56% and 2.5%.[4,5] Motor vehicle accidents, bicycle accidents, falls, and assaults often cause the blunt trauma that leads to TON.[6–10] However, some head injuries with profound visual loss can appear relatively innocuous (see Fig. 16.1).[11] The vast majority of the patients are young adult males; in one series 85% were males with an average age of 34.[10] A variety of features have been associated with a poorer outcome including immediate and complete loss of vision, initial presentation with no-light perception vision, and orbital fractures, particularly those located in the posterior orbit.[11–15]

The optimal treatment for TON remains unclear. Surgical decompression of the optic nerve and corticosteroids have been used individually and in combination as therapy. Evaluation of the efficacy of treatment is complicated by the fact that spontaneous recovery may occur in some cases. As a result, the impact of medical or surgical intervention is controversial and the prognosis for visual recovery both with treatment and observation varies in different studies and ranges from 31% to 66%.[6,10,14,16] Surgical intervention with canal decompression has been advocated in cases with delayed visual loss.[11,17,18] Steroids to reduce both optic nerve swelling and the chemical mediators of central nervous system injury have been used for the last 25 years in cases of TON.[11] Treatment regimens are not without potential complications. Complications from surgical treatment range from bleeding (including from the carotid), cerebral spinal fluid rhinorrhea and meningitis, telecanthus, hypertrophic scar, and synechia.[10,19–21]

High-dose steroids may increase the risk for infection but are thought to be safe with low risk of complications.[22,23] To date, there has not been a National Institutes of Health (NIH)-sponsored clinical trial to examine the question of whether treatment improves the outcome in TON and the available literature consists of level III evidence.

The Rationale for Treatment with Corticosteroids

Differing regimens and steroid preparations have been recommended for the treatment of TON.[9,10,24,25] The use of corticosteroids is based on research on animal models of neuronal injury as well as on clinical research in acute spinal injury. Anderson et al. first reported the use of high-dose steroids to treat traumatic optic nerve injuries.[11] Anderson et al. considered the use of megadose steroids because of the neurosurgical literature supporting steroid use in traumatically induced brain edema.[11] The strong rationale for steroid use in TON was further supported by the initial interpretation of the National Acute Spinal Cord Injury Studies (NASCIS) II and III.[24] The results of these studies led to the widespread use of methylprednisolone (MP) in acute spinal cord injuries.

The pathophysiology of visual loss in TON is thought to result from optic nerve axonal injury. Vascular injury from compression, contusion, and/or stretch of the optic nerve causes axonal ischemia.[11] Impact force to the facial bones in the frontal and malar region is transmitted to the optic canal.[11,26,27] This force propagation causes damage to the vessels supplying the optic nerve.[11] Color Doppler imaging studies have shown alterations in orbital blood flow in TON.[28,29] Primary injury to the optic nerve axons results in permanent loss of function without the possibility of recovery or regeneration. The resulting local ischemia and expression of biochemical mediators

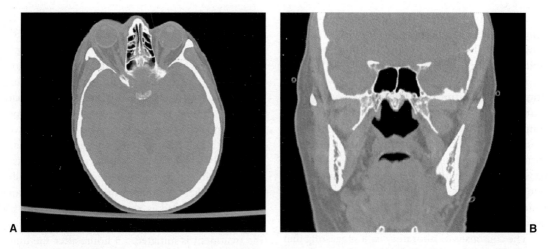

FIGURE 16.1 ▪ Axial and coronal computed tomography without evidence of optic canal fracture in a 75 year-old female with immediate loss of vision to light perception in the right eye after accidental fall on hardwood floor (wearing glasses). No loss of consciousness. Examination shows a right relative afferent pupillary defect OD, 2.5-cm laceration of the temporal brow; swelling and ecchymoses of the periorbita, subconjunctival hemorrhage, and an unremarkable dilated fundus examination. Vision improved to hand motions with observation. LP OD, light perception ocular dextra (right eye); OD, ocular dextra; DFE, dilated fundus exam; HM, hand motions.

of injury then causes additional secondary injury.[30] Ischemia and subsequent cellular depolarization leads to the opening of voltage-dependent ion channels and massive release of neurotransmitters such as glutamate. Increase in intracellular calcium leads to mitochondrial dysfunction, failure of aerobic energy metabolism, lactate accumulation, activation of mitochondrial and cytoplasmic nitric oxide synthase and nitric oxide production, and activation of phospholipase A2 with consequent cell damage by lipid peroxidation.[31,32] These chemical events occur within the first minutes, hours, and days after injury.[31] The progression of these cellular events becomes irreversible with time.[33] The secondary injury may be amenable to pharmacologic intervention with steroids, surgery, or other neuroprotective strategies.

The rationale for using glucocorticoids in the treatment of TON is based on neuroscience research. The theory of glucocorticoids for neuroprotection arose from their high lipid solubility and the possibility that they limit the propagation of lipid peroxidation chain reactions. In cats MP inhibited posttraumatic lipid peroxidation in spinal cord tissue at doses of 30 mg per kg but this effect was found to diminish at 60 mg per kg. Animal studies led to the following conclusions: Early treatment with large doses of steroids was required with constant intravenous infusion and therapy needed to be continued during the reaction phase of lipid peroxidative reactions (24 to 48 hours).[31]

Although evidence from animal models of neural injury treated with corticosteroids provides a rationale for therapy of TON, questions remain about the underlying basic science. Although rat optic nerve is commonly used as an animal model of both optic nerve disease and spinal cord injury[32,34], there are only three published studies examining the question of MP efficacy in TON.[35–37] One study showed no effect of treatment[35]; one resulted in a worsening of axonal loss[37]; and one showed that MP inhibits apoptosis after optic nerve crush.[36] A criticism leveled at similar spinal cord injury studies done on rats is that the complex pharmacokinetics of MP in rat models of spinal cord injuries has not been defined.[31,37] In fact, spinal cord literature suggests that there is a very short therapeutic window for MP treatment in rats and that both delayed treatment and excessive treatment can exacerbate loss.[38,39]

Another area of uncertainty relates to the different forms of corticosteroids available for usage. The different steroid preparations vary in biologic effect. Lipid peroxidative inhibition and anti-inflammatory potencies of glucocorticoids do not correlate; dexamethasone is five times more potent as a glucocorticoid than MP but inhibits lipid peroxidase only slightly more and carries greater steroid-related side effects. In addition, MP has greater antioxidant effect than dexamethasone.[31]

Although most research has been conducted using MP there is one rabbit model of TON that showed that high-dose dexamethasone improved orbital blood flow over nontreated controls.[40]

Extrapolation of animal studies provided the rationale for treatment of central nervous system injury with steroids. These studies have influenced the timing, dose, and duration of steroid treatment. There are significant difficulties extrapolating the results of animal studies to human optic nerve disease including whether treatment is given before the critical time point of irreversible cell death, the distance between the injury and the retinal ganglion cell, and the complexity of patient recruitment into treatment trials.[41]

The consensus of laboratory data suggesting that steroids might have a beneficial effect in acute spinal cord injury led to the NASCIS. The results of these studies lead to the use of MP in TON, and therefore, an understanding of these studies and their findings is important to the treating ophthalmologist.

The National Acute Spinal Cord Injury Studies

The NIH-sponsored NASCIS II trial was initiated in 1985 with three treatment groups for spinal cord injury patients. Within 12 hours of injury, one group received a loading dose of 30 mg per kg of MP, followed by a 5.4 mg/kg/h infusion for 23 hours; the second group received naloxone (an opiate receptor antagonist found to improve experimental spinal cord injury) 5.4 mg per kg bolus, followed by 4.0 mg/kg/h for 23 hours or placebo. The conclusion of the study was that patients treated with MP within 8 hours of injury had improvement in neurologic function over the other two groups at the 6-month and 1-year follow-up visit.[42,43] This study has been criticized because of the artificial time cut off of 8 hours, the failure to account for severity of injury, and the lack of measurement of functional recovery. A subsequent case–control study failed to demonstrate any benefit of MP.[44]

The NASCIS III was a double-blind randomized clinical trial comparing 24-hour MP to 48-hour MP administration and tirilazad mesylate administered for 48 hours.[45,46] This study was conducted to address whether extending the 24-hour high-dose steroid treatment, which was found effective in the NASCIS II, to 48 hours would result in better outcomes and whether treatment with tirilazad, a modified steroid molecule created to avoid the glucocorticoid effect and enhance the anti–lipid

peroxidase effect of steroids, was as effective as that with MP. The third question was whether initiation of treatment within 3 hours was more effective than when treatment was started 3 to 8 hours after injury. Results were similar at the 6-month and 1-year follow-up. When treatment was initiated within 3 hours, all three groups showed similar improvement. When therapy was started between 3 and 8 hours, the 48-hour MP group had better recovery but higher rates of infection. There was no difference in functional outcome. The investigators concluded that treatment within the first 3 hours is optimal, tirilazad is as effective as 24-hour MP, and that treatment for 48 hours is more effective if the treatment is initiated >3 hours after the injury. This study also suffered similar criticism as the North American Spinal Cord Injury Study (NASCIS II).[47]

The role of MP as standard of care for acute spinal cord injuries has been questioned, particularly the statistical analysis used in the NASCIS II and III. The subsequent conclusions have been criticized.[48–50] More recent neurosurgery literature argues that the harmful side effects of corticosteroids may be greater than the clinical benefit, specifically the risk for pneumonia and sepsis.[47] However, the difference in infection rates and death in the NASCIS II and III were only trends and were not statistically significant.[47] The argument against steroids relies most heavily on the failure to demonstrate a statistically significant difference in the functional outcome between the groups.[47] In spite of the criticisms, the primary investigator of the NASCIS supports the use of MP for acute spinal cord trauma because of the possible treatment benefit and the low risk of complication.[51] Bracken argues that a review of almost 2,500 patients in 51 trials indicated that MP is a safe treatment intervention.[22] He also argues that treatment with MP has a significant therapeutic effect if administered within 8 hours of injury.[47] The effect of treatment timing was also emphasized in a poststudy analysis of the NASCIS II data. This analysis showed that increased damage may result when the treatment is delayed >8 hours. This deleterious effect is speculated to result from glucocorticoid exacerbation of acute postischemic neuronal necrosis and inhibition of axonal sprouting.[52] The beneficial effect seen when treatment is given within 8 hours is thought to result from the inhibition of lipid peroxidation.[52] Although widely considered to be the standard of care in neurosurgery, MP is not registered for acute spinal cord injury in the United States.[31]

More recently, focus in the neurosciences has shifted to other emerging neuroprotective strategies for spinal cord injuries.[53] This spinal cord research has heightened the attention given to the possibility of neuroprotective intervention in optic neuropathies.[30,54] *In vitro* rat optic nerve studies have served as models of central white matter injury.[32,55] Extrapolation of *in vivo* spinal cord injury data may have clinical relevance for optic nerve injuries. The three rat model studies addressing the question of whether the use of high-dose steroids, as in acute spinal cord trauma, should be extended to optic nerve injuries. A dose-dependent, but statistically insignificant, decline in residual axons with increasing doses of MP was found by Steinsapir.[37] Alternatively, Sheng et al. found inhibition of apoptosis with MP treatment.[36]

Clinical Studies of the Treatment of Traumatic Optic Neuropathy

Corticosteroids

Very limited clinical studies have been conducted evaluating treatment interventions in TON. The bulk of the clinical data that exist includes retrospective case reports and case series. There are two primary difficulties with conducting studies on TON. Firstly, the incidence of TON is low with estimates between 0.1% and 6%.[3,4,56] As a result, study recruitment has been a major obstacle. Secondly, determining visual acuity (VA) and function as a primary outcome measure is often difficult in the setting of TON because of associated major trauma and head injury.[7] Difficulty in establishing visual loss in the unconscious patient further complicates the clinical decision process.

Surrogate outcome measures that are predictive of VA have been used in patients who are unconscious. Pupillary function and flash-evoked potentials have been shown to have a predictive value in determining final visual outcome.[57,58] Alford et al. found that patients with a 2.1 log unit or greater RAPD did not improve and all had final VA of 20/400 or worse.[57] Holmes et al. reported that VA never exceeded 20/300 if flash visual-evoked potential amplitude was <50% of the normal eye.[58] Additional variables associated with a poor outcome have been described: Blood within the posterior ethmoidal cells, age >40, loss of consciousness, and absence of recovery after 48 hours of steroid treatment (see Fig. 16.2).[59]

Most of the human TON studies (see Table 16.1) to date have looked at steroid treatment in a retrospective, observational manner. Conclusions regarding the efficacy of steroid therapy in these studies are often complicated because most of these studies have also included a surgical arm.

To better identify the best treatment for indirect TON, the International Optic Nerve Trauma Study (IONTS) was conducted. This study was originally designed as a randomized controlled pilot study comparing extracranial optic canal decompression combined with high-dose corticosteroids versus corticosteroids alone. The enrollment was insufficient and the study was converted to an observational

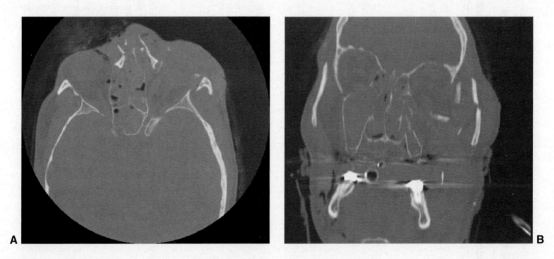

FIGURE 16.2 ▫ Axial and coronal computed tomography with extensive facial and orbital fractures and posterior ethmoid and sphenoid hemorrhage in a 52-year-old male with severe head injury secondary to a motor vehicle accident, altered MS, NLP vision OS, −4 motility in all fields of gaze, and RAPD OS. In spite of megadose steroids, final acuity NLP OS.

TABLE 16.1 ▪ Traumatic Optic Neuropathy Studies

Author (Date)	Study Design/Purpose	Study Participants	Treatment Protocol	Outcome	Conclusions/Limitations
Anderson (1982)[11]	Single-center, observational, retrospective review to evaluate indications and results of optic nerve decompression	7 patients with unilateral visual loss following head trauma	Dexamethasone varying from 20–60 mg q 6 h; 4/7 transethmoidal-sphenoid decompression	Visual acuity improvement: Observed in 1/4 surgical and steroids patients; 3/6 patients treated with steroids	Study concludes that megadose steroids are helpful in treatment and management decision. Limitations include no controls and variation in steroid dosing and amount
Matsuzaki (1982)[60]	Single-center, retrospective observational case series to compare medical vs. surgical treatment of TON	33 TON secondary to blunt head trauma	11/33 surgical decompression; 22/33 medical management with prednisolone, mannitol, urokinase, and vitamin B_{12}	Visual acuity improvement: No visual improvement in patients without vision initially (these patients excluded from analysis); improvement in 42.8% in surgery and 58.8% in medical groups	Study concludes that medical management preferable to surgical intervention. Limitations include unbalanced groups, lack of statistical analysis
Fujitani (1986)[61]	Single-center, retrospective observational case series to compare efficacy of steroid treatment to surgical decompression	110 indirect TON	43/110 steroids; 70/110 endonasal transethmoidal optic nerve decompression	Visual acuity improvement: 19/43 of the steroid group improved (44.2%); 34/70 of the surgical group improved (47.7%)	Study concludes that with complete visual loss found soon after injury, earliest possible surgery recommended. Limitations include unbalanced treatment groups and lack of statistical analysis
Lessell (1989)[6]	Single-center, retrospective observational case series to define clinical features that guide management	33 indirect optic nerve injury, excluded were those with chiasm or retinal-vitreous injury, penetrating orbital trauma, poor history, <1976, no follow-up	25/33 observation; 4/33 steroids, 4/33 steroids and transethmoidal decompression	Visual acuity improvement: 5/25 of observation group improved; 1/4 of steroids group improved; 3/4 of surgery group improved	Study notes that numbers too small to permit conclusions; limitations include unbalanced treatment groups. Dose and type of steroid not reported

Study	Study design	Population/Treatment	Results	Conclusions
Seiff (1990)[7]	Single-center, retrospective observational case series to compare steroid treatment with observation	36 indirect optic nerve injury; vision <20/20; RAPD, otherwise normal examination; 3/36 decompression; 5/36 had 1 mg/kg dexamethasone and decompression (4 transcranial, 3 transorbital, 1 lateral orbitotomy), 21/36 corticosteroids, and 15 untreated	Visual acuity improvement: No statistical difference in improvement between groups. Vision improved earlier in steroid-treated patients	Study concludes that n not large enough to show a significant difference between study groups. Limitations include unbalanced groups
Joseph (1990)[8]	Single-center, observational, retrospective review case series to report surgical technique and efficacy of extracranial decompression for TON	14 with TON within 1 wk of injury; excluded were comatose patients; other vision-limiting ocular lesions or orbital penetration; ipsilateral external ethmoidectomy 20 h, 5 d from injury; 8 patients on 10 mg dexamethasone intravenously for 1–2 d	Visual acuity improvement: 11/14 improved; 3/5 NLP improved 20/20 to counting fingers	Study recommends protocol of immediate administration of dexamethasone, surgical decompression if <7 d, and no contraindications to general anesthesia and no injury to globe. Limitations include uncontrolled series with small n.
Spoor (1990)[9]	2-center, comparative (nonrandomized) uncontrolled interventional study with dexamethasone at one center and MP at the second to report success of treatment with both high-dose and megadose steroids	21 patients with TON; complete neuro-ophthalmic evaluation and CT; patients excluded if associated concussive or penetrating ocular injury; 8/21 IV dexamethasone 20.0 mg q 6 h for 48 h (8.5 h to 15 d from injury); 13/21 IV methylprednisolone 30.0 mg/kg in 2 h followed by 15.0 mg/kg q 6 for 48 h, taper after 48 h; 3/13 MP had transcranial (1) or transethmoidal surgery	Visual acuity improvement: No difference between groups. 7/8 of dexamethasone group and 12/13 treated with MP improved. More rapid improvement with MP ($p = 0.008$)	Study concludes that high-dose or megadose steroids may be helpful and restore vision. Study uncontrolled with unbalanced treatment groups

(continued)

TABLE 16.1 ■ (Continued)

Author (Date)	Study Design/Purpose	Study Participants	Treatment Protocol	Outcome	Conclusions/Limitations
Mauriello (1992)[62]	Single-center, retrospective, noncomparative interventional case series to describe management protocol with MP followed by surgery if no improvement and CT identifiable pathology	23 patients with unilateral or bilateral TON within 48 h of trauma, visual loss, and RAPD; excluded if penetrating ocular injury or optic nerve avulsion	All received 1 g MP followed by 250 mg IV q 6 for 72 h; immediate canthotomy if increased orbital pressure; if vision did not improve after 24–48 h, decompression of nerve sheath hematoma or frontal craniotomy of optic canal if compression of canal by bone spicules seen on CT; if no surgically treatable pathology seen on CT then steroids tapered. If vision improved, steroids continued 5–7 d	Visual acuity improvement: 9/16 improved with steroids, 3/7 of surgery patients had some improvement; 7/10 with NLP had no improvement	Study concluded favorable prognosis associated with lucid interval and enlarged optic nerve sheath; poor prognosis if initial NLP vision, no lucid interval, large bone fragments against nerve and recommends decompression of sheath and canal in those patients who fail to respond to steroids. Limitations uncontrolled nonrandomized, small *n*
Girard (1992)[63]	Single-center, retrospective, observational case series to report outcome with surgery	11 patients with indirect TON	Tranethmoidal-sphenoid decompression up to 92 d after injury	Visual acuity improvement: 8/11 improved; 4 with NLP improved	Study concludes that transethmoid-sphenoid gives improvement with low morbidity. Limitations include small *n* and no controls
Levin (1994)[64]	Single-center, retrospective, observational, to identify factors associated with improvement in patients treated with canal decompression.	31 patients with TON after closed head trauma; excluded were patients with globe injury or alerted mentation	All treated with steroids and transethmoidal witnin 6 d of injury	Visual acuity improvement: 22/31 improved, greater improvement younger than 40	Study concluded that vision improved more in patients younger than 40 and that interval between injury and treatment, preoperative acuity and canal fracture did not affect outcome. Limitations include small *n* and uncontrolled study
Chou (1996)[13]	Single-center, retrospective, nonrandomized, observational study to evaluate the effect of steroids or steroids and surgery vs. no treatment.	58 patients with TON from blunt head injury	23 patients treated with oral or IV dexamethasone, 25 steroids and optic canal decompression, 10 patients no treatment	Visual acuity improvement: 13/23 medical treatment improved (*p* = 0.002), 15/25 medical and surgical improved (*p* = 0.002), no improvement in control group, NLP poorer outcome than >LP	Study concluded that optic canal fracture correlated with poor visual acuity and poor prognosis with best corrected vision of <20/200. Limitations include nonrandomized and small *n*.

Study	Study design	Patient population	Intervention	Results	Conclusions
Kuppersmith (1997)[65]	Two-center retrospective review, to describe combined transconjunctival/intranasal endoscopic approach to optic canal decompression	9 patients with TON caused by bone fragments or fractures impinging on optic nerve or visual deterioration despite high-dose MP	All 9 treated with both high-dose MP and combined transconjunctival/intranasal endoscopic optic nerve decompression	Visual acuity improvement: 5/9 with vision showed improvement of visual acuity; NLP failed to improve	Study concludes that this surgical method has improved exposure; Uncontrolled study with limited number of patients
Mine (1999)[66]	Single-center, retrospective, observational case series to identify factors affecting outcome and indications for surgery	36 patients with unilateral and bilateral indirect TON	12 patients treated with frontotemporal craniotomy; decompression of nerve and treatment with dexamethasone; 24 patients treated with only dexamethasone	Visual acuity improvement: 10/12 improved in surgery group; 14/24 in medical group	Study concludes that age and optic canal fracture are not correlated with visual improvement. Initial visual acuity is correlated with visual improvement (Surgery group $p < 0.0001$, medical group $p = 0.0268$) and improves significantly more in patients with initial visual acuity HM or better than LP only or worse. Visual improvement did not differ between surgery and medical treatment; however, in patients with initial visual acuity HM or better, surgery patients improved more ($p = 0.0009$). Limitations include nonrandomized study with unbalanced treatment groups, small n. Dose of dexamethasone not reported in study.

(continued)

TABLE 16.1 ☐ (Continued)

Author (Date)	Study Design/Purpose	Study Participants	Treatment Protocol	Outcome	Conclusions/Limitations
Levin (1999)[10]	Multicenter, comparative nonrandomized interventional study with concurrent treatment groups to assess whether visual outcome differed between treatment with corticosteroids, surgical intervention by optic canal decompression or observation	133 patients with TON and initial visual assessment within 3 d of injury. At least 1 mo follow-up.	Treatment: Untreated 9; corticosteroids 85; decompression 33	Visual acuity improvement: 3 lines or more improvement: 32% surgery, 57% untreated, 52% steroid; HM or worse to 20/40 or better: 1/3 untreated, 7/34 steroid group, 0/23 surgery group	Study unable to find a difference between treatment methods or with the untreated group. Initial visual acuity was a predictor of final visual acuity. Gender, age, canal fracture, and surgical approach did not correlate with outcome. Prognosis poor with initial NLP acuity. Methods not defined and varied in surgical approach and steroid dose. Examinations not standardized; not randomized, controlled, or masked; unbalanced treatment groups
Li (1999)[67]	Single-center, retrospective, consecutive, observational case series to report outcome of extracranial optic nerve decompression after 12–24 h steroids without improvement.	45 patients with TON	All treated with megadose steroids and extracranial optic nerve decompression	Visual acuity improvement: 32/45 improved.	Study recommends a treatment protocol of megadose steroids and optic nerve decompression. Limitations include no control or comparison group
Kountakis (2000)[68]	Single-center, retrospective, nonrandomized, interventional, observational case series to compare outcome of patients treated with steroids to those treated with surgery after failure to improve with steroids	42 patients with TON; 5 patients with ocular involvement excluded and 3 with loss of follow-up excluded	34 treated with MP 30 mg/kg IV followed after 45 min by 5.4 mg/kg/h for 47 h and H2 blockers; 11/34 improved; 17/23 not improved or worse after steroids treated with endoscopic optic nerve sheath decompression	Visual acuity improvement: 11/34 medical improved; 14/17 surgical patients improved. In those patients with initial acuity 20/400 or worse MP and surgery had better outcome. 8/11 NLP patients improved with surgery	Study concludes that patients treated with steroids and endoscopic decompression have better outcome than steroids alone ($p = 0.0007$). Limitations include no control group and small study size

Study	Design	Patients	Methods	Results	Conclusions
Wang (2001)[12]	Single-center, retrospective nonrandomized, observational case series to assess the effect of treatment options (steroids, surgical decompression, fracture repair, observation)	61 with sudden or progressive visual loss after penetrating and blunt facial trauma, comatose patients excluded	25/61 steroids; 7/61 surgical decompression, 13/61 no treatment; 21/61 fractures repaired	Visual acuity improvement: 22/61 patients improved. 18/40 with blunt trauma had improvement, 4/21 with penetrating trauma had improvement	Study concluded that presence of orbital fractures and initial NLP acuity negatively affected final acuity but age, fracture repair, or timing of repair did not affect final acuity. Study recommended aggressive medical and surgical treatment in blind patients. Limitations include treatment protocols not reported including dose of steroids and surgical approach
Lubben (2001)[20]	Single-center, retrospective, observational and interventional case series to study the efficacy of early optic nerve decompression in comatose and conscious patients	65 patients with indirect TON; 13/65 patients comatose	Fronto-orbital approach. All patients received high-dose IV steroids postoperatively. Surgery based on examination and CT findings of lesion inside optic canal or orbit apex. In comatose patients RAPD with disc edema with congestion of the vessels. In conscious patients posttraumatic decrease in vision, loss of vision with acuity 20/100 to 20/60 or increasing severe restriction of visual field	Visual acuity improvement: 30/52 (57.7%) conscious patients improved, 8/13 (61.5%) of comatose patients improved	The study concluded that final acuity correlated with preoperative acuity. No correlation between final acuity and location of fracture, time of injury to surgery, age, or gender of patient. Study recommends early decompression of the optic nerve. Limitations include nonreporting of steroid dose, no quantitative assessment of visual function in comatose patients, unbalanced treatment groups, limited n
Kitthaweesin (2001)[69]	Single-center, randomized, double-blind, observational and interventional study to compare the efficacy of dexamethasone to MP in indirect TON	21 patients with indirect TON. Injury to treatment within 7 d. 10/21 dexamethasone; 11/21 MP	Intravenous dexamethasone for 72 h or MP	Visual acuity improvement: 3 or more lines BCVA improvement 67% dexamethasone and 33.33% MP at 2 mo.	Study concluded no differences in visual improvement between the two groups, age, cause of injury, injury to treatment interval initial BCVA

(continued)

TABLE 16.1 □ (Continued)

Author (Date)	Study Design/Purpose	Study Participants	Treatment Protocol	Outcome	Conclusions/Limitations
Wohlrab (2002)[70]	Single-center, retrospective, study to describe results with surgical decompression	19 patients with indirect TON	Transethmoidal optic nerve decompression	Visual acuity improvement: 8/19 improved with surgery	Study concluded that surgery within 48 h beneficial. NLP initial vision can improve with surgery. Limitations included study size.
Yip (2002)[71]	Single-center, nonrandomized, retrospective study to compare efficacy of low-dose MP to conservative management	21 patients with indirect TON	9 patients treated with 125–250 mg MP q 6 h for 2–5 d; 12 patients on observation	Visual improvement: 44% of treated group improved, 33% of observation group improved ($p = 0.673$)	Study concluded that MP was not shown to improve outcome. Limitations include study size
Li (2002)[72]	Single-center, retrospective observational interventional study to report outcome with endoscopic optic nerve decompression	52 patients (53 eyes) with TON with follow-up 6 mo to 3 y	Steroid treatment and endonasal endoscopic optic nerve decompression	Visual acuity improvement: 21/53 eyes improved, 7 with only surgery, 14 surgery and steroids	Study concludes improved visual outcome with surgery. Limitations include uncontrolled study with small n and no standardized treatment protocol
Chuen-kongkaerw (2002)[73]	Single-center, prospective, randomized, observational and interventional study to compare TON outcomes, treating with high-dose dexamethasone vs. megadose methylprednisolone	44 patients with TON within 2 wk of injury	Intravenous high-dose dexamethasone or megadose methylprednisolone	Visual acuity improvement: 9/12 dexamethasone vs. 10/12 MP. No difference between initial and final visual acuity ($p = 0.60$)	Study concludes no difference in outcome between groups treatment with either steroid. Limitation study size

Study	Study design	Methods/Patients	Visual acuity outcome	Conclusions
Carta (2003)[59]	4-center, retrospective observational and interventional study to determine which initial signs correlate with final visual acuity	35 cases of TON after head trauma with at least 3 mo follow-up	Intravenous megadose MP within 72 h trauma according to NASCI 3 protocol. Steroids tapered after 1 wk	Visual acuity improvement: 12/35 improved after 48 h steroid treatment, 3/23 without improvement after 48 h improved. Immediate loss of vision was associated but did not reach statistical significance	Study concludes that blood within posterior ethmoid air cells (RR 2.25, 95% CI 1.25–4.04), age >40 (RR 1.79, 1.07–2.99), loss of consciousness (RR 2.21, 1.17–4.16), absence of recovery after 48 h steroids ($p < 0.01$) are poor prognostic signs for final outcome. Limitations include study size
Rajiniganth (2003)[19]	Single-center, prospective, nonrandomized, observational and interventional case series to assess outcome, treating with methylprednisolone and endoscopic nerve decompression	44 consecutive patients with unilateral indirect TON with minimum of 3 mo follow-up. 30/34 underwent surgery (4 did not because of optic atrophy)	Injection methylprednisolone 30 mg/kg per day. Endoscopic optic nerve decompression if no improvement after 72 h of MP, progressive loss during steroid treatment, total blindness with CT evidence of optic nerve compression	Visual acuity improvement: 10/44 improved with MP alone, 11/30 improved after surgery	Study concludes time lapse from injury to treatment ($p < 0.01$), degree of visual loss ($p < 0.01$), optic canal, or pericanal fracture ($p < 0.05$) significant prognostic factors. Recommends early surgery if total blindness with CT evidence of optic nerve compression. If vision present, treat medically first
Thakar (2003)[21]	Prospective, observational and interventional case series to study the efficacy of delayed optic nerve decompression in TON	35 with TON from blunt head injury and injury to surgery interval >2 wk	Surgery transethmoidal; if poor vision after treatment with 1 mg/kg prednisolone	Visual acuity improvement: 0/9 NLP patients improved; 20/26 with some vision improved.	Study concluded that poor prognostic factors include initial immediate blindness ($p = 0.02$). Age, presence of disc pallor, and type of visual field defect did not correlate with improvement. No significant difference in time of loss to surgery. Recommendations are for delayed surgery only in cases with some residual vision. Limitations include study size and no controls

(continued)

TABLE 16.1 ▢ (Continued)

Author (Date)	Study Design/Purpose	Study Participants	Treatment Protocol	Outcome	Conclusions/Limitations
Goldenberg-Cohen (2004)[74]	Single-center, retrospective, observational and interventional case series	40 patients <18 y at the time of injury, with unilateral and bilateral (3) TON from both blunt and penetrating trauma, excluded if ruptured globe; shaken-baby syndrome, no recorded vision at outcome. 22 patients with 1 mo follow-up and initial and final acuity documented	17 treated with either 1 mg/kg/d to 1,000 mg/d prednisone equivalent, one retrobulbar steroid injection, three optic nerve canal decompression, one optic nerve sheath fenestration	Visual acuity improvement: 9/22 improvement; Observation 3/7 improvement, 1/7 worse; Steroids 3/11 improvement, 3/11 worse; Surgery 3/4 improvement	Study concludes no difference in outcome between treated and untreated groups. Initial NLP vision poor prognostic sign. Limitation study size and unbalanced groups. No standardized steroid treatment. Study includes both blunt and penetrating trauma
Zhang (2004)[75]	Single-center retrospective, observational case series to discuss operative indications of transcranial optic nerve decompression	118 patients with optic nerve injury resulting from skull base fractures with 6 mo follow-up	Transcranial optic nerve decompression	Visual acuity improvement: 35/72 NLP improved, all 46 with residual vision improved	Study concludes that transcranial decompression should be recommended to patients with blindness <3 d, residual vision, and bilateral injury. Limitations include no control group
Yang (2004)[76]	Single-center, retrospective, observational case series to identify factors affecting final outcome and define treatment protocol	42 consecutive patients with TON after maxillofacial trauma, excluded if penetrating injury or optic nerve avulsion. Patients followed for 3 mo	Megadose steroid treatment (18), megadose steroid 30 mg/kg MP followed by 15 mg/kg every 6 h for 3 d and endoscopic assisted transorbital optic nerve decompression surgery (24) in those not improved with steroid	Visual acuity improvement 5/23 of NLP group improved, 13/19 of LP or better group improved; 10/24 of surgery group improved, 8/18 of no surgery group improved	Study concluded initial visual acuity (p = 0.006) correlated with outcome. Treatment within 7 d improved more but did not show statistical significance (p = 0.056). Surgery should be offered to patients NLP even >7 d from injury. Limitations include study size and nonrandomized

BCVA, best corrected visual acuity; HM, hand motions; NLP, no light perception; CT, computed tomography; IV, intravenous; MP, methylprednisolone; n, number of patients; NIH, National Institutes of Health; RAPD, relative afferent pupillary defect; TON, traumatic optic neuropathy.

study. This study is detailed in the subsequent text; the major conclusion was that there was no clear benefit to either intervention. Over 20 other retrospective series are briefly summarized in Table 16.1.

The IONTS addressed the question of whether visual outcome differed between treatment with corticosteroids, surgical intervention by optic canal decompression, or observation. The study was designed as a randomized controlled pilot study with two treatment arms, extracranial optic canal decompression combined with megadose steroids versus corticosteroids alone. The study was conducted from 1994–1997. After 2 years of attempted recruitment, with limited eligible patients, the study was transformed into an observational study. The study was a comparative, nonrandomized interventional study with concurrent treatment groups. Two hundred and six patients were included in the study. The average age was 34 ± 18 years and 85% were male. Motor vehicle accident was the most common cause of trauma. Visual loss was hand motions or worse in two thirds of eyes. Treatment decisions and methods were not defined nor were there standardized examinations. Data analysis excluded those patients without an ocular examination (15), penetrating injury (10), first visual assessment >3 days after injury (48) for a total of 127 unilateral and 6 bilateral injury patients. The study group was further reduced by 29 patients to 98 unilateral cases and 6 bilateral patients with at least 1 month follow-up. The bilateral injury group had a separate analysis. The 127 unilateral cases were grouped on the basis of intervention within 7 days of injury as no treatment (9), steroids (85) and surgery with or without steroids (33). Thirty-two of the 33 patients who underwent surgery received steroids. Steroid dose was classified by the initial dose of MP as megadose >5,400 mg (34), very high dose 2,000 to 5,399 mg (15), high dose 500 to 1,999 mg (16), moderate dose 100 to 499 mg (9) and low dose <100 mg (5) and unknown dose (7). Treatment began within 24 hours in 53 patients, 24 to 48 hours in 14, 48 to 72 hours in 8 and >72 hours in 7 and unreported time in 3. The surgery group had significantly more eyes that were NLP or LP ($p < 0.001$). This group also had more patients who had injury from a fall. There was not a significant difference in final VA between the surgery group and the untreated group and the steroid group after accounting for baseline acuity. The percentage of patients with improvement of three lines or more in VA were similar in the three groups.[10] Criticisms of the IONTS included the fact that different specialties performed the surgical decompressions with different approaches, techniques, and indications.[20] Major limitations of the study design limit the applicability of the results.

Surgery

Surgical decompression of the optic nerve in cases of TON is also considered in many cases. Consideration of surgical decompression of the optic canal in TON was suggested in 1963.[77] There are case reports in the literature before the 1980s that describe the successful return of vision with surgery alone.[18] The precise indications and efficacy of surgery remain unclear and lack evaluation with well-designed clinical trials. In addition, the treatment effect of surgery alone is difficult to determine given that most surgical series of optic canal decompression and optic nerve sheath fenestration are coupled with concurrent steroid treatment. Various surgical approaches have been used in the available studies: Transcranial, transethmoidal, endoscopy- assisted ethmoidal surgery, endoscopy-assisted transorbital, and frontal orbital surgery.[7,8,11,61−64,76] There are reports of improvement in VA with surgery even 92 days and 1 year after injury.[21,63]

Retrospective studies include Lubben's study, which evaluated the impact of canal decompression in both comatose and conscious patients. All patients received high-dose steroids. The surgical indications were CT scan findings of lesion inside the optic canal or the orbital apex coupled with ophthalmic examination. Six of 13 patients with preoperative, no-pupillary-light response had VA outcome of 20/50 or better.[20] Joseph et al. reported 14 patients with TON who were treated with both intravenous dexamethasone 8 to 10 mg and optic canal decompression through an external ethmoidectomy. Eleven of 14 patients had improvement in vision.[8] Yang et al. presented 42 consecutive patients, treated either with megadose MP (18) or with megadose MP and optic nerve decompression (24) through a subcaruncular transorbital approach. Three of 16 surgical group patients with initial VA no-light perception versus none of 7 nonsurgical group had improvement in vision. This was not statistically significant; however, the small sample size makes statistical inferences difficult.[76] Because these studies are uncontrolled and have small numbers of patients, it is difficult to base treatment decisions on this level of evidence.

Conclusions

There are no randomized controlled studies comparing either steroids or surgery to observation. Letters in the ophthalmic and head and neck literature highlight the controversy regarding treatment options.

In general, treatment recommendations are made on a case-by-case basis because of a lack of clear treatment guidelines. One suggested approach is to treat all patients with indirect TON with megadose steroids, and patients who do not improve after a trial of megadose steroids, cannot be weaned without visual loss, or who have a surgically treatable lesion on imaging are offered optic canal decompression surgery.[78] There is no evidence in the literature to either support or contradict this approach.[79] The conclusion that patients with TON must be treated with a combined therapy protocol including surgery and steroids to achieve a better visual outcome is also unsupported by the literature.[80] Many authors feel that each case should be managed on an individual basis.[81]

Although there are reports of visual improvement with surgery alone, most the patients who undergo surgery have poor initial acuity and have failed to improve with initial steroid therapy. The most common surgical decompression is extracranial through a transethmoidal approach. There is no evidence available to conclude that surgical intervention improves outcome; however most patients treated with surgery had worse initial acuity and there are reports of improvement after surgery even up to a year after trauma.[21] Extrapolation of both animal models and spinal cord human studies suggest that treatment with high-dose steroids may be beneficial if started immediately after injury. There is no evidence that proves that steroid treatment improves outcome in TON. The failure to show a difference in the treatment options of observation, steroids, or surgery is most likely a factor of study design and small numbers of study subjects. Because of the lack of data, practice recommendations cannot be reliably made on the basis of the available literature.

Late Treatment

Caution should be taken in the initiation of megadose steroid treatment after the 8-hour window determined by the NASCIS II as there is no evidence to suggest this is helpful. Extrapolation of the spinal cord data and basic science experiments suggest that it may be harmful compared to observation. Improvement of VA following surgical intervention is reported as long as 1 year after injury.

Duration of Treatment

If treatment is started after 3 hours but before 8 hours from the time of injury, the 48-hour MP regimen may be a preferred duration of treatment. The 48-hour regimen may carry some risk of sepsis and pneumonia.

Method of Treatment

If there is no improvement after 48 hours of megadose steroids, surgical intervention could be considered if the VA is 20/400 or worse or if clinical judgment determines possible benefit. There is not enough evidence in the literature to support the benefit of surgical intervention.

References

1. Apte R, Scheufele T, Blomquist P. Etiology of blindness in an urban community hospital setting. *Ophthalmology*. 2001;108(4):693–696.
2. Walsh F, Hoyt W. *Clinical neuroophthalmology*, 3rd ed. Vol. Baltimore, MD: Lippincott Williams & Wilkins; 1969;3:2375–2381.
3. Dancey A, Perry M, Silva D. Blindness after blunt facial trauma: Are there any clinical clues to early recognition? *J Trauma*. 2003;58:328–335.
4. al-Qurainy IA, Stassen LF, Dutton GN, et al. The characteristics of midfacial fractures and the association with ocular injury: A prospective study. *Br J Oral Maxillofac Surg*. 1991;29(5): 291–301.
5. Ansari M. Blindness after facial fractures: A 19 year retrospective study. *J Oral Maxillofac Surg*. 2005;63:229–237.
6. Lessell S. Indirect optic nerve trauma. *Arch Ophthalmol*. 1989;107(3):382–386.
7. Seiff S. High dose corticosteroids for treatment of vision loss due to indirect injury to the optic nerve. *Ophthalmic Surg*. 1990;21:389–395.
8. Joseph MP, Lessell S, Rizzo J, et al. Extracranial optic nerve decompression for traumatic optic neuropathy. *Arch Ophthalmol*. 1990;108(8):1091–1093.
9. Spoor TC, Hartel WCLensink DB, et al. Treatment of traumatic optic neuropathy with corticosteroids. *Am J Ophthalmol*. 1990;110(6): 665–669.
10. Levin LA, Beck RW, Joseph MP, et al. The treatment of traumatic optic neuropathy: The International Optic Nerve Trauma Study. *Ophthalmology*. 1999;106(7):1268–1277.
11. Anderson R, Panje W, Gross C. Optic nerve blindness following blunt forehead trauma. *Ophthalmology*. 1982;89:445.
12. Wang BH, Robertson BC, Girotto JA, et al. Traumatic optic neuropathy: A review of 61 patients. *Plast Reconstr Surg*. 2001;107(7):1655–1664.

13. Chou P, Sadam A, Chen Y, et al. Clinical experiences in the management of traumatic optic neuropathy. *Neuroophthalmol.* 1996;16:325.

14. Cook MW, Levin LA, Joseph MP, et al. Traumatic optic neuropathy. A meta-analysis. *Arch Otolaryngol Head Neck Surg.* 1996;122(4):389–392.

15. Tsai HH, Jeng SF, Lin TS, et al. Predictive value of computed tomography in visual outcome in indirect traumatic optic neuropathy complicated with periorbital facial bone fracture. *Clin Neurol Neurosurg.* 2005;107(3):200–206.

16. Hughes B. Indirect injury of the optic nerves and chiasma. *Bull Johns Hopkins Hosp.* 1962;111:98–126.

17. Hooper R. Orbital complications of head injury. *Br J surg.* 1951;39:126–138.

18. Kennerdell J, Amsbaugh G, Myers E. Transantral ethmoidal decompression of optic canal fracture. *Arch Ophthalmol.* 1976;94:1040–1043.

19. Rajiniganth MG, Gupta AK, Gupta A, et al. Traumatic optic neuropathy: Visual outcome following combined therapy protocol. *Arch Otolaryngol Head Neck Surg.* 2003;129(11):1203–1206.

20. Lubben B, Stoll W, Grenzebach U. Optic nerve decompression in the comatose and conscious patients after trauma. *Laryngoscope.* 2001;111(2):320–328.

21. Thakar A, Mahapatra AK, Tandon DA. Delayed optic nerve decompression for indirect optic nerve injury. *Laryngoscope.* 2003;113(1):112–119.

22. Bracken M. Methylprednisolione and acute spinal cord injury: An update of the randomized evidence. *Spine.* 2001;26(24S):S47–S54.

23. Wing P, Nance P, Connell D, et al. Risk of avascular necrosis following short term megadose methylprednisolone treatment. *Spinal Cord.* 1998;36:633–636.

24. Steinsapir KD, Goldberg RA. Traumatic optic neuropathy. *Surv Ophthalmol.* 1994;38(6):487–518.

25. Steinsapir KD. Traumatic optic neuropathy. *Curr Opin Ophthalmol.* 1999;10(5):340–342.

26. Gross C, DeKock J, Panje W, et al. Evidence for orbital deformation that may contribute to monocular blindness following minor frontal head trauma. *J Neurosurg.* 1981;55:963–966.

27. Turner J. Indirect injuries of the optic nerve. *Brain.* 1943;66:140–151.

28. Mariak Z, Obuchowska I, Ustymowicz A, et al. Color Doppler ultrasonography in diagnosis of post-traumatic optic neuropathy. *Klin Oczna.* 1999;101(2):105–110.

29. Mariak Z, Obuchowska I, Ustymowicz A, et al. The role of vascular factors in the development of traumatic optic neuropathy in course of closed head injury. *Klin Oczna.* 2002;104(5–6):384–390.

30. Yoles E, Schwartz M. Potential neuroprotective therapy for glaucomatous optic neuropathy. *Surv Ophthalmol.* 1998;42(4):367–372.

31. Hall E, Springer J. Neuroprotection and acute spinal cord injury: A reappraisal. *NeuroRX.* 2004;1:80–100.

32. Stys P. Anoxic and Ischemic injury of myelinated axons in CNS white matter: From mechanistic concepts to therapeutics. *J Cereb Blood Flow Metab.* 1998;18:2–25.

33. Walsh F. Pathological-clinical correlations. I: Indirect trauma to the optic nerves and chiasm. II: Certain cerebral involvements associated with defective blood supply. *Invest Ophthalmol.* 1966;5(5):433–449.

34. Levkovitch-Verbin H. Animal models of optic nerve diseases. *Eye.* 2004;18:1066–1074.

35. Ohlsson M, Westerlund U, Langmoen I, et al. Methylprednisolone treatment does not influence axonal regeneration or degeneration following optic nerve injury in the adult rat. *J Neuroophthalmol.* 2004;24(1):11–18.

36. Sheng Y, Zhu Y, Wu L. Effect of high dosage of methylprednisolone on rat retinal ganglion cell apoptosis after optic nerve crush. *Yan Ke Xue Bao.* 2004;20(3):181–186.

37. Steinsapir KD, Goldberg RA, Sinha S, et al. Methylprednisolone exacerbates axonal loss following optic nerve trauma in rats. *Restor Neurol Neurosci.* 2000;17(4):157–163.

38. Hall E. The neuroprotective pharmacology of methylprednisolone. *J Neurosurg.* 1992;76:13–22.

39. Yoon D, Kim Y, Young W. Therapeutic time window for methylprednisolone in spinal cord injured rat. *Yonsei Med J.* 1999;40(4):313–320.

40. Lew H, Lee SY, Jang JW, et al. The effects of high-dose corticosteroid therapy on optic nerve head blood flow in experimental traumatic optic neuropathy. *Ophthalmic Res.* 1999;31(6):463–470.

41. Levin L. Extrapolation of animal models of optic nerve injury to clinical trial design. *J Glaucoma.* 2004;13(1):1–5.

42. Bracken M, Shepard M, Collins W, et al. A randomized, controlled trial of methylprednisolone or nalaxone in the treatment of acute spinal cord injury: Results of the Second National Acute Spinal Cord Injury Study (NASCIS-2). *N Engl J Med*. 1990;322:1405–1411.

43. Bracken M, Shepard M, Collins WJ, et al. Methylprednisolone or naloxone treatment after acute spinal cord injury: 1-year follow-up data. Results of the Second National Acute Spinal Cord Injury Study. *J Neurosurg*. 1992;76(1): 23–31.

44. Poyton A, O'Farrell D, Shannon F, et al. An evaluation of the factors affecting neurological recovery following spinal cord injury. *Injury*. 1997;28:545–548.

45. Bracken M, Shepard M, Holford T, et al. Administration of methylprednisolone for 24 or 48 hours or tirilazad mesylate for 48 hours in the treatment of acute spinal cord injury. Results of the Third National Acute Spinal Cord Injury Randomized Controlled Trial. National Acute Spinal Cord Injury Study. *JAMA*. 1997;277:1597–1604.

46. Bracken MBSM, Holford TR, Leo-Summers L, et al. Methylprednisolone or tirilazad mesylate administration after acute spinal cord injury: 1-year follow up. Results of the third National Acute Spinal Cord Injury randomized controlled trial. *J Neurosurg*. 1998;89(5):699–706.

47. Hadley MN, Walters BC, Grabb PA, et al. Pharmacological therapy after acute cervical spinal cord injury. *Neurosurgery*. 2002; 50(3 Suppl):S63–S72.

48. Hurlbert R. Methylprednisolone for acute spinal cord injury: An inappropriate standard of care. *J Neurosurg*. 2000;93:1–7.

49. Coleman W, Benzel D, Cahill D, et al. A critical appraisal of the reporting of the National Acute Spinal Cord Injury Studies (II and III)of methylprednisolone in acute spinal cord injury. *J Spinal Disord*. 2000;13:185–199.

50. Short D, El Masry W, PW J. High dose methylprednisolone in the management of acute spinal cord injury: A systematic review from a clinical perspective. *Spinal Cord*. 2000;38:273–286.

51. Bracken M. High Dose methylprednisolone must be given for 24 or 48 hours after acute spinal cord injury. *Br Med J*. 2001;322(7290): 862–863.

52. Bracken M, Holford T. Effects of timing of methylprednisolone or naloxone administration on recovery of segmental and long-tract neurological function in NASCIS 2. *J Neurosurg*. 1993;79(4):500–507.

53. Kwon B, Fisher C, Dvorak M, et al. Strategies to promote neural repair and regeneration after spinal cord injury. *Spine*. 2005;30(17S): S3–S13.

54. Heiduschka P, Fischer D, Thanos S. Neuroprotection and regeneration after traumatic lesion of the optic nerve. *Klin Monatsbl Augenheilkd*. 2004;221(8):684–701.

55. Jette N, Coderre E, Nikolaeva M, et al. Spatiotemporal distribution of spectrin breakdown products induced by anoxia in adult rat optic nerve *in vitro*. *J Cereb Blood Flow Metab*. 2006;26:777–786.

56. Joseph E, Zak R, Smith S, Best WR, et al. Predictors of blinding or serious eye injury in blunt trauma. *J Trauma*. 1992;33(1):19–24.

57. Alford MA, Nerad JA, Carter KD. Predictive value of the initial quantified relative afferent pupillary defect in 19 consecutive patients with traumatic optic neuropathy. *Ophthal Plast Reconstr Surg*. 2001;17(5):323–327.

58. Holmes MD, Sires BS. Flash visual evoked potentials predict visual outcome in traumatic optic neuropathy. *Ophthal Plast Reconstr Surg*. 2004;20(5):342–346.

59. Carta A, Ferrigno L, Salvo M, et al. Visual prognosis after indirect traumatic optic neuropathy. *J Neurol Neurosurg Psychiatry*. 2003;74(2): 246–248.

60. Matsuzaki H, Kunita M, Kawai K. Optic nerve damage in head trauma: Clinical and experimental studies. *Jpn J Ophthalmol*. 1982;26(4): 447–461.

61. Fujitani T, Inoue K, Takahashi T, et al. Indirect traumatic optic neuropathy-visual outcome of operative and nonoperative cases. *Jpn J Ophthalmol*. 1986;30(1):125–134.

62. Mauriello JA, DeLuca J, Krieger A, et al. Management of traumatic optic neuropathy-a study of 23 patients. *Br J Ophthalmol*. 1992;76(6):349–352.

63. Girard BC, Bouzas EA, Lamas G, et al. Visual improvement after transethmoid-sphenoid decompression in optic nerve injuries. *J Clin Neuroophthalmol*. 1992;12(3):142–148.

64. Levin L, Joseph M, Rizzo JF Jr. Optic canal decompression in indirect optic nerve trauma. *Ophthalmology*. 1994;101(3):566–569.

65. Kuppersmith RB, Alford EL, Patrinely JR, et al. Combined transconjunctival/intranasal endoscopic approach to the optic canal in traumatic optic neuropathy. *Laryngoscope*. 1997;107(3): 311–315.

66. Mine S, Yamakami I, Yamaura A, et al. Outcome of traumatic optic neuropathy. Comparison between surgical and nonsurgical treatment. *Acta Neurochir (Wien)*. 1999;141(1):27–30.

67. Li KK, Teknos TN, Lai A, et al. Traumatic optic neuropathy: Result in 45 consecutive surgically treated patients. *Otolaryngol Head Neck Surg*. 1999;120(1):5–11.

68. Kountakis SE, Maillard AA, El-Harazi SM, et al. Endoscopic optic nerve decompression for traumatic blindness. *Otolaryngol Head Neck Surg*. 2000;123(1 Pt 1):34–37.

69. Kitthaweesin K, Yospaiboon Y. Dexamethasone and methylprednisolone in treatment of indirect traumatic optic neuropathy. *J Med Assoc Thai*. 2001;84(5):628–634.

70. Wohlrab TM, Maas S, de Carpentier JP. Surgical decompression in traumatic optic neuropathy. *Acta Ophthalmol Scand*. 2002;80(3):287–293.

71. Yip CC, Chng NW, Au Eong KG, et al. Low-dose intravenous methylprednisolone or conservative treatment in the management of traumatic optic neuropathy. *Eur J Ophthalmol*. 2002;12(4):309–314.

72. Li Y, Xu G, Xie M, et al. Traumatic optic neuropathy: Importance and result of surgical treatment. *Zhonghua Er Bi Yan Hou Ke Za Zhi*. 2002;37(3):206–209.

73. Chuenkongkaew W, Chirapapaisan N. A prospective randomized trial of megadose methylprednisolone and high dose dexamethasone for traumatic optic neuropathy. *J Med Assoc Thai*. 2002;85(5):597–603.

74. Goldenberg-Cohen N, Miller NR, Repka MX. Traumatic optic neuropathy in children and adolescents. *J AAPOS*. 2004;8(1):20–27.

75. Zhang TM, Yin DL, Fu JD, et al. Transcranial optic nerve decompression for optic nerve injury. *Zhonghua Yi Xue Za Zhi*. 2004;84(2):130–133.

76. Yang WG, Chen CT, Tsay PK, et al. Outcome for traumatic optic neuropathy-surgical versus nonsurgical treatment. *Ann Plast Surg*. 2004;52(1):36–42.

77. Seitz R. Etiology and genesis of acute blindness as a consequence of blunt cephalic traumas: A contribution of an exploratory opening of the optic canal. *Klin Monatsbl Augenheilkd*. 1963;143:414–428.

78. Lee AG. Traumatic optic neuropathy. *Ophthalmology*. 2000;107(5):814.

79. Levin LA, Beck RW, Joseph MP, et al. Traumatic optic neuropathy. *Ophthalmology*. 2000;107(5):814. Author's reply.

80. Perry JD. Treatment of traumatic optic neuropathy remains controversial. *Arch Otolaryngol Head Neck Surg*. 2004;130(8):1000, author reply –1.

81. Gupta A. Treatment of traumatic optic neuropathy remains controversial—reply. *Arch Otolaryngol Head Neck Surg*. 2004;130(8):1000–1001.

GLOSSARY

5-FU	5 Fluorouracil	DS	Deep sclerectomy
ACEI	Angiotensin converting enzyme inhibitors	EDIC	Epidemiology of Diabetes Interventions and Complications
ACV	Acyclovir		
AGIS	Advanced Glaucoma Intervention Study	EFP	Extra-retinal fibrovascular proliferation
AK	Astigmatic keratotomy	EGPS	European Glaucoma Prevention Study
ALT	Argon laser trabeculoplasty	EKT	Epithelial Keratitis Trial
AMD	Age-related macular degeneration	ERG	Electroretinogram
AMS	Antigen Matching Study	ETDRS	Early Treatment Diabetic Retinopathy Study
APT	Acyclovir Prevention Trial	EVA	Electronic visual acuity
AREDS	Age-Related Eye Disease Study	EVS	Endophthalmitis Vitrectomy Study
ARR	Absolute risk reduction	FAZ	Foveal avascular zone
ASVD	Acute severe vision decrease	FDA	Food and Drug Administration
ATS	Amblyopia Treatment Study	FFSS	Fluorouracil Filtering Surgery Study
ATT	Argon laser trabeculoplasty-trabeculotomy-trabeculotomy	FNAB	Fine Needle Aspiration Biopsy
		FT4	Free thyroxine
BCVA	Best-corrected visual acuity	FVPED	Fibrovascular pigment epithelial detachment
BRVO	Branch Retinal Vein Occlusion	GLD	Greatest linear diameter
BVOS	Branch Vein Occlusion Study	GLT	Glaucoma Laser Trial
C_3F_8	Perfluoropropane	GLTS	Glaucoma Laser Trial Studies
CBA	Cost–benefit analysis	HDLs	High-density lipoproteins
CCT	central corneal thickness	HEDS	Herpetic Eye Disease Studies
CCTS	Collaborative Corneal Transplantation Studies	HHDC	High human development countries
CDMS	Clinically Definite Multiple Sclerosis	HLA	Histocompatibility
CDS	Cornea Donor Study	HMO	Health Maintenance Organization
CEA	Cost-effective analysis	HRC	High-risk characteristics
CI	Confidence interval	HRQL	Health-related quality of life
CIGTS	Collaborative Initial Glaucoma Treatment Study	HSV-1	Herpes Simplex Virus Type 1
		ICER	Incremental Cost-Effectiveness Ratio
CK	Conductive keratoplasty	ICG	Indocyanine green
CLE	Clear lens exchange	ICRs	Intracorneal rings
CLEK	Collaborative Longitudinal Evaluation of Keratoconus	ICL	Implantable Collamer Lens
		IGF-1	Insulin-like growth factor-1
CMA	Cost-minimization analysis	ILM	Internal limiting membrane
CME	Cystoid Macular Edema	IMAs	Immune-modulating agents
CNTGS	Collaborative Normal-Tension Glaucoma Study	IOLs	Intraocular lens
		IONTS	International Optic Nerve Trauma Study
CNV	Choroidal neovascular membrane	IOP	Intraocular pressure
COMS	Collaborative Ocular Melanoma Study	IRMA	Intraretinal Microvascular Abnormalities
CRA	Chorioretinal anastomosis	IRT	Iridocyclitis, receiving topical steroid
CRP	C-reactive protein	ISIS	Intravitreous Steroid Injection Study
CRVO	Central Retinal Vein Occlusion	IVMP	Intravenous methylprednisolone
CS	Corticosteroid	KC	Keratoconus
CS	Crossmatch Study	LALES	Los Angeles Latino Eye Study
CSDME	Clinically Significant Diabetic Macular Edema	LAR	Long-acting repeatable
CT	Computed Tomography	LASEK	Laser epithelial keratomileusis
CUA	Cost–utility analysis	LASIK	Laser In Situ Keratomileusis
CVOS	Central Vein Occlusion Study	LDLs	Low-density lipoproteins
D5W	Dextrose 5% in water	LHDC	Lower human development countries
DCCT	Diabetes Control and Complications Trial	LOCS	Lens Opacities Classification System
DCNVA	Distance corrected near visual acuity	LTK	Laser Thermal Keratoplasty
DME	Diabetic Macular Edema	MD	Mean deviation
DRS	Diabetic Retinopathy Study	MHDC	Middle human development countries
DRVS	Diabetic Retinopathy Vitrectomy Study	MIC	Minimum inhibitory

MIRA-1 trial	Multicenter Investigation of Rheopheresis for AMD
MMC	Mitomycin C
MP	Methylprednisolone
MPS	Macular Photocoagulation Study
MRI	Magnetic Resonance Imaging
MS	Multiple Sclerosis
MVR	Microvitreoretinal
NASCIS	National Acute Spinal Cord Injury Studies
NEI/NIH	National Eye Institute of the United States National Institutes of Health
NIDDM	Noninsulin-Dependent Diabetes Mellitus
NIH	National Institutes of Health
NNT	Number needed to treat
NPDR	Nonproliferative diabetic retinopathy
NVA	Neovascularization of the angle
NVD	Neovascularization of the disc
NVE	Neovascularization elsewhere
NVI	Neovascularization of the iris
OCT	Optical coherence tomography
OH	Ocular hypertension
OHTS	Ocular Hypertension Treatment Study
ONSD	Optic nerve sheath decompression
ONTT	Optic Neuritis Treatment Trial
OP	Oral prednisone
OR	Odds Ratio
PARD	Pseudophakic and aphakic retinal detachment
PAS	Peripheral anterior synechiae
PBK	Pseudophakic Bullous Keratopathy
PCS	Prospective Cohort Studies
PDR	Proliferative Diabetic Retinopathy
PDT	Photodynamic Therapy
PED	Pigment epithelial detachment
PEDIG	Pediatric Eye Disease Investigator Group
PEG	Polyethylene-glycol
PERK	Prospective Evaluation of Radial Keratotomy
PFO	Perfluoro-n-octane
PKC-DMES	Protein Kinase C β Inhibitor Diabetic Macular Edema Study
PKC-DRS	Protein Kinase C β Diabetic Retinopathy Study
PKC-DRS2	Protein Kinase C β Inhibitor Diabetic Retinopathy Study 2
PKC	Protein kinase C
PKP	Penetrating keratoplasty
PMA	Postmenstrual age
POAG	Primary open-angle glaucoma
PPPV	Primary pars plana vitrectomy
PPV	Pars plana vitrectomy
PRK	Photorefractive keratectomy
PRP	Panretinal photocoagulation
PRR	Prevalence Rate Ratio
PSD	Pattern standard deviation

PVD	Posterior vitreous detachment
PVR	Proliferative Vitreoretinopathy
QALY	Quality adjusted life year
QOL	Quality of life
RCS	Retrospective Cohort Studies
RCT	Randomized Controlled Trials
RD	Retinal detachment
RFS	Recurrence Factor Study
RGP	Rigid gas-permeable lenses
RK	Radial keratotomy
RL	Refractive lensectomy
RM-ROP	Risk-Model Retinopathy of Prematurity
RON	Radial optic neurotomy
ROP	Retinopathy of prematurity
RRMS	Relapsing-remitting multiple sclerosis
RRR	Relative Risk Ratio
rt-PA	Plasminogen activator
SAP	Standard achromatic perimetry
SB	Scleral buckling
SCORE	Standard of Care versus Corticosteroid for Retinal Vein Occlusion
SELEX	Systematic Evolution of Ligands by EXponential enrichment
SF_6	Sulfur hexafluoride
SKN	Stromal keratitis, not on the steroid
SKS	Stromal keratitis, on steroid treatment
SLT	Selective Laser Trabeculoplasty
SMAS	Specular Microscopy Ancillary Study
SOC	Standard of care
SRF	Subretinal fluid
SRG	Standard reference gamble
T3	Tri-iodothyronine
TAT	Trabeculotomy-argon laser trabeculoplasty-trabeculotomy
TED	Thyroid eye disease
TON	Traumatic optic neuropathy
TSH	Thyroid-stimulating hormone
TTO	Time trade-off
TTT	Transpupillary thermotherapy
UBM	Ultrasound biomicroscopy
UCVA	Uncorrected visual acuity
VA	Visual acuity
VC	Viscocanalostomy
VEGF	Vascular endothelial growth factor
VFQ	Visual Function Questionnaire
VFs	Visual fields
VIM	Verteporfin In Minimally Classic
VIO	Verteporfin In Occult (VIO) Choroidal Neovascularization
VIP	Verteporfin in Photodynamic Therapy
WESDR	Wisconsin Epidemiologic Study of Diabetic Retinopathy

INDEX

Note: Page numbers followed by *f* indicate figures; those followed by *t* indicate tables.